# Nutrition Curriculum Activities Kit Level 2

Paul E. Bell, D.Ed.
Carol Byrd-Bredbenner, Ph.D.
Lily Hsu, M.S.
Idamarie Laquatra, Ph.D.
James Rye, M.S.
Karin Rosander Sargrad, M.S.

Illustrated by Eileen Gerne Ciavarella

THE CENTER FOR APPLIED RESEARCH IN EDUCATION, INC.
West Nyack, New York 10995

## Acknowledgments

This curriculum has been a collaborative effort of the College of Human Development and the College of Education at The Pennsylvania State University; it was sponsored by the Nutrition Foundation and supported by the Heinz Endowment. The School Nutrition Education Curriculum Study was conducted under the direction of Helen Guthrie and Barbara Shannon.

Many individuals, too numerous to mention by name, have contributed to the development of the nutrition education materials in this kit. We would like to acknowledge their contributions and hope that they are as excited as we are to see the fruits of their labor in print. A special thanks goes to JoAnn Daehler and to Lisa Oesterling for technical assistance. A very special thank-you goes to Norma Woika for the preparation of the manuscript and for her never-failing optimism about this project.

10 9 8 7 6 5 4 3

**Library of Congress Cataloging-in-Publication Data**

Nutrition curriculum activities kit.

1. Nutrition—Study and teaching (Elementary)
2. Diet—Study and teaching (Elementary) I. Bell, Paul E. [DNLM: 1. Child Nutrition—Education. 2. 2. Curriculum. WS 18 N9767]
TX364.N87 1986 372,3′7 86-4203

ISBN 0-87628-617-1 (level 1)

ISBN 0-87628-618-X (level 2)

Printed in the United States of America

# About the Authors

The *Nutrition Curriculum Activities Kits, Level 1* and *Level 2,* are based on the nationwide "Pennsylvania State University Nutrition Education Project" conducted from 1974 to the present. The Project consisted of several studies, done at each grade level, that examined nutrition knowledge and attitudes, and also the dietary behavior changes that occurred because of nutrition education. The content material was field-tested in Pennsylvania public schools. Authors of the materials are:

Paul E. Bell, D.Ed., Curriculum and Supervision, is an Associate Professor of Science Education at The Pennsylvania State University. Dr. Bell has many years of experience in elementary and secondary science education, curriculum development, and supervision. An active lecturer and consultant, he has made presentations to the Association for Supervision and Curriculum Development, the School Science and Math Association, the National Science Teachers Association, and the California Dairy Council. He has also contributed nutrition education articles to *Today's Education* and the *Journal of Nutrition Education.*

Carol Byrd-Bredbenner, Ph.D., Home Economics Education, is an Assistant Professor of Nutrition at Montclair State College, Montclair, New Jersey. She is an ADA Registered Dietitian and a member of the American Home Economics Association and the Society for Nutrition Education. Dr. Byrd-Bredbenner has presented research papers to the Society for Nutrition Education, the American Home Economics Association, the International Congress of Nutrition, and the American Dietetic Association. Her nutrition education articles have been published in the *Journal of Nutrition Education, Thresholds in Education,* and the *Home Economics Research Journal.*

Lily Hsu, M.S., Nutrition, is an Instructor in Nutrition at The Pennsylvania State University. She is an ADA Registered Dietitian and a member of both the Society for Nutrition Education and the International Reading Association. Ms. Hsu has made nutrition education presentations to the Society for Nutrition Education and the International Reading Association and has published nutrition articles in the *Journal of Nutrition Education, Thresholds in Education,* and *Highlights for Children.*

Idamarie Laquatra, Ph.D., Applied Nutrition, is a Corporate Nutritionist with the Heinz Corporation. She is a frequent nutrition counseling workshop leader and speaker. She is an ADA Registered Dietitian and a member of the Society for Nutrition Education. Dr. Laquatra has published articles in the *Journal of the American Dietetic Association* and the *Journal of the Medical Society of New Jersey.* She has presented papers at the American Dietetic Association and for the New Jersey and the New York affiliates of the American Heart Association.

James Rye, M.S., Nutrition, is Chairperson of the Dietetics Department at Viterbo College in LaCrosse, Wisconsin. He is an ADA Registered Dietitian and a member of the Society for Nutrition Education. Mr. Rye was a team member responsible for delivering the

Special Supplemental Feeding Program for Women, Infants, and Children throughout Arizona and has helped to implement a cardiovascular risk factor intervention program. His nutrition articles have been published in the *Journal of Nutrition Education* and the *Journal of the American Dietetic Association.*

Karin Rosander Sargrad, M.S. Nutrition, is a Nutritionist at The Pennsylvania State University. She has extensive experience counseling pregnant and breast-feeding women, mothers of infants and children, and children. She is involved in a variety of nutrition education projects, including nutrition courses by correspondence. Ms. Sargrad is a member of the Society for Nutrition Education and is an ADA Registered Dietitian. She has published nutrition research articles in the *Journal of Nutrition Education* and has made presentations to the Society for Nutrition Education.

# About the *Nutrition Curriculum Activities Kits*

The *Nutrition Curriculum Activities Kits, Level 1* and *Level 2,* are unique aids designed to provide a complete nutrition education activities program for grades 5 through 12 in two self-contained kits. The kit for Level 2 includes twenty carefully planned nutrition-teaching lesson/units for grades 9 through 12 with over 140 pages of reproducible lesson materials composed of nutrition information, student worksheet activities, tables, tests, and other evaluation devices.

The scope and sequence of the kits were developed to provide students with the knowledge and skills necessary to make personal dietary decisions. The basic premise of the kits is that nutrition education should encompass three aspects of learning: cognitive, affective, and psychomotor. In order to improve their eating habits, students must understand certain nutrition information (cognitive), must choose and apply these ideas within their personal value systems (affective), and must develop the skills to carry out these tasks (psychomotor). In this spirit, the first units in Level 1 of the kits introduce basic nutrition concepts as a firm foundation on which to teach subsequent units in diet planning, special diets, meal planning and preparation, and nutrition issues. In Level 1, the emphasis is on nutrition knowledge, while Level 2 emphasizes the application of nutrition knowledge and skills in higher-level lessons.

In the beginning, students accumulate firsthand experiences through the lesson/units in order to broaden their perspective on food and nutrition. Attention is also given to the development of sensory skills, to familiarity with food variety, to the nutrient content of food, and to the relationship of food to various social settings. Students also learn the food sources of several nutrients as well as how their bodies use nutrients. Here the focus is on the individual and on his or her food choices. Finally, the units deal with nutrition issues and controversies and with the application of nutrition knowledge. Topics of interest to teenagers are presented in order to spark their interest and to encourage them to explore nutrition. In Level 2, topics like the vegetarian diet, the interpretation of ingredient labels, and special diets for various life stages are among those included.

The *Nutrition Curriculum Activities Kits* offer several unique features. The kits were developed to encompass the nutrition concepts that were identified in a nationwide survey conducted by recognized nutrition educators and that should be studied in grades 5 through 12. Going beyond an introduction to the Basic Food Groups, the kits include teaching units devoted to nutrients and to their food sources and also to the application of nutrition knowledge and skills in personal diet decision making.

Each lesson/unit in the kits provides:

- A detailed teacher's guide that includes all of the background information and step-by-step directions needed for teaching the unit. Discussed also are "Concepts" the unit will develop, the specific learning "Objectives" of the unit, and a "Teacher's Unit Introduction" that can be used, as is, to present the unit in class. The guide also provides reproducible student nutrition information sheets that open the unit topic for class discussion and it includes tips on classroom implementation to help maximize learning.
- A "Basic Activity," in an easy-to-follow lesson plan format, that spells out the "Time Needed," the "Materials Needed," and step-by-step procedures for carrying out the activity in class. All materials for teaching the unit are provided within the pages of the spiral-bound kit, including student worksheet, table, information, and evaluation pages designed to be copied directly, for immediate distribution, with no additional teacher preparation.
- Full-page, reproducible student worksheet activities pages, which students use to apply the nutrition knowledge and skills learned in the "Basic Activity." These activities give students practice in interpreting the various nutrition tables and charts included in the kit.
- "Advanced" and "Follow-Up" activities for students who want to learn more about the unit topic. These activities give students the opportunity to become involved in activities like interviewing, library research, and out-of-class preparation for presentations such as demonstrations and food fairs.
- An "Evaluation" device for each unit with a complete "Answer Key" (printed at the end of the kit). The devices include a wide range of formats such as multiple-choice and short-answer tests, attitude scales, writing exercises, word searches, and crossword puzzles. The "Evaluation" devices may be used for a pre- or post-assessment of student understanding of the unit material.

In short, each teaching unit provides all of the elements required for a well-organized, easy-to-use nutrition lesson. All you need to do to get started is either to reproduce the student materials for classroom distribution or to make acetate copies for projection on an overhead projector.

The following chart defines the scope and sequence of the *Nutrition Curriculum Activities Kits, Level 1* and *Level 2*.

## Nutrition Curriculum Activities Kit Level 1

### Section I Basic Nutrition Concepts

Unit 1 Nutrition Overview: Proteins, Carbohydrates, and Fats
Unit 2 Nutrition Overview: Vitamins, Minerals, and Water
Unit 3 RDA Doorway to Good Health
Unit 4 RDA Meterstick to Good Nutrition
Unit 5 The Three Bs: Meeting Your RDAs
Unit 6 Your RDA for Energy
Unit 7 RDA in the U.S.A.
Unit 8 Identifying Nutrient-Rich Foods
Unit 9 Determining Nutrient Density in Food

### Section II Diet Planning

Unit 10 Eating Right, Feeling Well
Unit 11 How Do You Stack Up Nutritionally?
Unit 12 Start the Day Better with Breakfast
Unit 13 Your School Lunch
Unit 14 The Good Goodies
Unit 15 Designing a Personal Diet Plan
Unit 16 Discovering Foods with Your Senses

### Section III Special Diets

Unit 17 Energy Balance and Fad Diets
Unit 18 The Athlete's Diet

### Section IV Meal Planning and Preparation

Unit 19 Interpreting Ingredient Labels

### Section V Nutrition Issues

Unit 20 A Close Look at Food Advertising

## Nutrition Curriculum Activities Kit Level 2

### Section I Basic Nutrition Concepts

Unit 1 Metabolism: Calories In, Calories Out
Unit 2 Metabolism: Balancing Energy Input and Energy Output

### Section II Diet Planning

Unit 3 How Food Patterns Develop
Unit 4 Analyzing Your Food Intake

### Section III Special Diets

Unit 5 The Vegetarian Way of Life
Unit 6 Nutrition for the Expectant Mother
Unit 7 Nutrition for Infants and Children
Unit 8 Nutrition for Adolescents, Adults, and the Aged

### Section IV Meal Planning and Preparation

Unit 9 Interpreting Ingredient Labels: Nutritive Food Additives
Unit 10 Interpreting Ingredient Labels: Cosmetic Food Additives
Unit 11 Getting the Most for Your Food Dollar
Unit 12 Storing Foods to Preserve Nutrients
Unit 13 Budgeting Resources in Meal Planning
Unit 14 Menu Planning Using the "Daily Food Guide"
Unit 15 Menu Planning for the Family

### Section V Nutrition Issues

Unit 16 Evaluating Nutrition Information
Unit 17 Diet and Disease: Obesity
Unit 18 Diet and Disease: World Health Problems
Unit 19 Dietary Guidelines for Americans
Unit 20 Designing a National Nutrition Policy

# How to Use This Resource

### Using the *Nutrition Curriculum Activities Kits* in Your Program

The *Nutrition Curriculum Activities Kits, Level 1* and *Level 2,* are designed to facilitate and promote nutrition in grades 5 through 12. These kits will save lesson preparation time and energy by providing imaginative, new nutrition units ready for immediate use in the classroom. The kit for Level 2 contains twenty ready-to-use, self-contained nutrition lesson/units complete with student worksheets, charts, information sheets, and evaluation devices to be reproduced by copier for distribution to students.

The two kits comprise a full sequential nutrition education curriculum for grades 5 through 12. Ideally, students would begin their exposure to nutrition education at the preschool level and continue through the twelfth grade. Since this continuity is not always possible within a school district, a review of the basic nutrition content usually presented in the earlier grades is provided in the first two units of *Level 1:* "Nutrition Overview: Proteins, Carbohydrates, and Fats" and "Nutrition Overview: Vitamins, Minerals, and Water." These two units serve as an introduction to nutrition for students who have had little or no exposure to nutrition education. These units also serve as a review for students who have been taught nutrition in earlier grades, thus providing a common starting point for all students in the class.

### CLASSROOM IMPLEMENTATION OF THE NUTRITION UNITS

The nutrition units can be used in sequence to provide a complete nutrition education program, or they can be used to supplement the existing curriculum. The units are equally appropriate for individuals, small groups, or the entire class.

Each unit follows the same easy-to-use format:

- The "Unit Title" introduces the unit.
- Specific "Concepts" to be developed in the unit are listed. Generally, a unit addresses several related concepts, encompassing both nutrition content and practical applications.
- Specific behavioral "Objectives" that students should be able to achieve throughout the unit are listed. There are also several objectives and concepts for each unit including both affective and cognitive goals.
- The "Teacher's Unit Introduction" provides background information on the nutrition topic of the unit and may be used, as is, to introduce students to the unit. Although the information presented is not comprehensive, enough material has been provided to spark students' interest in the topic and to facilitate the teaching of the unit. Further

investigation of the topic is encouraged. The thorough "References/Resources" section at the end of this kit offers sources of additional materials (books, booklets, audiovisuals, software, and other printed matter) pertinent to each unit. Following each "Teacher's Unit Introduction" are specific implementation tips and suggestions for the unit, along with references to materials in other units in *Level 2* that may be useful in instruction.

- The core of each unit is found in the sections entitled "Basic Activity," "Advanced Activity," and "Follow-Up Activities." The "Basic Activity" and "Advanced Activity" appear in the same easy-to-follow format which indicates the "Time Needed," "Materials Needed," and numbered step-by-step procedures for carrying out the activity in class. The "Basic Activity" is designed for students who have little or no background in the nutrition topic, and the "Advanced Activity" and "Follow-Up Activities" are for students who want further study or challenges in the topic area. Generally the "Advanced Activity" requires additional reading, writing, or intellectual skills and may require out-of-class assignments. The "Follow-Up Activities" consist of short descriptions of teaching ideas that may be used in addition to either the "Basic Activity" or the "Advanced Activity." Due to their supplemental nature, the "Follow-Up Activities" do not contain as much detail and are not as fully developed as either of the other two activity types.

The following activities are presented in a wide variety of formats to stimulate student interest and expression:

taste-testing parties
field trips
puzzles and games
library research
learning centers
bulletin board preparation
lab experiments
contests
unique meal planning and preparation
attitude surveys
interviews
panel discussions
guest speakers
debates
diet and activity diaries
roleplaying
case studies
demonstrations
ad writing
practice shopping
menu planning

- Following the step-by-step activity directions is a section of reproducible student materials, including information sheets, charts, worksheets, and evaluation devices. Each of these appears on a full page and may be photocopied directly from the kit pages for distribution to the class. "Answer Keys" for worksheets and evaluation devices are located at the end of this kit.

- Reproducible "Student Charts and Tables" are also located at the end of this kit. Within the nutrition units, you will find references to these charts and tables. As the need arises, provide students with individual copies of them and instruct students to keep them on hand for reference.

The student reference charts and tables include:

| | |
|---|---|
| Chart A | Recommended Dietary Allowances |
| Chart B | Daily Food Guide |
| Chart C | Key Nutrients in Food |
| Chart D | Food Composition Table for Selected Nutrients |
| Chart E | Dietary Calculation Chart |
| Chart F | Height/Weight and Recommended Energy Intake |
| Chart G | Calorie Expenditure by Activity |

The *Nutrition Curriculum Activities Kits* promote a well-rounded study of nutrition, in new and interesting ways, in order to stimulate student involvement. The nutrition skills taught in these units will serve your students for a lifetime!

# Contents



This section completes the groundwork for all other nutrition instruction that was begun in the BASIC NUTRITION CONCEPTS introduced in *Level I* by focusing on metabolism and the maintenance of energy balance. The information presented in this section will facilitate the students' application of nutrition knowledge in personal diet decision-making.



This section gives students experience in applying basic nutrition concepts when making snacking and meal decisions. These units help students explore how an individual's food selection is influenced and observe associations between eating habits and good health.



This section expands the concepts introduced in Section II by examining the special dietary needs of vegetarians, the expectant mother, and all persons through all life stages from infancy to old age.

## SECTION IV MEAL PLANNING AND PREPARATION 123

This section focuses on nutrition consumerism and the food supply. The increasing number of new food products marketed each year causes consumers to be faced with more and more food decisions. In order to make wise food choices, students continue nutrition label-reading activities begun in *Level I* and develop skills in purchasing and storing foods and in menu planning.



## SECTION V NUTRITION ISSUES 225

This section promotes critical thinking and the application of nutrition knowledge and skills. The skills developed in this section will help students discriminate between nutrition information and misinformation and prepare them to deal with other nutrition-related controversies outside the classroom.



## APPENDICES 281

**Reproducible Student Charts and Tables**

# SECTION I

# BASIC NUTRITION CONCEPTS

*Unit 1 Metabolism: Calories In, Calories Out*
*Unit 2 Metabolism: Balancing Energy Input and Energy Output*

# Unit 1: Metabolism: Calories In, Calories Out

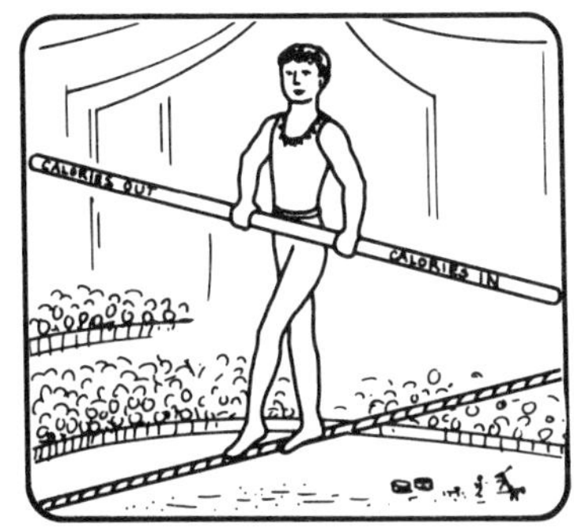


## CONCEPTS

–Energy metabolism refers to the conversion of food energy to body-function energy.

–Calories are used by the body for basal metabolism, for the digestion of food, and for physical activity.

## OBJECTIVES

–Students will account for total daily calorie intake in terms of calories used for basal metabolism, for digestion of food, and for physical activity.

## TEACHER'S UNIT INTRODUCTION

The term "calorie" gets a lot of use these days, mainly because people are so concerned about weight control. In fact, it has been estimated that 10 to 20 million Americans are currently dieting to lose weight. But, what exactly *is* a calorie? A *calorie* is a unit of heat that expresses the energy value of food. Properly speaking, one calorie is the amount of heat necessary to increase the temperature of 1 gram of water by 1° centigrade. The energy value of food is actually measured in terms of "kilocalories," or 1,000 calories. Thus, when we say that a glass of milk contains 120 "calories," in reality it contains 120,000 calories. We use the term "kilocalories" to simplify the numbers.

To a scientist, the words "calorie" and kilocalorie" are very different, but most people use the more familiar term "calorie" to mean "kilocalorie." In this kit, we will use the more familiar term "calorie" instead of "kilocalorie."

**Calories In.** The sole source of incoming calories is from food. More specifically, the four components in food that provide calories are protein, fat, carbohydrate, and alcohol. In Unit 2 you will learn more about the calories in food. You will learn about the variety of food sources that provide your body with calories.

**Calories Out.** To accurately estimate total energy used by the body, three factors are measured: (1) basal metabolic rate (BMR), (2) physical activity, and (3) the digestion of food.

*Basal metabolic rate* (BMR) is the amount of energy required by the body to carry on its vital processes while at rest. We are usually unaware of these processes, which include respiration, circulation, glandular activity, cellular metabolism, and the maintenance of body temperature. An estimate of BMR can be calculated by allowing one calorie per kilogram of body weight per hour. Since BMR is calculated on a daily basis, the calculation is simply 24 times the body weight in kilograms (weight in kilograms = weight in pounds ÷ by 2.2).

According to many surveys, it has been determined that 16 to 18 hours a day are spent in various forms of physical activity. The energy required for physical activity is a function of the type of activity, the duration of the activity, and the size of the individual. Numerous experiments have enabled scientists to compile tables of calorie expenditures for a wide range of activities. Chart G, "Calorie Expenditure by Activity," is an example of this type of table. An estimate of the energy a person expends in physical activity can be obtained by keeping a minute-by-minute diary of activities for one day. Remember, however, these figures are only rough estimates of actual energy expenditures.

Energy used in the digestion of food must also be included in the calculation of energy expenditure because the energy for BMR allows only for energy the body uses at complete physical and digestive rest. The digestion of food encompasses the activity processes of the breakdown, absorption, and assimilation of food. It is generally assumed that the effect of food digestion amounts to 10 percent of the total energy needs for basal metabolism and physical activity:

$$(\text{BMR calories} + \text{physical activity calories}) \times 10\% = \text{calories needed to digest and absorb food}$$

To obtain an estimate of total calorie output, add the calories for BMR, the calories for physical activity, and the calories for food digestion and absorption.

**Balancing Input and Output.** The state of energy balance reflects the relationship between incoming and outgoing calories. Three relationships are possible:

$$\text{input} = \text{output}$$
$$\text{input} > \text{output}$$
$$\text{input} < \text{output}$$

The effect on body weight in each instance is easy to see. The first case illustrates equilibrium, a state of body weight maintenance. When calorie intake exceeds (>) expenditure, weight is gained. Conversely, when intake fails to meet (<) the calorie needs of the body, weight is lost.

---

The activities in Unit 1 will help students gain an understanding of calories and energy balance. The "Basic Activity" demonstrates how the calorie values of food are determined. The equipment for the experiment in this activity is usually available in the science laboratory. It may be necessary to make arrangements for some of the equipment listed under "Materials Needed."

Also note that Chart G, "Calorie Expenditure by Activity," located at the end of this kit, lists caloric expenditures for many daily and sports activities. Since basal metabolic functions and, for the most part, digestion of food, are continuous throughout a 24-hour period, the calorie figures given for these activities *include* calories being expended simultaneously for basal metabolism and digestion. The concept of basal metabolism introduced in this unit is explored in detail in Unit 2.

## BASIC ACTIVITY

**Time Needed:** Three class periods

**Materials Needed:** Small bag of cheese puff snacks *or* marshmallows
Graduated cylinder
Gram scale
6-ounce metal juice can
Water
Centigrade thermometer
Paper clip
Ball of clay
Wire mesh
Ring stand
Fireproof mat
Kitchen matches
Sheet 1-1: "The Case of the Burning Cheese Puff Calculation Sheet"
Sheets 1-2 through 1-5: "The Survival Mission"
Chart D: "Food Composition Table for Selected Nutrients"
Chart G: "Calorie Expenditure by Activity"
Quiz Sheet 1-1

### Class Period 1

1. The first part of this activity is a teacher demonstration. Distribute copies of Sheet 1-1, "The Case of the Burning Cheese Puff Calculation Sheet," to the students and have them complete it as you perform the experiment.[1] The procedure follows here:

a. Set up the equipment as illustrated on top of a fireproof mat.

b. Randomly select three cheese puff samples (or marshmallows) and determine the total weight in grams. Students should record this weight on Sheet 1-1.

---

[1]From *Creative Sciencing: Ideas and Activities for Teachers and Children.* DeVito, A. and Krockover, D. H. Little, Brown and Company, Boston, MA, 1980.

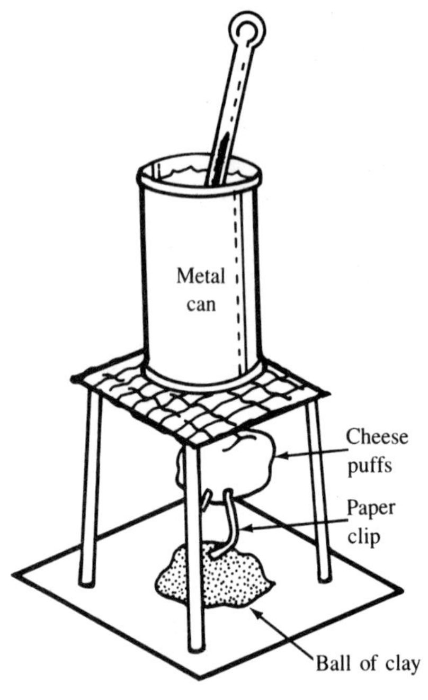


c. Pour a measured amount (in milliliters) of water to nearly fill a 6-ounce metal juice can. Students should record this volume in milliliters and convert it to liters following the hint on the worksheet if necessary.

d. State the initial temperature (centigrade) of the water and have the students record this. Remove the thermometer from the can.

e. As illustrated, place the three cheese puffs under the juice can full of water. Position the juice can on a piece of wire mesh arranged on top of a ring stand. Hold the cheese puffs in place with a bent paper clip stuck into a ball of clay for support. Strike a kitchen match and light the cheese puffs.

f. After the cheese puffs have burned completely, reinsert the thermometer in the water and have the students record the temperature of the heated water. They should then calculate the temperature change.

g. By filling the appropriate numbers in the formula in on their sheets, the students can now calculate the number of calories of heat given off by the cheese puffs to heat the water. The calculation is based on the density of water (1 gram/milliliter) and on the heat capacity of water (1 calorie/gram-degree). Their calculations should result in an answer in calories.

2. Explain that the students have measured the approximate amount of energy (calories) that the cheese puffs provide when they are burned. Note that this amount is not exact because some heat was lost to the air since the apparatus was not enclosed. The students should be made aware of this heat loss. The experiment shows approximately the amount of calories the body burns when a human being eats three cheese puffs.

3. Ask the students the following questions:

a. Why does the body need calories? (*Answer:* To provide energy for BMR, for physical activity, and for digestion and absorption.)

b. Which burns more calories: walking to school or riding the bus to school? (*Answer: Walking.)*

c. What do you think would happen if you ate more calories than you burned over a long period of time? (*Answer:* Gain weight.) What if you burned more calories than you ate? (*Answer:* Lose weight.)

d. How could you maintain your weight? (*Answer:* Balance input and output by eating and burning the same number of calories.)

**Class Period 2**

1. The next part of the "Basic Activity" requires that students work on their own but cooperate to share needed information. Distribute Sheets 1-2 through 1-5, "The Survival Mission." Also distribute, or make available, a number of copies of Chart D, "Food

Composition Table for Selected Nutrients," and Chart G, "Calorie Expenditure by Activity," since the students will need these charts as references.

2. The activity is self-explanatory, but students may need some encouragement and some tips on handling the work involved. When students reach the section that requires checking activity calories and food calories, the work may be divided in a number of ways: (1) a "search" person could be put in charge of looking up the calories and announcing them to the whole class; (2) students could work in pairs, with one member working on input and the other on output; or (3) half the class could work on input and half on output. Note that if students work individually on the entire activity, they are not likely to complete it by the end of the class period. In this case, the remainder of the work could be assigned as a homework project.

**Class Period 3**

1. Conduct a review session to summarize the concepts in this unit. Begin the discussion by asking, "Do you think Jim and Joe will get paid $100 each?" Compare and contrast answers both for calorie input and calorie output, and also for the consequences of the imbalance. Encourage students to give their solutions to the imbalance.

2. As a final area of discussion, ask students for their answers to question #9 on Sheet 1-5. See if they can come up with solutions to the problems they found. (*For example:* Using freeze-dried foods instead of canned or fresh foods; adding food to increase calories; adding an extra glass of milk to meet daily requirements.)

3. Proceed with the "Advanced Activity" if you wish; otherwise use the quiz mentioned in step 4.

4. **Evaluation:** Distribute Quiz Sheet 1-1 and have students complete it independently. Or, use the sheet as a guide in a final summary discussion of the unit.

## ADVANCED ACTIVITY

**Time Needed:** Two class periods

**Materials Needed:** Sheet 1-6: "24-Hour Intake Record"
Sheet 1-7: "24-Hour Activity Record"
Chart D: "Food Composition Table for Selected Nutrients"
Chart G: "Calorie Expenditure by Activity"
*Optional:* other Food Composition Tables (*see* "References/Resources")
Quiz Sheet 1-1

**Class Period 1**

1. Distribute Sheet 1-6, "24-Hour Intake Record." Have students complete the worksheet by recording all of the food and beverages consumed in a 24-hour period and also the amounts consumed.

2. Distribute Chart D, "Food Composition Table for Selected Nutrients." Because Chart D is only a partial listing of foods, you may need to provide additional food

composition tables such as the ones listed in "References/Resources" at the end of this kit. Using Chart D, have students calculate the number of calories consumed on the day that they recorded their intake.

3. Distribute Sheet 1-7, "24-Hour Activity Record," and Chart G, "Calorie Expenditure by Activity." For homework, have the students keep a detailed activity record for one 24-hour period.

**Class Period 2**

1. Using Sheet 1-7 and Chart G, students should calculate the calories they expended for each activity. Since Chart G is not comprehensive, students may need to choose an activity on the chart that is similar to the one they engaged in. Point out that the chart lists average values. Have each student total his or her calorie output and compare this with the calorie input on Sheet 1-6.

2. Ask the students to come up with reasons why calorie input does not exactly balance calorie output. Remind them that these calculations are not exact, but only approximations. Will they maintain weight, gain weight, or lose weight with this kind of regimen?

3. **Evaluation:** Distribute Quiz Sheet 1-1 and have students complete it independently. Discuss the answers as a class.

## FOLLOW-UP ACTIVITIES

1. Have the students design a bulletin board that shows methods for increasing daily activity by comparing pairs of activities where one is active and the other sedentary. Using Chart G, have students record also the calories used per pound for one hour of each of the compared activities.

| For example: | walking upstairs<br>6.8 calories/minute | *vs.* | taking the elevator (like standing) 0.6 calories/minute |
|---|---|---|---|
| | bicycling<br>3.2 calories/minute | *vs.* | watching TV<br>0.4 calories/minute |

You might have students multiply the figures by an average weight for the age of the students in order for them to make a more realistic comparison. Or, they might subtract the sedentary calories from the more active calories for comparative activities in order to show the difference that the increase in activity makes.

2. Discuss the changes in BMR that come with age. Encourage the students to give their ideas about the consequences of maintaining the same calorie intake throughout life, while physical activity remains constant or decreases. Ask how they can maintain a comfortable weight throughout their life. (*Answer:* By decreasing input or increasing output.)

3. Have students investigate their town or city to find out the types of physical activities available. (*Examples:* YMCA and YWCA clubs, tennis clubs, health spas.)

Name ______________________________ Sheet 1-1

# THE CASE OF THE BURNING CHEESE PUFF
# CALCULATION SHEET

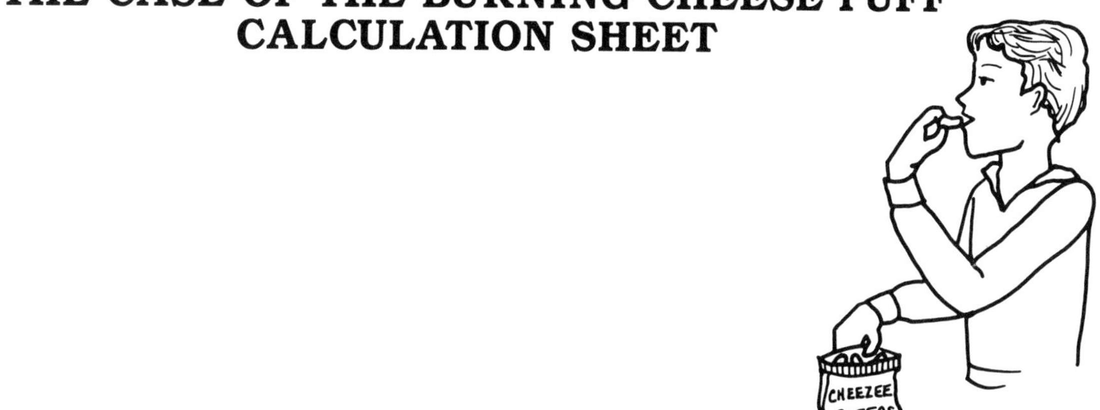


A *calorie* is a measure of the heat energy in food. This experiment shows how many calories are available in three cheese puffs. (These calories are similar to, but not exactly the same as, the number of calories your body can burn when you *eat* three cheese puffs.)



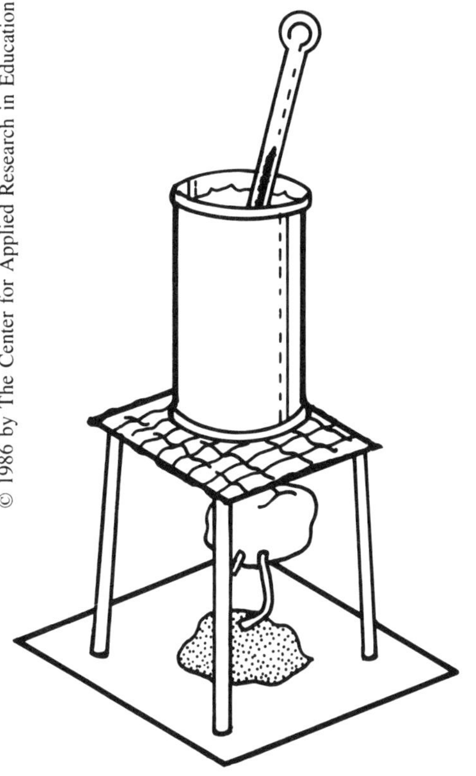

1. What is the weight of three cheese puffs? __________ grams

2. How much water is in the can? ______________ milliliters
   Convert this to liters: __________ liters
   (Hint: There are 1,000 milliliters in a liter.)

3. What is the initial temperature of the water?
   __________ degrees centigrade

4. What is the final temperature of the water?
   __________ degrees centigrade

5. What is the temperature change? ______________ degrees centigrade (Hint: Subtract the answer in #3 from the answer in #4.)

6. How many calories were given off as heat by the cheese puffs:

$$\left[\frac{\text{\_\_\_\_ liters of water (see \#2)}}{1}\right] \times \left[\frac{\text{\_\_\_\_ degrees centigrade (see \#5)}}{1}\right] \times \left[\frac{\text{1 kilogram}}{\text{1 liter of water}}\right] \times \left[\frac{\text{1 calorie}}{\text{1 kilogram-1 degree centigrade}}\right] = \text{\_\_\_\_ calories}$$

Name ______________________________ Sheet 1-2

# THE SURVIVAL MISSION

Jim and Joe, identical twins, were reading the Saturday morning paper. Jim came across an ad that read: "Our firm is seeking people to go on a survival mission. For more information, call 291-0050."

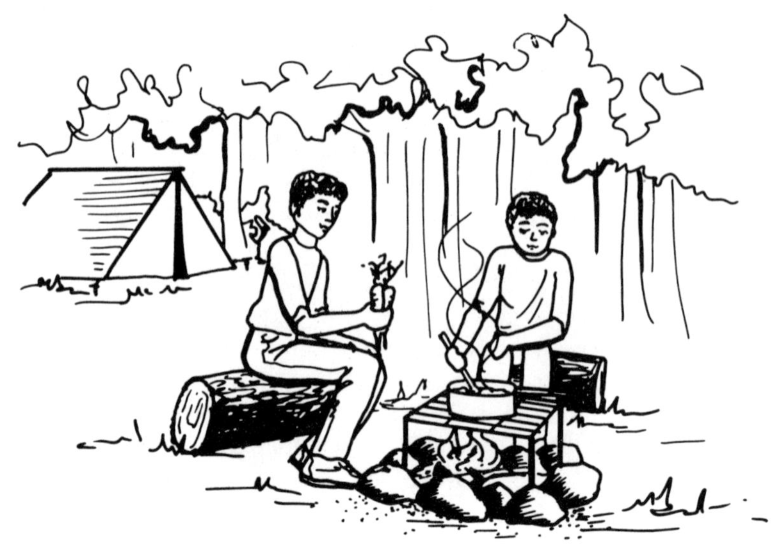

"Hey, Joe!" Jim exclaimed. "Did you see this? What do you think?"

Quickly reading it, Joe replied, "I'm all for it!"

Jim called the phone number, and a woman answered after two rings. "This is Calorie Balance Associates. May I help you?" Jim spoke to her for a long time and Joe was getting impatient.

"What is she saying? What is she saying?" he kept asking. Finally, Jim hung up the phone and let Joe in on all the details.

"Well," Jim started, "it sounds like fun . . . but it is risky. It's a survival mission all right—in Limestone National Park. The mission lasts for one week, and we will have to camp out and do a lot of walking and climbing. The company wants to check and see how well we make it through the week, so they will do all kinds of tests on us before and after the mission. We'll each get $100 if we complete it successfully."

Joe laughed. "Jim, you sound so nervous! We've camped out lots of times before. What's the problem?"

"Here's the catch," Jim answered in a low voice. "They're only going to give us the exact amount of food we'll need for the whole trip. We'll have to plan our calorie intake carefully so that we don't gain or lose weight on the mission, because if we don't maintain our weights we won't get paid a cent! We will have to submit the number of calories we need, and the company will supply us with just that amount of food—and no more."

"Hmmm," Joe muttered thoughtfully. "I think we can do it. All we have to do is balance our calorie input and output. Since we weigh the same, that should be easy."

So, the two of them started planning. Joe appointed himself as the person in charge of calorie output. Jim worked on calorie input.

Joe knew that the body uses calories in three ways. The first way is through the Basal Metabolic Rate, also called the BMR. Joe read that BMR means the amount of energy the body uses to carry on life processes that we do not usually think about. Activities like breathing, blood circulation, and even wound healing are included under BMR. Joe also read that BMR is always measured when a person is awake but in a resting state.

The second way that the body burns calories is through food digestion. Joe remembered from science class that it takes energy to break down and absorb food. Even though the amount of energy needed for food digestion is not very high, Joe knew that he would have to consider it or his calculation of energy output would be too low.

Name ____________________ Sheet 1-3

The final way the body uses calories is through physical activity. At first, Joe thought the category of physical activity included only activities like swimming, running, or playing basketball. He talked to his health teacher and found out that sitting, standing, writing, and even dressing used calories!

"How am I ever going to figure out how many calories we will burn each day on our trip?" Joe thought, and he worried about this until he came up with a great idea.

"See you later!" Joe called to Jim, who was busily working on calorie input.

"Where are you going?" Jim asked, afraid that Joe had given up on the job.

"To the library," Joe answered. "I'll be back before dinner." And off Joe went. The walk to the library usually took twenty minutes, but it was chilly and Joe wanted to get there fast, so he ran. He thought as he ran, "Gee, I'm burning calories right now in all three ways at once! The scratch on my knee is healing—that's BMR. At the same time, I know my food from lunch is being digested and absorbed—that would be considered energy needed for digestion. Also, I am not in a resting state, so I am using more calories than just for my BMR, and that would be physical activity. If all three ways that the body burns calories occur at once, I'll have to find some kind of chart that tells me the *combined* calories burned."

Joe arrived at the library breathless and excited. He searched and quickly found just what he wanted: a list of activities that combined BMR calories, food digestion calories, and physical activity calories. The chart was called "Calorie Expenditure by Activity."

In order to use the chart, Joe first had to put together a daily activity record for the mission. He spent almost an hour working on it, and this is the final version:

| ACTIVITY | TIME SPENT IN ACTIVITY | CALORIES PER POUND |
|---|---|---|
| Sleeping | 9 hours | ____________ |
| Personal care (total) | 1/2 hour | ____________ |
| Dressing | 15 minutes | ____________ |
| Packing up and unpacking sleeping bags (like housework) | 15 minutes | ____________ |
| Swimming | 1 hour, 45 minutes | ____________ |
| Eating: Breakfast | 1/2 hour | ____________ |
| Lunch | 1/2 hour | ____________ |
| Snacks (total) | 15 minutes | ____________ |
| Dinner | 1 hour | ____________ |
| Preparation and cleanup for meals (like housework) | 1 hour | ____________ |
| Writing in daily diary | 15 minutes | ____________ |
| Walking (3 mph) | 4 hours | ____________ |

Name ______________________________ **Sheet 1-4**

| ACTIVITY | TIME SPENT IN ACTIVITY | CALORIES PER POUND |
|---|---|---|
| Mountain climbing | 1 hour | ______ |
| Setting up camp (like housework) | 1 hour | ______ |
| Conversing | 2 hours | ______ |
| Standing (no activity) for a rest | 45 minutes | ______ |
| TOTAL: | 24 hours | TOTAL: ______ |

1. Using Chart G, "Calorie Expenditure by Activity," determine how many calories Joe used in each of the physical activities listed above. Put your answer in the column marked "Calories Per Pound."
2. Multiply the number of total calories in this column by Joe's weight (100 pounds). What was Joe's total calorie output for the whole day? ______________________________
3. Meanwhile, Jim had been working for hours preparing menus for the week. He decided to run a calorie check on a typical day. Jim's menu looked like the one below:

| FOOD | | AMOUNT | CALORIES |
|---|---|---|---|
| Breakfast: | Cereal, ready-to-eat | 1 ounce | ______ |
| | Grape juice | 4 ounces | ______ |
| | Orange | 1 | ______ |
| | Bread, whole wheat (toasted) | 1 slice | ______ |
| | Butter | 1/2 tablespoon | ______ |
| | Egg, scrambled with butter | 1 | ______ |
| Lunch: | Sandwich: | | |
| | Bread, whole wheat | 2 slices | ______ |
| | Peanut butter | 2 tablespoons | ______ |
| | Chocolate chip cookies | 2 | ______ |
| | Apricots, dried | 1/2 cup | ______ |
| | Milk, nonfat dry powder | 1/3 cup with water | ______ |
| Snack: | Apple | 1 | ______ |
| Dinner: | Tuna cassserole: | | |
| | Tuna, canned | 1/2 cup | ______ |
| | Noodles, enriched | 1 cup | ______ |
| | Peas, canned | 1/2 cup | ______ |
| Dinner: | Carrots, raw | 1 whole | ______ |
| | Milk, nonfat dry powder | 1/3 cup with water | ______ |
| | Doughnut, cake | 1 | ______ |
| Snack: | Popcorn (prepopped in hot air) with salt | 3 cups | ______ |
| | | TOTAL: | ______ |

Use Chart D, "Food Composition Table for Selected Nutrients," to determine how many calories are in Jim's menu. Put your answers in the column marked "calories."

4. How many calories will come from food in one day? ______________________________
   This is what Jim calls calorie "input."

Joe and Jim meet to compare the calorie input and calorie output they researched. Fill in their totals below:

5. Calorie input = ______________

   Calorie output = ______________

6. How do these compare? ______________________________

   ______________________________

7. Will Jim and Joe gain weight, lose weight, or stay the same on their survival mission? (Remember, they both start out weighing the same.) ______________________________

8. If they stay the same, skip this question. If you found that they will gain or lose weight, what do you think they will have to do to balance calorie input and calorie output? (Be specific.) ______________

   ______________________________

   ______________________________

9. Can you see any problems with the kind of menu Jim prepared for camping out?

   ______________________________

   ______________________________

   ______________________________

Name ______________________________ 

# 24-HOUR INTAKE RECORD

**Directions:** Record all of the food and beverages you consume in an average 24-hour period. Be sure to include soft drinks, gum, snacks, and condiments (ketchup, mustard, mayonnaise).

| FOOD EATEN | AMOUNTS | CALORIES |
|---|---|---|
| | | |
| | TOTAL CALORIE INPUT: | |

Name ____________________ Sheet 1-7

# 24-HOUR ACTIVITY RECORD

**Directions:** Record all of your activities in an average 24-hour period. Try to record each activity in 15- , 30- , 45- , or 60-minute blocks of time. Use Chart G, "Calorie Expenditure by Activity," for your calculations.

| TIME OF DAY | ACTIVITY | MINUTES SPENT | CALORIES USED |
|---|---|---|---|
| | | | |
| | | TOTAL CALORIES USED PER POUND: | |

Total Calorie Output = ____________ (TOTAL CALORIES USED PER POUND) × ____________ (YOUR WEIGHT IN POUNDS) = ____________ CALORIES

# QUIZ
# METABOLISM: CALORIES IN, CALORIES OUT

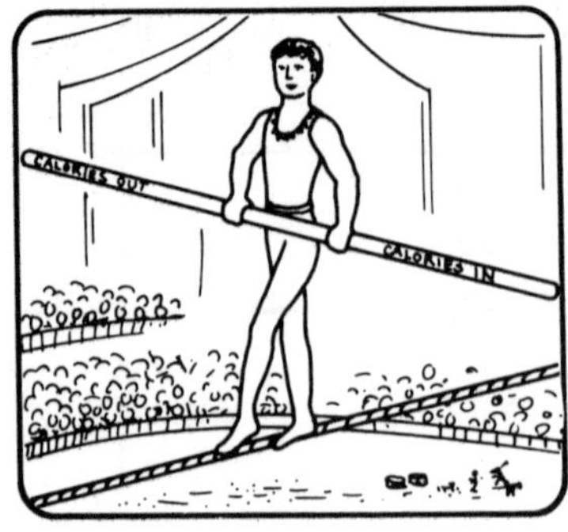


____ 1. The three main ways our body uses energy are:
- a. Basal metabolism, food digestion, and physical activity.
- b. Basal metabolism, physiological state, and physical activity.
- c. Food absorption/digestion, physiological state, and basal metabolism.
- d. Physiological state, physical activity, and chemical activity.

____ 2. Calories measure:
- a. Body weight.
- b. Food energy.
- c. Fatness.
- d. All of the above.

____ 3. What would happen if your calorie input was greater than your calorie output?
- a. I would lose weight.
- b. I would gain weight.
- c. I would stay the same weight.
- d. Nothing would happen to me.

4. In one short paragraph, answer the following question: What is a calorie? (Make sure to include in your answer (a) a definition of the word "calorie," (b) sources of calories in the diet, and (c) uses of calories by the body.)

______________________________________________

______________________________________________

______________________________________________

______________________________________________

______________________________________________

______________________________________________

______________________________________________

______________________________________________

______________________________________________

______________________________________________

# *Unit 2: Metabolism: Balancing Energy Input and Energy Output*

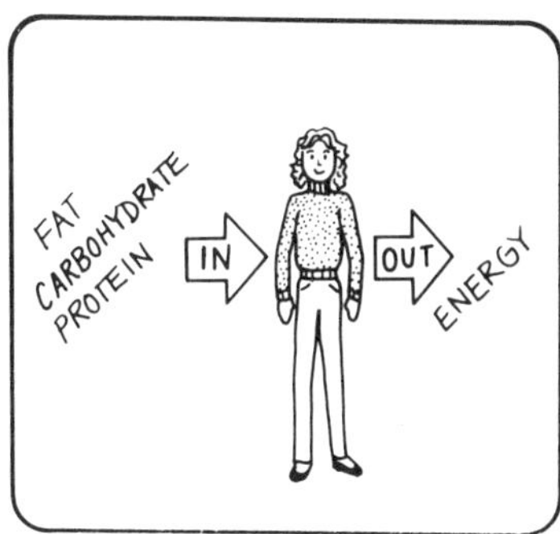


## CONCEPTS

–Fuel for the body is obtained from carbohydrate, protein, and fat.

–The amount of energy needed for basal metabolism, physical activity, and the digestion of food is influenced by body size, sex, age, environment, physiological state, and life style.

## OBJECTIVES

–Students will be able to identify protein, carbohydrate, and fat as sources of food energy.

–Students will examine how various factors influence energy needs.

## TEACHER'S UNIT INTRODUCTION

Most people are aware that the body needs energy to operate. Body weight is maintained by balancing energy input and energy output. When energy input equals energy output, weight is held constant. Weight is gained if energy input is greater than energy output, and weight is lost if energy input is less than energy output. Attempts to change body weight should evaluate both energy input and energy output.

Almost everyone knows that energy input refers to the energy derived from the food we eat. Energy from food is measured in calories. Remember from Unit 1 that a "calorie" is a measure of heat. One calorie is the amount of heat necessary to raise the temperature of one gram of water 1° centigrade.

We are all aware that some foods contain more calories than others. The difference in the number of calories is due to how much protein, fat, carbohydrate, and (if present) alcohol the food contains. Protein, fat, carbohydrate, and alcohol are the only components in food that provide calories. One gram (which is about the weight of a raisin) of protein or carbohydrate provides four calories, one gram of fat provides nine calories, and one gram of alcohol provides seven calories. As you can see, fat has more than twice the calories of protein or carbohydrate. The consequences of adding fat to food are shown in the following table. [The table may be shown on an overhead or opaque projector.]

**Caloric Effect of Adding Fat to Food**

| Food | Weight | Protein (grams) | Fat (grams) | Carbohydrate (grams) | Calories |
|---|---|---|---|---|---|
| Baked Potato (one plain) | 3 oz. | 2 | 0 | 17 | 74 |
| Baked Potato with 2 Tbsp. Sour Cream | 3 oz. | 3 | 6 | 18 | 136 |
| French Fries (20 pieces) | 3 oz. | 3 | 11 | 30 | 229 |
| Potato Chips (42 chips) | 3 oz. | 4 | 33 | 42 | 480 |

Unfortunately, carbohydrates often take the blame for what fat does because people believe that carbohydrates are high in calories. Actually, it is the fat that adds calories most quickly to foods.

The calorie content of any food can be determined by knowing the number of grams of protein, carbohydrate, and fat contained in the food.* For example, eight ounces of whole milk contain eight grams of protein, nine grams of fat, and eleven grams of carbohydrate. The total number of calories in the cup of milk is 157. This total was derived from these calculations:

| | | |
|---|---|---|
| 8 grams protein × 4 calories/gram of protein | = | 32 calories |
| 9 grams fat × 9 calories/gram of fat | = | 81 calories |
| 11 grams carbohydrate × 4 calories/gram carbohydrate | = | 44 calories |
| Total | = | 157 calories |

*Alcohol is generally not included in these food calculations because it is not a normal component of most foods. However, keep in mind that alcohol does provide the body with calories.

Because the number of grams of protein, carbohydrate, and fat have been rounded to the nearest whole number, the total of 157 calories may not correspond exactly to values listed in food composition tables. However, this method for determining calories in food will provide a close approximation. Calorie intake (or energy input) for an entire day can be measured by simply keeping track of the total grams of protein, fat, carbohydrate, and alcohol consumed.

After we take in energy, our bodies turn to the task of using it. In Unit 1 you learned that energy output is usually divided into three categories: basal metabolism, physical activity, and the digestion of food.

Not everyone uses the same amount of energy for these three processes. The amount of energy expended depends on the following factors: body size and composition, sex, age, the environment, the physiological state, and the personal life style of the individual.

**Body Size and Composition.** The greater the body size, the more energy is needed for body movements. Energy needs for basal metabolism are also increased because larger bodies have more tissues to maintain. Obese individuals thus expend more energy in exercising than do lean persons. Unfortunately, many obese persons are very sedentary, so that the decreased physical activity compensates for the increased body size. The energy expended for basal metabolism in the obese person may be lower per unit of body weight than a lean person's. This is due to a higher proportion of fat tissue to muscle tissue in the obese person. It takes less energy to maintain the integrity of fat tissue than muscle tissue and, therefore, basal metabolism is lower.

**Sex.** The sex of a person affects basal metabolism. Body size and composition usually differ between the sexes. Females are usually smaller than males and have a higher proportion of body fat. As a result, females have a five- to-ten percent lower basal metabolism than males.

**Age.** Growing older has some definite effects on basal metabolism. During infancy, childhood, and adolescence, basal energy needs are high. During adulthood, basal metabolism begins to decline. After twenty years of age, the approximate rate of decline of basal metabolism is two percent per decade. For example, a 19-year-old male, 5 feet 10 inches tall and weighing 154 pounds, would need approximately 1,800 calories for basal metabolism. (*Note:* This is *not* total energy output, because it does not include calories for physical activity or food digestion.) By age 50, the energy needed for the basal metabolism of this male will decrease to about 1,700 calories. [Display the calculation below.]

50 years − 20 years (approximate time that decline starts) = 30 years
30 years ÷ 10 years = 3 decades
3 decades × .02 (decline per decade) = .06
1,800 calories × .06 = 108 calories
1,800 calories − 108 calories = 1,692 or approximately 1,700 calories

The difference is approximately 100 calories. Because one pound of body fat represents 3,500 stored calories, eating an extra 100 calories a day can add more than ten pounds in one year! This phenomenon explains in part why many people gain weight during middle age. If physical activity remains the same, total energy input will need to decrease in order to maintain weight because of a decline in basal metabolism. Unfortunately, physical activity also tends to decline as people age, resulting in an even lower energy output.

There are two exceptions to the decline in basal metabolism with advancing age: during pregnancy and during breast-feeding. Pregnant women have higher energy needs than nonpregnant females of the same age because they are undergoing a "growth" period. Pregnancy involves the growth of the mother's tissues and the growth of the fetus. Women who breast-feed also have a higher basal metabolism because milk production costs calories.

**Environment.** Extremes in environmental temperatures can affect the amount of energy required to keep a constant body temperature of 98.6° F. At temperatures below 57° F, the body has to expend more calories to maintain 98.6° if it is inadequately clothed. Even when clothing is adequate, it has been found that the energy cost of physical activity is greater in a colder environment. In addition, there is an increased energy use due to carrying the extra weight of winter clothing. Both of these factors can cause a seven- to-ten percent increase in total calorie need.

In tropical climates, the basal metabolism slows down and may be five- to-twenty percent lower than the basal metabolism of people in a temperate climate. If strenuous activity is undertaken in extreme heat, total energy expenditure will increase slightly. The increased output is due to the activity of the cooling systems of the body. The cooling systems are the sweat glands. When sweat reaches the surface of the skin, it evaporates and a cooling effect results. If sweating did not occur, the body temperature would rise uncontrollably and death would result.

**Physiological State.** Illness can rapidly change energy expenditure. For example, cancer increases basal metabolism as a result of the rapid growth of cancer cells. It is extremely difficult to encourage weight maintenance in cancer patients due to the increased energy needs and an often decreased appetite.

Fever also increases basal metabolism. When a person has a fever, more heat than usual is produced by the body. It takes calories to produce that heat, and a common estimate is a seven percent increase in basal metabolism for every one-degree Fahrenheit increase in body temperature. Going back to our 19-year-old male, at a body temperature of 98.6° F, 1,800 calories are required for basal metabolism. If he has a fever, and his body temperature rises to 102°F, the calories needed for basal metabolism will increase to approximately 2,200 calories. [Display the calculations below.]

102° − 98.6° = 3.4°
3.4° × .07 (increase per degree F) = .238
1,800 calories × .238 = 428.4 calories
1,800 calories + 428.4 calories = 2,228.4 or about 2,200 calories

**Personal Life Style.** Sedentary individuals expend fewer calories than active individuals, and this is true for both basal metabolism and for activity. Athletes tend to maintain a higher BMR than nonathletes; athletes also require more calories for their strenuous activities.

The total calories expended for physical activity in one day can be estimated by first determining the basic activity level most typical of the individual. This table lists physical activities in four classifications. [Display the table.]

**Classification of Activities**

| SEDENTARY | LIGHT | MODERATE | VERY ACTIVE |
|---|---|---|---|
| Doing homework | Activities done while standing | Carpentry work | Basketball |
| Eating | Dishwashing | Gardening | Bicycling (13 mph) |
| Listening to the radio | Making beds | Heavy housework | Cheerleading |
| Other sitting types of activity that are not strenuous | Mopping | Walking moderately fast | Cross-country skiing |
| Playing cards | Personal care | Window washing | Dancing, fast |
| Reading | Preparing food | | Football |
| Sewing | Sweeping | | Running (7 mph) |
| Sitting in class | Walking slowly | | Skiing |
| Typing | | | Swimming |
| Watching T.V. | | | Tennis |
| Writing | | | |

When an individual's activity level is determined, the following formulas may be used, along with the basal metabolism requirement, to estimate the total calories expended for physical activity in one day:

For "sedentary" individuals:
calories for basal metabolism × 20% = calories for physical activity

For "light activity" individuals:
calories for basal metabolism × 30% = calories for physical activity

For "moderate activity" individuals:
calories for basal metabolism × 40% = calories for physical activity

For "very active" individuals:
calories for basal metabolism × 50% = calories for physical activity

An example will illustrate the profound impact of personal life style on energy needs. Again, we will use our 19-year-old male who is 5 feet 10 inches and 154 pounds. Remember that total energy needs must include calories spent for basal metabolism, for physical activity, and for digestion of food.

| SEDENTARY | | VERY ACTIVE | |
|---|---|---|---|
| • calories expended for basal metabolism: | 1,800 | • calories expended for basal metabolism: | 1,800 |
| • calories expended for physical activity (1,800 × .20 = 360) | + 360 | • calories expended for physical activity (1,800 × .50 = 900) | + 900 |
| SUBTOTAL | 2,160 | SUBTOTAL | 2,700 |
| • calories expended for food digestion (2,160 × .10 = 216) | + 216 | • calories expended for food digestion (2,700 × .10 = 270) | + 270 |
| Total Energy Expenditure | 2,376 | Total Energy Expenditure | 2,970 |

If the sedentary male eats 2,970 calories each day instead of 2,376, he will gain almost 62 pounds in a single year!

The many factors that affect energy expenditure rarely occur in isolation. This makes an accurate calculation of energy expenditure very difficult, if not impossible. A close approximation, however, can be made using the steps outlined in this unit.

---

This unit builds on Unit 1 by providing more information on basal metabolic rate and on the factors that can affect it. Prior to beginning this unit, it may be useful to review with students the concepts in Unit 1. When presenting the information in the "Teacher's Unit Introduction," it will be helpful to demonstrate problems on the chalkboard.

The activities in this unit require some basic math skills. It may be helpful, depending on the level of your class, to review basic addition, subtraction, multiplication, and division principles. Students with weak math skills could be paired with students having well-developed skills. Go over the examples of each mathematical equation and problem encountered in this unit.

## BASIC ACTIVITY

**Time Needed:** One class period

**Materials Needed:** Sheet 2-1: "Nomogram"
Sheet 2-2: "Basal Metabolism Calories"
Sheet 2-3: "Calculating Energy Needs"
*Optional:* Tape measure and scale
Quiz Sheet 2-1

1. Distribute copies of Sheet 2-1, "Nomogram," Sheet 2-2, "Basal Metabolism Calories," and Sheet 2-3, "Calculating Energy Needs," to each student. In the spaces provided on Sheet 2-3 each student should record his or her height in feet and inches and weight in pounds. If students do not know their measurement or weight, have them measure and weigh each other. (*Note:* Some students in the class may be reluctant to be weighed due to over- or underweight. Be sensitive to the needs of your students and allow students to estimate their weights if necessary.)

2. On Sheet 2-1, "Nomogram," students mark their height in the column labeled "Height" and their weight in the column labeled "Weight." They then draw a ruled line to connect the two marks. The example on the sheet illustrates the case of a female who is 5′3″ tall and weighs 110 pounds. The "Nomogram" line intersects the "Surface Area" line at 1.5 square meters. Students should enter their "Surface Area" statistic on Sheet 2-3.

3. After determining their "Surface Area," students use Sheet 2-2, "Basal Metabolism Calories." Each student should locate his or her age and sex, and should multiply the calories/square meter/hour figure for it by the square meter "Surface Area" value determined in step 2.

4. Next, students follow the steps for calculating calories for basal metabolism provided on Sheet 2-3, "Calculating Energy Needs," and round off numbers at each step. Following are the calculations for a 16-year-old female with a Surface Area of 1.5 square meters:

| | | |
|---|---|---|
| 1.5 square meters | × 37.2 cal/sq. m/hr | = 56 calories/hour |
| 56 calories/hour | × 24 hours/day | = 1,344 calories/day |

This girl needs about 1,340 calories each day for basal metabolism alone.

5. Next, students calculate physical activity calories. Display the "Classification of Activities" table from the "Teacher's Unit Introduction" on the chalkboard or use an opaque projector or overhead projector. Also supply the percentage of calories for basal metabolism for each of the four activity levels, which follows the table. Students should determine their overall activity level: sedentary, light, moderate, or very active, and should calculate their physical activity calories by multiplying the calories determined in step 4 by the appropriate percentage. Continuing with our example, assume that the female is moderately active:

1,340 basal metabolism calories × 40% = 536 physical activity calories

This girl needs about 540 calories (rounded off) each day for physical activity.

6. Finally, have the students calculate food digestion calories by multiplying the sum of their basal metabolism calories and physical activity calories by 10 percent. This figure (rounded) is then added to the sum of the first two calorie categories to determine the total energy needs for one day. To complete the example:

| | | | | |
|---|---|---|---|---|
| 1,340 + 540 | | | = | 1,880 calories |
| 1,880 calories × 10% | | | = | 188 food digestion calories, rounded to 190 calories |
| 1,340 | + 540 | + 190 | = | 2,070 |
| basal metabolism calories | + physical activity calories | + food digestion/ absorption calories | = | total calories needed each day |

7. After students have completed Sheet 2-3, discuss how body size, sex, age, and physical activity affect total calorie needs by comparing the values the students obtained.

8. Proceed with the "Advanced Activity" if you wish. Otherwise, use the quiz mentioned in step 9.

9. **Evaluation:** Distribute Quiz Sheet 2-1 and have students complete it independently, or use it as the basis of a group discussion.

## ADVANCED ACTIVITY

**Time Needed:** Two class periods

**Materials Needed:** Sheet 2-1: "Nomogram"
Sheet 2-2: "Basal Metabolism Calories"
Sheet 2-3: "Calculating Energy Needs"
Sheets 2-4 through 2-6: "What Is the Energy Output?"
Sheet 2-7: "Energy Input/Output Facts"
Quiz Sheet 2-1

### Class Period 1

1. Students must complete the "Basic Activity" in order to do the "Advanced Activity." Allow one class period for the "Basic Activity" and the following period for the "Advanced Activity."

### Class Period 2

1. Give each student copies of Sheets 2-4 through 2-6, "What Is the Energy Output?" and Sheet 2-7, "Energy Input/Output Facts," and have them work independently. Or, divide the class into groups and assign one case to each group.

2. After completing Sheets 2-4 through 2-6, have the students write a short description of their cases with the derived Total Energy Output. Have them briefly discuss how the Total Energy Output undergoes changes for each specific case due to changes in life style,

environment, age, and physiological state. How could each person cope with these changes through nutrition?

3. Conduct a class discussion using the following questions along with Sheet 2-7:

- Who had the least energy output? (*Answer:* Tomchuk) The most? (*Answer:* Sinwa)
- What factors caused the lowest output? (*Answer:* being female) The highest? (*Answer:* being male; having a fever)
- What factors increase basal metabolism calories? (*Answer:* cold climate, active life style, fever, large body size)
- What factors increased basal metabolism calories? (*Answer:* cold climate, active life style, fever, large body size)
- How does physical activity affect total energy output? (*Answer:* more physical activity leads to increased energy output)
- How could you classify most Americans in terms of physical activity? (*Answer:* sedentary)

4. After students have completed Sheet 2-3, "Calculating Energy Needs," and Sheets 2-4 through 2-6, "What Is the Energy Output?" discuss how body size, sex, age, and physical activity affect total calorie needs by comparing the values students obtained.

5. **Evaluation:** Distribute Quiz Sheet 2-1 and have students complete it independently. Discuss the answers as a class.

## FOLLOW-UP ACTIVITIES

1. Have students keep a food diary for one 24-hour period. The headings of the diary should look like this:

FOOD DIARY

| Food | Description | Amount | TOTAL GRAMS | | |
|---|---|---|---|---|---|
| | | | Protein | Carbohydrate | Fat |
| | | | | | |

Have students use a food composition table to calculate the total grams of protein, carbohydrates, and fat they consumed (*see* "References/Resources").

2. Have students use Chart G, "Calorie Expenditure by Activity," and food composition tables to develop a bulletin board that shows how much time must be spent in specific activities to work off calories from particular foods.

Name ____________________

Sheet 2-1

# NOMOGRAM*

**Directions:** To use the Nomogram, place a dot on the left graph for your height. Then place a dot on the right graph for your weight. Using a straight edge, draw a line from the left dot to the right one. The point where your ruled line crosses the middle graph indicates your "Surface Area" in square meters. Be sure to use the precise place where the line crosses the graph in your computations.

**EXAMPLE:** A female 5′3″ tall and weighing 110 pounds has a Surface Area of 1.5 square meters.

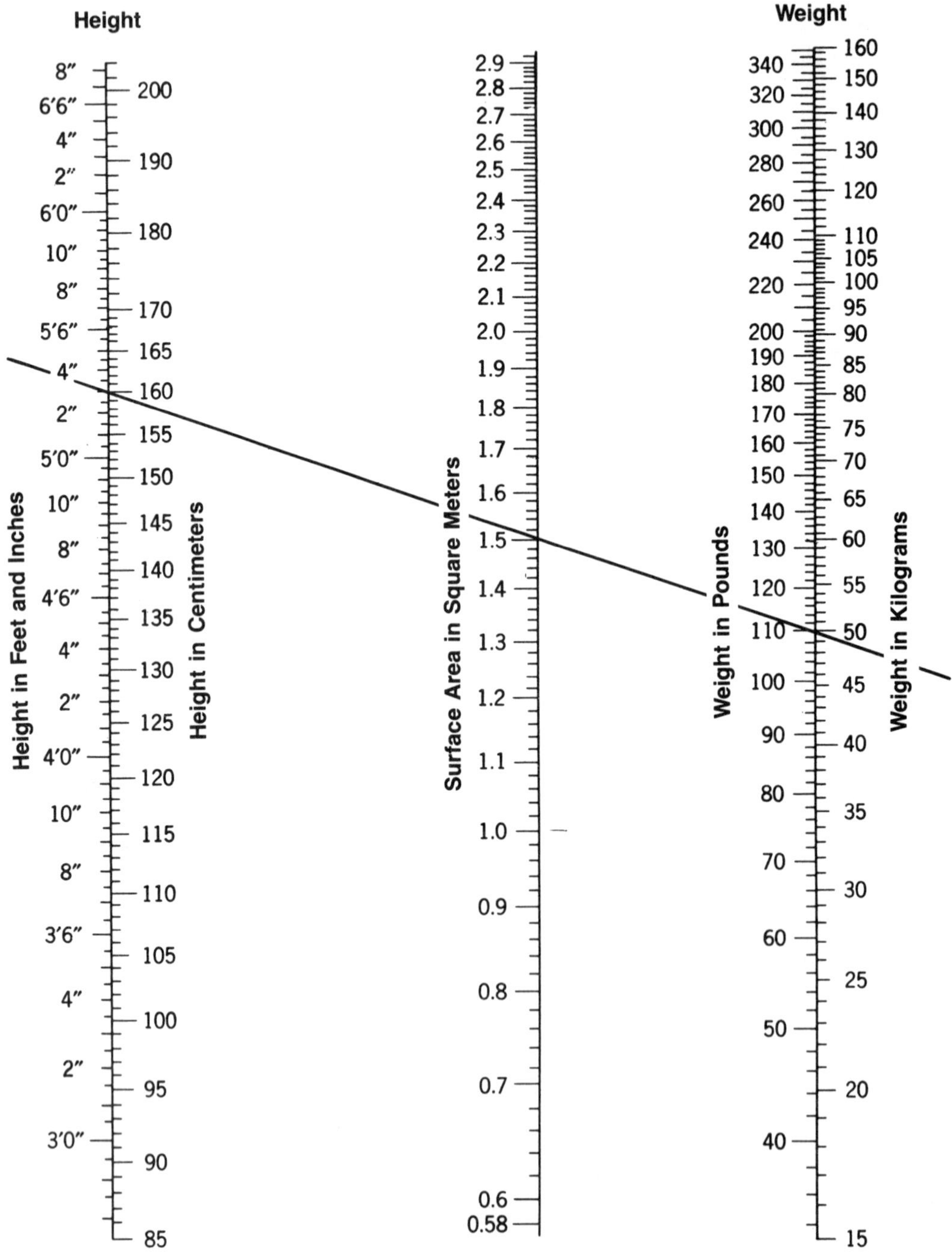




*From Boothby, W. M., Berkson, J., and Dunn, H. L. "Studies of the energy of normal individuals: A standard for basal metabolism, with a nomogram for clinical application." *American Journal of Physiology* 116:468, 1936.

Name ________________________________ Sheet 2-2

# BASAL METABOLISM CALORIES*

**Directions:** To find your basal metabolism calories for a day, locate your age on this chart and find the number of calories per square meter per hour for your sex. Multiply this figure by your body Surface Area in square meters (from Sheet 2-1) and then multiply by 24 (hours in a day).

| Age (yr) | Males (cal/sq m/hr) | Females (cal/sq m/hr) | Age (yr) | Males (cal/sq m/hr) | Females (cal/sq m/hr) |
|---|---|---|---|---|---|
| 3 | 60.1 | 54.5 | 26 | 38.2 | 35.0 |
| 4 | 57.9 | 53.9 | 27 | 38.0 | 35.0 |
| 5 | 56.3 | 53.0 | | | |
| 6 | 54.0 | 51.2 | 28 | 37.8 | 35.0 |
| 7 | 52.3 | 49.7 | 29 | 37.7 | 35.0 |
| | | | 30 | 37.6 | 35.0 |
| 8 | 50.8 | 48.0 | 31 | 37.4 | 35.0 |
| 9 | 49.5 | 46.2 | 32 | 37.2 | 34.9 |
| 10 | 47.7 | 44.9 | | | |
| 11 | 46.5 | 43.5 | 33 | 37.1 | 34.9 |
| 12 | 45.3 | 42.0 | 34 | 37.0 | 34.9 |
| | | | 35 | 36.9 | 34.8 |
| 13 | 44.5 | 40.5 | 36 | 36.8 | 34.7 |
| 14 | 43.8 | 39.2 | 37 | 36.7 | 34.6 |
| 15 | 42.9 | 38.3 | | | |
| 16 | 42.0 | 37.2 | 38 | 36.7 | 34.5 |
| 17 | 41.5 | 36.4 | 39 | 36.6 | 34.4 |
| | | | 40–44 | 36.4 | 34.1 |
| 18 | 40.8 | 35.8 | 45–49 | 36.2 | 33.8 |
| 19 | 40.5 | 35.4 | 50–54 | 35.8 | 33.1 |
| 20 | 39.9 | 35.3 | | | |
| 21 | 39.5 | 35.2 | 55–59 | 35.1 | 32.8 |
| 22 | 39.2 | 35.2 | 60–64 | 34.5 | 32.0 |
| | | | 65–69 | 33.5 | 31.6 |
| 23 | 39.0 | 35.2 | 70–74 | 32.7 | 31.1 |
| 24 | 38.7 | 35.1 | 75+ | 31.8 | |
| 25 | 38.4 | 35.1 | | | |

*From *Handbook of Biological Data,* Boothby, W. M. W. B. Saunders Company, Philadelphia, PA, 1956.

# CALCULATING ENERGY NEEDS

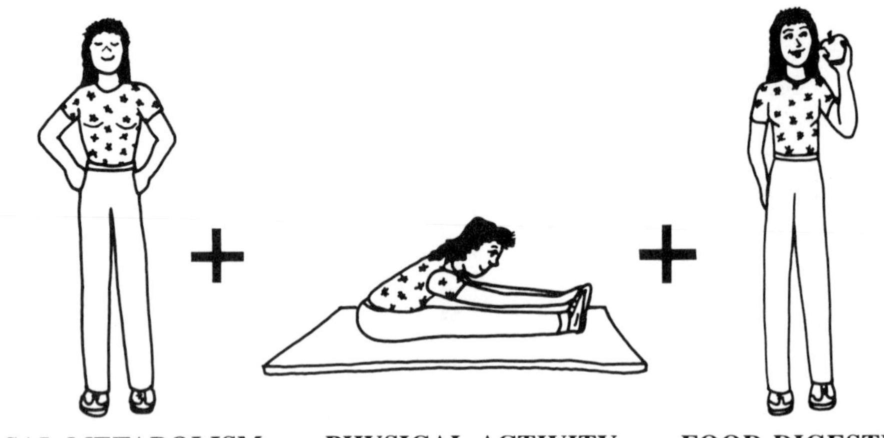

**BASAL METABOLISM** + **PHYSICAL ACTIVITY** + **FOOD DIGESTION**

**BASAL METABOLISM CALORIES:**

Your height = ______________________

Your weight = ______________________ pounds

Your surface area (from Sheet 2-1) = ______________________ square meters

1. ______________ (your surface area) × ______________ (calories/square meter/hour for your age & sex from Sheet 2-2) = ______________ (calories/hour)

2. For one day, your basal metabolism calories are:

______________ (calories/hour from #1 above) × 24 (hours/day) = ______________ (basal metabolism calories/day)

**PHYSICAL ACTIVITY CALORIES:**

| | |
|---|---|
| Sedentary: | 20% |
| Light: | 30% |
| Moderate: | 40% |
| Very Active: | 50% |

3. Multiply your basal metabolism calories from step #2 by the percentage that best describes your overall activity level.

______________ (basal metabolism calories) × ________% = ______________ (physical activity calories)

**FOOD DIGESTION CALORIES:**

4. Add your: basal metabolism calories to your ______________

physical activity calories + ______________

Multiply the total × 10% Total: ______________ × 10% = ______________ (food digestion calories)

**TOTAL ENERGY NEEDS:**

5. ______________ (basal metabolism calories) + ______________ (physical activity calories) + ______________ (food digestion calories) = ______________ (total calories needed each day)

Name ______________________ Sheet 2-4

# WHAT IS THE ENERGY OUTPUT?

## CASE #1

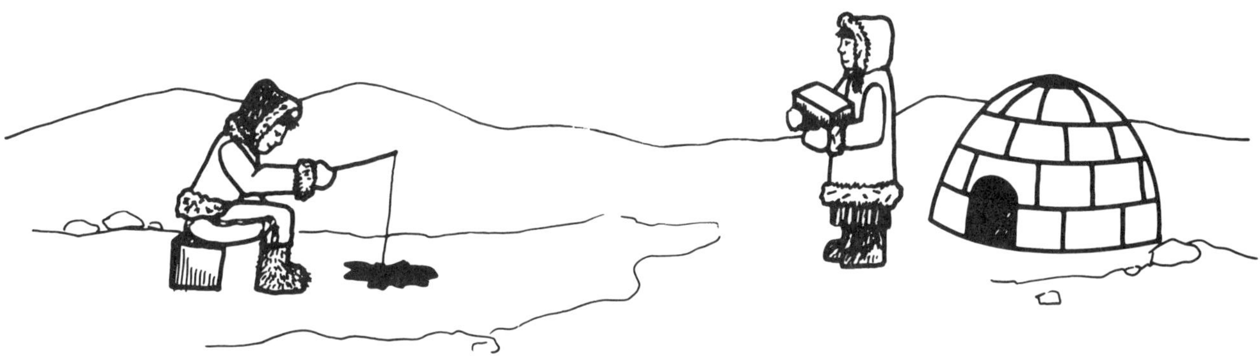

Tomchuk is a 40-year-old Eskimo woman who lives in the Arctic. She stands 5′5″ tall and weighs 136 pounds. The basal metabolism calories for Tomchuk are:

(a) ______________________
(basal metabolism calories)

Tomchuk spends most of her time doing housework and carrying heavy items. To calculate the number of calories she expends in physical activity, multiply (b) __________% by the answer determined in (a). Your answer is:

______________ × ______________ = (c) ______________
(answer from a) (answer from b) (physical activity calories)

Because of the frigid temperatures, Tomchuk wears heavy, thick clothing and she uses more energy to walk around. Her physical activity calories are increased by (d) __________%.

To calculate the additional calories needed for physical activity, multiply the answer in (d) by the answer in (c):

______________ × ______________ = (e) ______________
(answer from d) (answer from c) (additional physical activity calories in cold temperatures)

The total calories Tomchuk expends for physical activity is:

______________ + ______________ = (f) ______________
(answer from c) (answer from e) (total physical activity calories)

Determine the number of calories Tomchuk needs for food digestion by:

[ ______________ + ______________ ] × 10% = (g) ______________
(answer from a) (answer from f) (food digestion calories)

Tomchuk's total energy output is:

______________ + ______________ + ______________ = (h) ______________
(answer from a) (answer from f) (answer from g) (total energy output)

Name ______________________________ **Sheet 2-5**

# WHAT IS THE ENERGY OUTPUT?

### CASE #2

Sinwa is 16 years old and lives on an island near the equator. He is 5′5″ tall and weighs 136 pounds. The basal metabolism calories for Sinwa are:

(a) ______________________________
(basal metabolism calories)

Because Sinwa lives in a tropical climate, his basal metabolism requires about

(b) __________% less energy than someone of his age and sex living in a temperate climate. A better estimate of Sinwa's basal metabolism energy needs is:

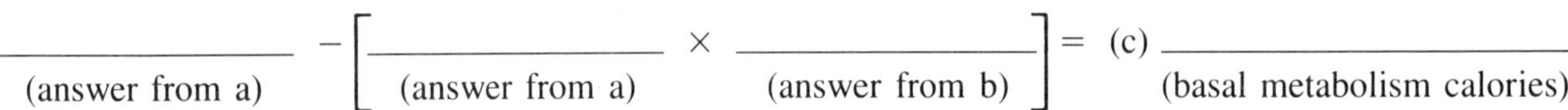

______________ − [ ______________ × ______________ ] = (c) ______________
(answer from a) [ (answer from a) (answer from b) ] (basal metabolism calories)

This morning Sinwa awoke feeling ill and discovered he had a temperature of 102°F. His basal metabolism calories are affected by his fever. Every degree Fahrenheit over 98.6°F. increases Sinwa's basal metabolism calories by (d) __________%. Calculate the basal metabolism calories Sinwa needs while he has a fever:

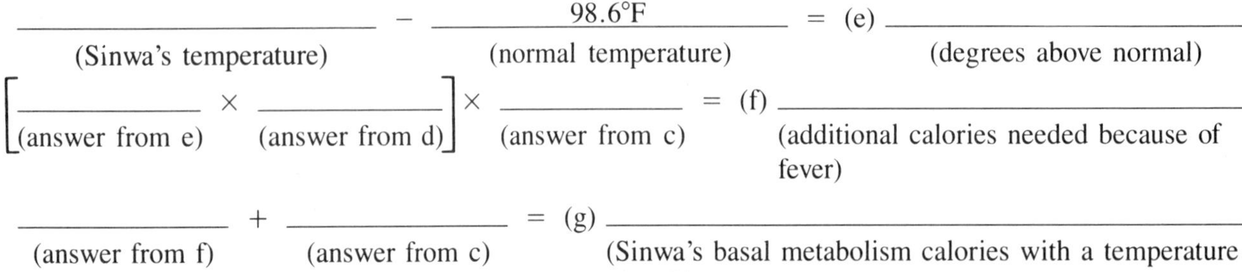

______________ − 98.6°F = (e) ______________
(Sinwa's temperature) (normal temperature) (degrees above normal)

[ ______________ × ______________ ] × ______________ = (f) ______________
[(answer from e) (answer from d)] (answer from c) (additional calories needed because of fever)

______________ + ______________ = (g) ______________
(answer from f) (answer from c) (Sinwa's basal metabolism calories with a temperature of 102°F.)

Sinwa is in bed because he is so sick. His activity level would, therefore, be classified as (h)

______________________________________________.

The calories needed for physical activity would be:

______________ × 20% = (i) ______________
(answer from g) (physical activity calories)

Determine the number of calories Sinwa needs for food digestion by:

[ ______________ + ______________ ] × 10% = (j) ______________
[ (answer from g) (answer from i) ] (food digestion calories)

Sinwa's total energy output is:

______________ + ______________ + ______________ = (k) ______________
(answer from g) (answer from i) (answer from j) (total energy output)

Name ____________________ Sheet 2-6

# WHAT IS THE ENERGY OUTPUT?

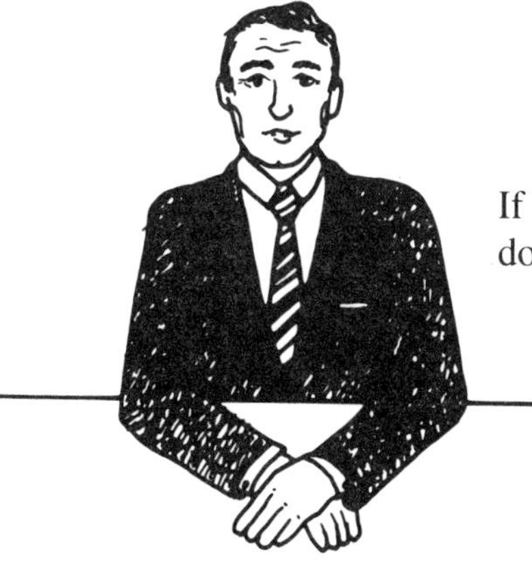

**CASE #3**

Mr. Robertson is 50 years old. He is 5′10″ tall and weighs 175 pounds. If his basal metabolism calories at age 20 were 1,877, how many calories does he now need for basal metabolism?

(a) ______ (his age) − 20 years = (b) ______ (years)

or (c) ______ (number of decades)

1,877 − [( ______ (answer from c) × 2% (rate of decrease for basal metabolism calories per decade) ) × 1,877] = (d) ______ (basal metabolism calories for Mr. Robertson)

Mr. Robertson works in an office and sits most of the day. How would you classify his activity level?

(e) ______

How many calories does Mr. Robertson expend in physical activity?

______ (answer from d) × ______% (physical activity factor) = (f) ______ (physical activity calories)

How many calories does Mr. Robertson need for food digestion?

[ ______ (answer from d) + ______ (answer from f) ] × 10% = (g) ______ (food digestion calories)

Mr. Robertson's total energy output is:

______ (answer from d) + ______ (answer from f) + ______ (answer from g) = (h) ______ (total energy output)

Name ______________________________ Sheet 2-7

# ENERGY INPUT/OUTPUT FACTS

1. The basal metabolism calories of a female are on the average about 8 percent less than the basal metabolism calories of a male.
2. For every ten years over the age of 20, basal metabolism calories decrease by 2 percent. Therefore, if an 18 year old needs 1,800 calories for basal metabolism, a 70-year-old person would need:

$$70 - 20 = 50 \text{ years} \div 10 = 5 \text{ decades}$$
$$5 \times 2\% = 10\%$$
$$1{,}800 \text{ calories} \times 10\% = 180 \text{ calories}$$
$$1{,}800 \text{ calories} - 180 \text{ calories} = \underline{1{,}620 \text{ calories}}$$

3. Cold temperatures mean an average increase of about 9 percent in physical activity calorie needs because it takes more energy to work in the cold and to carry the extra clothing.
4. In tropical climates, basal metabolism slows down. It decreases an average of 13 percent.
5. When a person has a fever, basal metabolism increases. For every degree Fahrenheit over 98.6° F (normal body temperature), there is a 7 percent increase in calories needed for basal metabolism. For example, John normally needs 1,800 calories for basal metabolism, but if he had a fever of 100° F, he would require:

$$100° \text{ F} - 98.6° \text{ F} = 1.4° \text{ F}$$
$$1.4° \text{ F} \times .07 = .098$$
$$1{,}800 \text{ calories} \times .098 = 176.4 \text{ calories}$$
$$1{,}800 \text{ calories} + 176 \text{ calories} = 1{,}976 \text{ calories}$$

6. Activity level plays an important part in the total number of calories a person needs each day. If a person is *sedentary,* multiply his or her basal metabolism calories by *20 percent,* then add this to his or her basal metabolism calories:

   1,800 × 20% = 360 (physical activity calories)
   1,800 + 360 = 2,160 calories needed for basal metabolism and sedentary activity

   If a person does *light activity, use 30 percent.*
   If a person is *moderately active, use 40 percent.*
   If a person is *very active, use 50 percent.*

7. Calories needed for the digestion and absorption of food can be calculated by adding the calories for basal metabolism to the calories for physical activity and then multiplying the sum by 10 percent.

   (basal metabolism calories + physical activity calories) × 10% = food digestion calories

8. Total energy output is the sum of calories needed for basal metabolism, physical activity, and food digestion.

   basal metabolism calories + physical activity calories + food digestion calories = total energy output

# QUIZ
# BALANCING ENERGY INPUT AND ENERGY OUTPUT

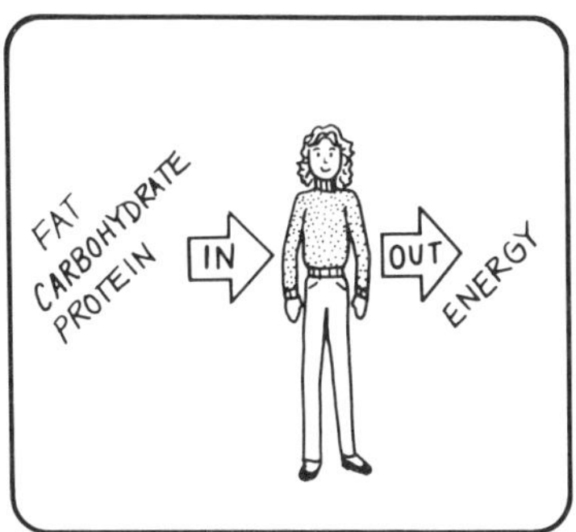


_____ 1. Which nutrient has more than twice the calories as the same amount of protein?
- a. Carbohydrate.
- b. Fat.
- c. Vitamins.
- d. Minerals.

_____ 2. As a person grows older, his or her basal metabolism
- a. Increases.
- b. Decreases.
- c. Stays the same.
- d. Not enough information to answer.

_____ 3. If all of the following have the same body weight, who would need the most calories?
- a. An 18-year-old female who lives in North America and is sedentary.
- b. An 18-year-old male who lives in North America and is moderately active.
- c. An 18-year-old female who lives in the tropics and is moderately active.
- d. An 18-year-old male who lives in the Arctic and is moderately active.

_____ 4. Of the total calories needed each day, most are used for:
- a. Basal metabolism.
- b. Physical activity.
- c. Digestion of food.
- d. Absorption of food.

_____ 5. Which is true?
- a. The greater the body size, the greater the energy expended.
- b. A person with a fever expends less energy than a person without a fever.
- c. During adult life there is a steady increase in caloric needs.
- d. Pregnant women have a lower basal metabolic rate than nonpregnant women.

_____ 6. To increase the total number of calories expended each day you could:
- a. Eat more food.
- b. Eat less food.
- c. Increase physical activity.
- d. Increase basal metabolism.

# SECTION II

# DIET PLANNING

# Unit 3: How Food Patterns Develop

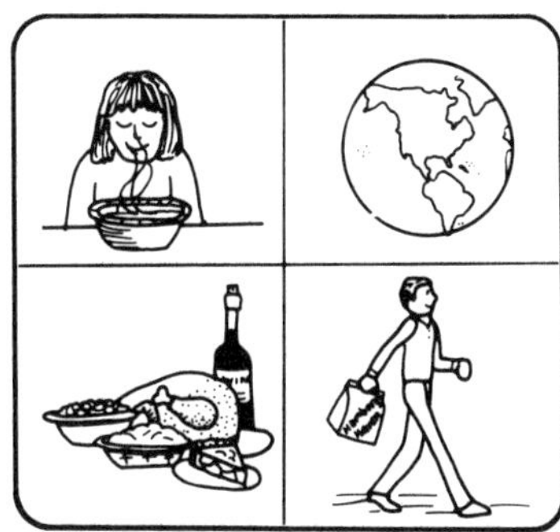

## CONCEPTS

–Traditional and common foods in our diet originate from various parts of the world.

–The significance of these foods can be measured by their nutrient contribution, availability, and social meaning.

## OBJECTIVES

–Students will list and explain the factors influencing the development of food patterns.

–Students will evaluate the nutritional contribution of various traditional foods.

## TEACHER'S UNIT INTRODUCTION

What we eat depends on a number of factors. These factors cause us to choose different foods, to have different preferences, and consequently to have different eating patterns. Food habits, which begin developing early in life, are the result of many influences, including ethnic and family customs, food availability, life style, and personal preferences. The saying "you are what you eat" is often true because the foods you eat reflect the combination of these factors and help to make you the unique person that you are. Let's take a closer look at some of these factors.

**Psychological Factors.** Food often has psychological meaning. The attachment of an emotional meaning to food is often the result of an association of a time, place, person, or situation with a particular food. This emotional tie gives the food more meaning to the individual than can be explained by its taste or nutritional value alone. For example, when a child became sick, he or she may always have been given homemade chicken soup. Thereafter, the child may associate security with the soup. And, when the child is older, he or she may desire chicken soup whenever stricken with illness, because it symbolizes security. Another example of this phenomenon may be the smell of homemade bread evoking memories of an individual's childhood when special days were spent in the kitchen while mother baked bread. Oftentimes, foods used repeatedly in the same social context develop some psychological meaning. Foods can be associated with a wide variety of feelings: security, reward, punishment, or happiness. These feelings are often unique to the individual or family.

**Cultural Factors.** Food patterns are strongly influenced by a person's culture. "Culture" includes the way people behave and also their thoughts, speech, customary beliefs, and social acts. Most cultural food patterns are based on geographic location, religious beliefs, social traditions, and life style. Cultural traditions related to food are usually so strong that people take their food traditions with them when they leave their native land, as did many of the immigrants who came to America. For example, individuals of Italian descent may still begin their evening meal with an antipasto and may also have some pasta as a side dish. Likewise, people of Mexican descent may include a large variety of dishes incorporating beans in their daily diet.

Today in the United States there are numerous examples of food customs that originated in other countries and that have become traditional foods. As a result, the American diet has become a wonderful mixture, or "melting pot," of foods from many cultural backgrounds.

**Geographic Factors.** The geography of a country has a large impact on the development of food patterns. The climate and soil of a country determine the foods that are eaten in that area. Even though international trade has made once exotic foods available in lands where they are not native, countries continue to depend on locally grown, raised, or caught foods. These foods often become staple foods. Since people learn to depend on foods in plentiful supply, food patterns are built around what is available, and people acquire a taste for foods that are familiar.

Many examples show the effect of geography on the typical foods eaten by people around the world. Rice grows well in hot, humid climates, and wheat grows best in more moderate, drier conditions. Thus, rice is a staple in Oriental countries, and wheat is a staple in the United States and Europe where climatic conditions are favorable to each food. In countries that have large coastal regions, such as Japan, England, and Greece, fish is a basic food. Where grazing land is abundant, cattle are often raised for beef and dairy products. If pastureland is either hilly or not plentiful, raising sheep and goats is more successful than raising cattle. For this reason, lamb and goat are important foods in many Mediterranean countries.

Differences in food habits due to geography can be seen even in the United States. In New England, where coastal waters are abundant and farmland is rocky and limited in area, seafood is frequently used in the diet. A preference for cornbread is noted in the South where corn grows well. Potatoes are a common addition to many dinner tables in the Midwest and in the northern states due to the excellent growing conditions for potatoes in these regions.

**Religious Factors.** Religious traditions influence the foods we eat in that some religious doctrines prohibit certain foods, either completely or on specific occasions. Many religions hold to dietary guidelines. For example, Hindus avoid all meat, onions, garlic, and turnips. Seventh Day Adventists are *ovolacto* vegetarians, and individuals of the Jewish faith often do not eat pork or shellfish and do not eat dairy/meat food combinations.

**Social and Family Factors.** Two other factors influencing the development of food patterns are social and family traditions. Many food customs are founded on social occasions and special events such as birth, marriage, anniversaries, and national and religious holidays. It would be hard to imagine a birthday party without a cake and ice cream, or a Thanksgiving without turkey, or a 4th of July picnic without hotdogs and hamburgers. Foods have become associated with special occasions for a variety of reasons. One reason may be to relive a particular event; many of the traditional foods that grace the modern Thanksgiving table are the same ones shared by the Indians and Pilgrims. In the past, many foods were too scarce or expensive for everyday use, so they were saved for special holidays. This was particularly true of sugar in early Colonial days and may offer an explanation for the use of cakes and sweets to celebrate special occasions like birthdays, weddings, and holidays.

Food is also a sign of hospitality. In most cultures, the offering of food and beverage to visitors is a sign of welcome. This custom probably comes from the fact that visitors were often weary and hungry after traveling long distances in what today would be primitive circumstances. Some foods in particular have become traditional welcome foods, such as tea or coffee in the United States and bread and cheese in many European countries.

Family traditions may also color one's food patterns. Families tend to hold on to favorite and familiar foods typical of their ethnic backgrounds. The food customs of your grandparents and great-grandparents influence the foods your family eats now. This is because the food customs of a family are taught to the children as a part of eating habits. Examples of the family's influence in determining food habits might include: (1) a particular meal that is served on a certain night of the week; (2) a certain combination of dishes that becomes a traditional meal; or (3) a special way of preparing a dish that was handed down from one generation to the next.

**Life Style Factors.** One's life style can often dictate the types of food that make up one's diet. People who live "on-the-run" and who do not spend much time at home preparing or eating their meals may choose a food pattern consisting largely of convenience foods, frozen foods, or foods from fast-food restaurants. In contrast, someone who has a more leisurely life style may have a completely different meal pattern, which might include homemade breads, fresh garden vegetables, and foods that involve more preparation time.

**Individual Preference Factors.** Individual likes and dislikes also help to determine one's food pattern. Traditional or common foods may be deleted from one's diet because of personal taste. New foods from other cultures or areas of the world might be added to one's food customs if they are agreeable to an individual's tastes.

**Nutritional Factors.** One last point that should be noted is that many of the traditional foods in our diet make a significant contribution to our nutritional needs. Oftentimes, the combination of ingredients or dishes in a meal provides the variety of nutrients that are an important part of a nutritious diet and that help us maintain health. These food patterns have survived and have become traditional probably because the individuals who ate these foods survived and passed them down in their family.

It is interesting to observe that different foods are relied upon to provide the same nutrients in various cultures. An example of this is the use of yams in the southern United States and of tomatoes in Italian cuisine to provide Vitamin A. Another example is the typical glass of orange juice at breakfast in the United States and a selection of assorted fresh fruits in the diets of people from tropical countries, both of which supply Vitamin C.

---

While the discussion of food patterns is an interesting activity, many misconceptions and biases may surface. Students must be reminded that generalizations cannot be made based upon limited exposure to various cultures. In addition, the individual habits and patterns of each student can be personal issues. Discussion leaders should be sensitive to students' privacy.

## BASIC ACTIVITY

**Time Needed:** One class period

**Materials Needed:** Sheet 3-1: "Foods I Eat"
Sheet 3-2: "Nutrients in Food Dishes"
Chart B: "Daily Food Guide"
Sheet 3-3: "Survey: How Food Patterns Develop"

1. Discuss the variety of food patterns that exist. Use the following questions as guidelines for the discussion:

- How do food patterns of people in this country differ?
- How do foods from various cultures differ?
- Why would food patterns be different?

2. Distribute copies of Sheet 3-1, "Foods I Eat," and have the students complete the sheet independently.

3. As a class, discuss the factors affecting individual food patterns (psychological, cultural, geographical, religious, social and family traditions, life style, individual preferences, nutritional, and any others that would apply).

4. Encourage students to share personal food associations by posing questions like these:

- Are the emotions associated with foods always positive emotions? Why?
- How do people develop an emotional association with certain foods?
- How do foods get passed down through the generations in a family? Give examples from your own family.
- How do foods become common in a country other than where they originated?
- What social occasions or holidays are associated with particular foods?

- What are some of the foods that are plentiful in this part of the country and that are important in our diet?
- How do family food customs develop? Give some examples from your own family.
- How do different life styles affect food patterns? How could you alter your life style to improve your eating habits?
- How or why do foods become common or traditional for different meals during the course of a day?

5. Divide the class into groups of four students apiece and give each student a copy of Sheet 3-2, "Nutrients in Food Dishes." Assign each group one set of foods to analyze for nutrients. They may look up the foods in Chart B, "Daily Food Guide," as a group or they may divide the task among the group members.

6. Each group should list the major nutrients (protein, carbohydrate, fat, and specific vitamins and minerals) contributed by each food in each main dish. Then have students rate the four dishes from low to high as contributors of major nutrients.

7. Have each group present its results. Then have the whole class discuss the different sources of protein, carbohydrate, fat, and specific vitamins and minerals in the various foods and have them also discuss the assigned ratings.

8. **Evaluation:** Distribute Sheet 3-3 and have students complete it independently. Then discuss their answers as a class.

## ADVANCED ACTIVITY

**Time Needed:** Two class periods

**Materials Needed:** Resource materials in the library

### Class Period 1

1. Have students divide into groups of three to five and choose a particular culture of interest to them.

2. Have each group research the food customs and habits of the chosen culture. Students should look for information to answer the following questions:

- What are the traditional foods of the area?
- Why do you suppose the foods are traditional?
- Are there any special occasions or holidays that are celebrated with traditional foods? How are they celebrated?
- What are the particular factors that affect the food availability and choices of the people in that area?

### Class Period 2

1. Have students share the information they find with the class in whatever format they choose: oral report, demonstration, food fair, play, and so forth. Compare and contrast the

food patterns of various cultures and regions; look for similarities and differences, and try to propose reasons for them.

## FOLLOW-UP ACTIVITIES

1. Have students prepare a meal or dish that is a family favorite. Ask them to bring to class recipes for the foods. The recipes can then be compiled into a class booklet called "Family Favorites."

2. Have students research food taboos. Have them determine how the food taboos might contribute to malnutrition.

Name ______________________________ 

# FOODS I EAT

**Directions:** Write your own food associations by filling in each category below.

Foods that have some emotional meaning to me: ______________________________

______________________________

Foods that my ancestors ate and that my family still eats: ______________________________

______________________________

Foods I eat because of social traditions: ______________________________

______________________________

Foods I eat or avoid because of religious beliefs: ______________________________

______________________________

Foods I eat because they are plentiful where I live: ______________________________

______________________________

Foods I eat because of my family customs: ______________________________

______________________________

Foods I eat because of my life style: ______________________________

______________________________

Foods I eat that originated in another country: ______________________________

______________________________

Foods I eat with friends: ______________________________

______________________________

Foods that my family (friends) like, but that I do not care for (or vice versa): ______________________________

______________________________

Foods I eat for other reasons (specify):

______________________________

______________________________

______________________________

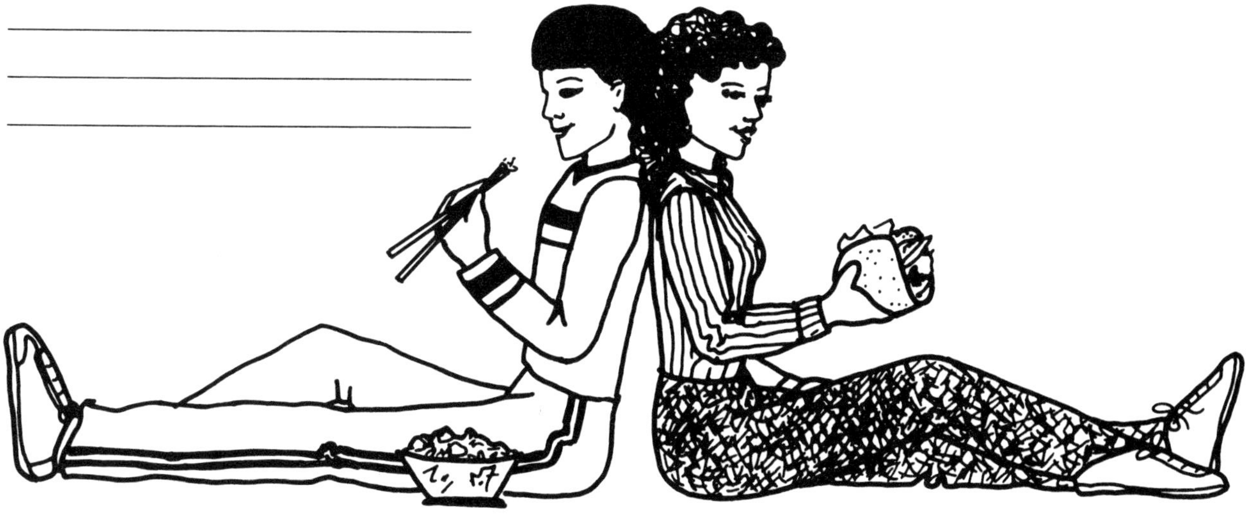

Name ______________________________ 

# NUTRIENTS IN FOOD DISHES

**Directions:** Choose one set of food dishes below and use Chart B, "Daily Food Guide," to analyze the major nutrients contributed by each food in the dish. Write each food with its nutrients in the appropriate columns below. Continue on the back of this sheet if necessary.

SET 1
- Mexican Taco—cornmeal taco shell filled with tomatoes, lettuce, and cheese
- Southern Spoon Bread—soft cornmeal bread eaten with a spoon
- New England Clam Chowder—clams and potatoes in a soup broth made of clam juice, water, and milk
- Pennsylvania Dutch Scrapple—pork cooked with cornmeal and seasonings

SET 2
- Chili con Carne—hamburger, kidney beans, and onions in a spicy tomato sauce
- Quiche Lorraine—pie shell filled with a custard/egg mixture and flavored with onion, cheese, and bacon
- Cheese Ravioli—pasta squares filled with cheese in tomato sauce
- Irish Stew—lamb cooked with potatoes, onions, and carrots

SET 3
- Beef Stroganoff—sliced beef with mushrooms and onions in a sour cream sauce and served over noodles
- Shrimp Egg Rolls—egg roll shell filled with shrimp and shredded vegetables
- Curried Chicken—sliced chicken in a spicy cream sauce served over rice
- Beans with Rice—cooked kidney beans mixed with rice

SET 4
- Macaroni and Cheese—baked casserole of tube macaroni, cheese, and milk sauce
- Bean Tostadas—mashed beans on a crisp, round cornmeal tortilla, topped with tomatoes and grated cheese
- Candied Yams—sliced yams baked in a brown sugar/butter sauce
- Carrot and Raisin Salad—shredded carrots and raisins mixed with salad dressing

| | |
|---|---|
| **FRUIT-VEGETABLE GROUP:** | **MILK-CHEESE GROUP:** |
| | **MEAT-POULTRY-FISH-BEANS GROUP:** |
| **BREAD-CEREAL GROUP:** | **FATS-SWEETS-ALCOHOL GROUP:** |

Name ______________________________ Sheet 3-3

# SURVEY: HOW FOOD PATTERNS DEVELOP

**Directions:** List below the eight factors that influence our individual eating patterns. Next to each factor, give at least one example of how that factor has influenced *your* eating patterns.

| FACTORS | EXAMPLES |
|---|---|
| 1. ______________________ | ______________________ |
| | ______________________ |
| 2. ______________________ | ______________________ |
| | ______________________ |
| 3. ______________________ | ______________________ |
| | ______________________ |
| 4. ______________________ | ______________________ |
| | ______________________ |
| 5. ______________________ | ______________________ |
| | ______________________ |
| 6. ______________________ | ______________________ |
| | ______________________ |
| 7. ______________________ | ______________________ |
| | ______________________ |
| 8. ______________________ | ______________________ |
| | ______________________ |

# Unit 4: Analyzing Your Food Intake

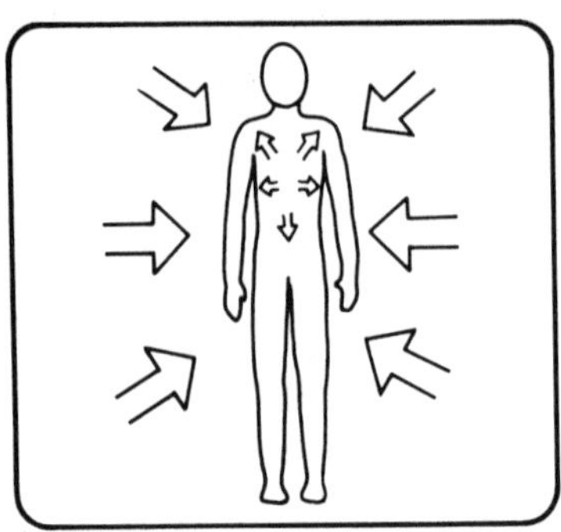

## CONCEPTS

–Food intake is regulated and influenced by a combination of internal and external factors.

## OBJECTIVES

–Students will be able to identify internal and external factors that influence food intake.

–Students will examine how their own eating behaviors are influenced by internal and external factors.

–Students will be able to list the possible health consequences that result when internal and external factors do not function properly.

## TEACHER'S UNIT INTRODUCTION

Why do people eat? How do people maintain an energy balance? Much research has been devoted to answering these two questions. Nutritionists currently believe that the regulation of food intake is influenced by an interplay of internal and external factors. Internal factors refer to the processes that occur inside the body and that create hunger. External factors refer to environmental influences and may be thought of as occurring outside the body. These environmental influences typically create an appetite that may or may not coincide with hunger.

Although hunger and appetite are often experienced together, they are not the same. *Hunger* is the response to the body's need for nutrients and calories. *Appetite* is a response shaped by experiences in the environment and is not always associated with a physical need. Knowing the difference between hunger and appetite may help a person change eating behavior in order to maintain desirable body weight.

**Internal Factors.** There are several theories that try to explain how internal factors regulate food intake. One theory states that the brain always creates hunger signals that begin your eating behaviors. When the physical need for nutrients has been met, hormonal or nerve signals overpower the hunger signals, which results in a feeling of fullness. Another theory states that hour-to-hour changes in sugar or glucose concentration in the blood affect how often and how much food is eaten. When blood glucose levels are too low, the brain signals us to eat. Another theory of food intake regulation states that your eating behaviors are regulated by the number and size of the fat cells in your body. According to this theory, the body closely watches how much fat it has and works to maintain that amount of fat (adipose tissue). This theory of food intake regulation is concerned with gradual adjustments in food intake to maintain weight. This may explain why some people appear to maintain a certain weight over a long period of time regardless of their activity level or of what they eat. These are only a few of the theories that suggest how internal factors influence food intake regulation.

**External Factors.** People eat in response not only to what is occurring inside of their bodies, but also in response to what is occurring in the environment. Everyone has experienced an appetite for a particular food when he or she was not hungry. This experience is often due to an external cue. Some of these external factors have been listed in this table. [The table shown below should be shown using an opaque or overhead projector.]

External Factors Influencing Food Intake

| External Factors | Description |
|---|---|
| 1. The taste of food | Foods are often eaten because they taste good, not always because we are hungry. For example, we may eat an extra helping of dressing at Thanksgiving dinner or a piece of pumpkin pie even after a large Thanksgiving meal. |
| 2. Food availability | Many foods are made to eat on the run. Fast-food restaurants offer these foods. Supermarkets also sell many instant or ready-to-eat foods, which are easier and faster to prepare than foods made from scratch. |
| 3. Time of day | Many individuals become accustomed to eating at a particular time of day. We respond to "It is noon and therefore time to eat" rather than "I am hungry and so I will eat." |
| 4. Social gatherings | Eating is an integral part of social life. Who would think of giving a party without food or beverages? How many of us crave a hotdog at a baseball game or popcorn at the movies? |

External Factors Influencing Food Intake

| External Factors | Description |
|---|---|
| 5. Sight and smell of food | Billboards, magazines, newspapers, and television and radio commercials constantly tell us about all of the foods we can eat and how tasty they are. How many of us can resist the urge to buy pastries when passing a bakery window or to buy bread just out of the oven? |
| 6. Emotional outlet | When people are bored, tense, angry, frustrated, or happy, eating may be relied upon to pull them through the experience or to celebrate the occasion. For example, you might eat a whole box of cookies while studying for an exam or have cheesecake to celebrate losing five pounds. |

Our environment bombards us with cues to stimulate appetite and promote eating. To say that we eat simply because we are hungry is not true. Because we are social beings, external cues work with physical needs to influence eating behavior.

What happens when internal factors or external factors fail to regulate food intake according to physical needs? When food intake regulation breaks down, individuals will become overweight or underweight and are at risk of developing other health problems. For example, being underweight may increase an individual's susceptibility to infection. On the other hand, consumption of calories in excess of body needs over a long period of time will result in obesity. Excess body fat seriously affects the organs and systems of the body. Associated with obesity are decreased life expectancy, kidney problems, heart disease, gall bladder disease, increased blood pressure, diabetes, and arthritis. Oftentimes the cause of obesity cannot be explained by a physical problem such as an underactive thyroid condition. To achieve and maintain a desirable body weight, most overweight people may need to exert greater control over the external factors that influence their food intake. A heightened sensitivity to these cues may help to avoid future weight problems.

---

When teaching this unit, keep in mind the main question that students are trying to answer: Why do we eat? Each student has a variety of individual reasons for eating. These reasons can change dramatically from day to day, even from moment to moment. The most important aspect of this unit is the students' exploration of the various internal and external factors that affect their eating habits and patterns. If students are having difficulty with the discussions and brainstorming sessions, suggest that they discuss their reasons for eating a particular meal—for example, the breakfast of that morning or the dinner of the previous day. Alternatively, have students pair off and sit with their partner at lunch time. Have each pair of students share their reasons for eating that particular lunch. The discussions may also be encouraged by giving your own personal reasons for eating.

## BASIC ACTIVITY

**Time Needed:** One class period

**Materials Needed:** Sheet 4-1: "Eating Under the Influence"
Quiz Sheet 4-1

1. Distribute Sheet 4-1, "Eating Under the Influence," to all students.
2. Discuss with students how food intake can be regulated and influenced by internal and external factors.
3. Have students record on Sheet 4-1 all of the foods and beverages they consumed in one 24-hour period. For each food eaten, students should also specify the time of day it was consumed and identify which factor or factors (internal, external, or a combination of the two) influenced them to eat that food. By figuring their percentages of "I," "E," and "C" factors, students should then determine whether their eating behavior was motivated more by internal or external cues.
4. Conduct a class discussion of the activity using the following as guidelines:

- How many students were influenced more by external factors?
- What was the average external factor percentage for the class?
- How many students were influenced primarily by internal factors?
- What was the average internal factor percentage for the class?
- How many students were influenced primarily by a combination of both factors?
- What was the average combination factor percentage for the class?
- How do the average values compare?
- Do the students feel that their calculated averages reflect the typical eating pattern of the entire country?
- What nutrition problems do the students believe are being aggravated by the number of external factors influencing food intake?
- How many students would like to change their response to external influences? How could they do this?

5. Divide the students into six groups. Assign each group to one of the external factors listed in the "Teacher's Unit Introduction."
6. Have each group list examples of how food intake is influenced by the external factor assigned to their group. For example, the group assigned to "social gathering" might list Easter as a time when many people desire chocolate, candy, or roast lamb.
7. Have students brainstorm how these influences on food intake could be changed to limit nutritional problems like obesity.
8. Conclude the activity by having a spokesperson from each group present the group's examples and ideas.
9. Proceed with the "Advanced Activity" if you wish; otherwise use the quiz mentioned in step 10.

10. **Evaluation:** Distribute Quiz Sheet 4-1 and have students complete it independently during class or as a homework assignment. Discuss the answers as a class.

## ADVANCED ACTIVITY

**Time Needed:** One class period

**Materials Needed:** Sheet 4-2: "External Eating Influences"
Quiz Sheet 4-1

1. Distribute Sheet 4-2, "External Eating Influences," at least one day in advance of the classroom activity. Have students keep a record of all of the external influences on their food intake that they observe in one 24-hour period. They should record the location of the external cue (the particular social gathering, billboard, TV or radio commercial, magazine or newspaper advertisement or article, and so on).

2. Following completion of Sheet 4-2, have students answer these questions:

- Why do advertisers appeal to external influences on food intake regulation?
- What would happen if internal factors were emphasized by advertisers?
- How can people strike a comfortable balance between internal and external regulation of food intake?

3. Divide the class into groups of four and have each group design an advertisement for broadcast or print media that appeals to internal factors.

4. Have each group present their advertisement and report the problems they encountered in developing it.

5. **Evaluation:** Distribute Quiz Sheet 4-1 and have students complete it as a homework assignment. Discuss the answers as a class.

## FOLLOW-UP ACTIVITIES

1. Have students design a bulletin board with magazine ads that emphasize external cues. Students should identify the cues involved in each ad.

2. Invite a dietitian to class to talk about behavior modification for weight loss, which is a regimen based on the control of external influences.

Name ______________________________ 



# EATING UNDER THE INFLUENCE

When you feel hunger, your body is telling you to eat because it needs nutrients. There are many theories that attempt to explain how internal body processes regulate hunger and food intake. Sometimes you eat because you are influenced by external factors, or cues, in the environment such as the time of day, food availability, the taste of food, social gatherings, the sight and smell of food, and food as an emotional outlet.

**Directions:** Record below each food and beverage you consume in one 24-hour period. Write down the time at which you consumed the food. For the column labeled "Factor":

—Write *I* if the intake of food was primarily influenced by hunger (internal factor).

—Write *E* if the intake of food was primarily influenced by an external factor.

—Write *C* if a combination of internal and external factors influenced your eating.

Continue your record on the back of this sheet if necessary. When the sheet is complete, do the calculations at the bottom of the page.

| TIME | FOOD | FACTOR | TIME | FOOD | FACTOR |
|---|---|---|---|---|---|
| | | | | | |

1. What percentage of food intake was regulated primarily by hunger or by other internal factors?
   (Number of *I* items ÷ total number of factors) × 100% = ____________%
2. What percentage of food intake was regulated primarily by external factors?
   (Number of *E* items ÷ total number of factors) × 100% = ____________%
3. What percentage of food intake was regulated by a combination of factors?
   (Number of *C* items ÷ total number of factors) × 100% = ____________%

Name ______________________________ 

# EXTERNAL EATING INFLUENCES

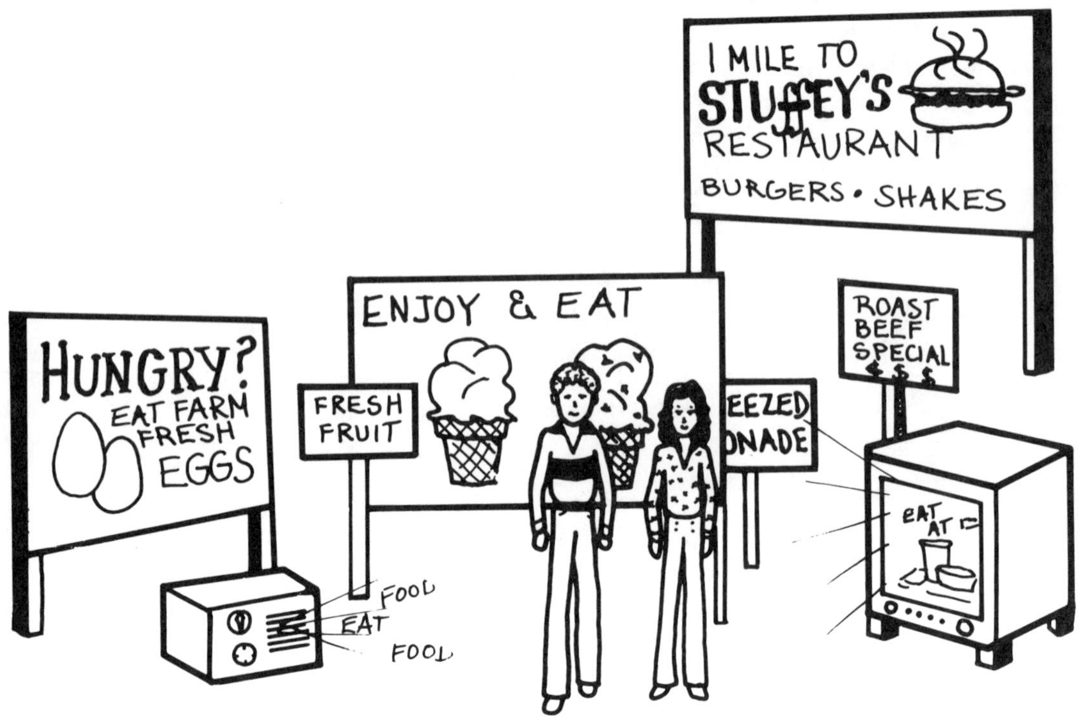


**Directions:** For one 24-hour period, record each external factor that may influence your food intake. Be sure to include the location of the external influence and describe the external factor emphasized. Use the back of this sheet to continue your record if necessary.

| LOCATION | EXTERNAL FACTOR EMPHASIZED |
|---|---|
| | |

Name ________________________________ Quiz Sheet 4-1

# QUIZ
# ANALYZING YOUR FOOD INTAKE

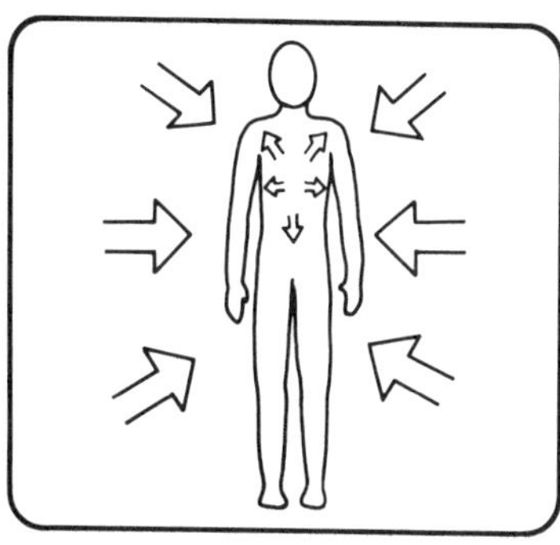

1. Food intake is regulated by two main factors. Name the factors.

________________________________________

________________________________________

________________________________________

________________________________________

2. Give at least four examples of things that affect *your* eating behaviors.

________________________________________

________________________________________

________________________________________

________________________________________

________________________________________

________________________________________

3. List at least three health consequences that result when food intake regulation does not function properly.

________________________________________

________________________________________

________________________________________

________________________________________

________________________________________

________________________________________

________________________________________

________________________________________

________________________________________

________________________________________

________________________________________

________________________________________

# SECTION III

# SPECIAL DIETS

# Unit 5: The Vegetarian Way of Life

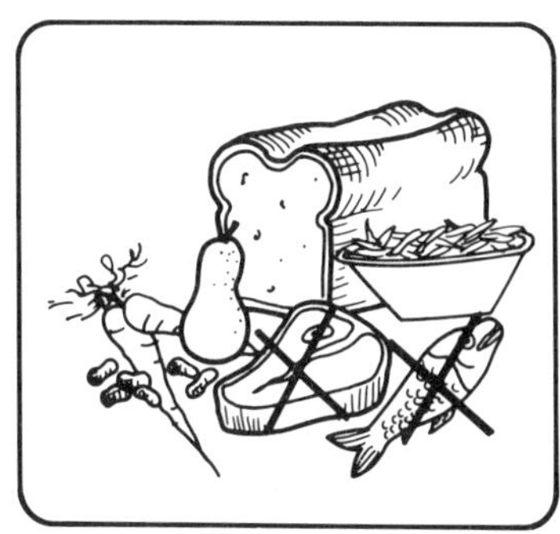

## CONCEPTS

–All diets may be placed on a continuum, from a diet consisting entirely of foods of animal origins to a diet consisting entirely of foods of plant origins.

–A vegetarian diet consists mainly of foods of plaint origin. Some vegetarian diets include foods of animal origin, especially milk, milk products, and/or eggs.

–There are a variety of vegetarian diets ranging from the vegan diet (no foods of animal origin) to the ovolacto vegetarian diet (includes milk, milk products, and eggs).

–A vegetarian diet can be planned using an adaptation of the Daily Food Guide.

## OBJECTIVES

–Students will be able to define several types of vegetarian diets (vegan, lacto vegetarian, ovolacto vegetarian) and will be able to list foods that are included in each type of diet.

–Students will be able to plan a nutritious vegetarian diet using an adaptation of the "Daily Food Guide."

–Students will be able to judge their own diets by placing themselves on a continuum of diets (from inclusion of all meats to exclusion of all meats and animal products).

## TEACHER'S UNIT INTRODUCTION

The vegetarian diet is as old as time itself, though in recent years it has gained a popular and modern appeal. Vegetarianism is practiced for various reasons. Some people are vegetarians for nutritional reasons. They believe that a vegetarian diet is more nutritious and beneficial to their health. Many people are vegetarians for economic reasons, in that a meat-based diet is usually an expensive diet. Others are vegetarians for environmental or political reasons, because they believe both that the world's arable land and other resources cannot support meat-eating populations and also that meat-eating populations consume more than their share of the world's energy and resources. Still other people are vegetarians for moral or ethical reasons; they believe that it is wrong to kill animals for human consumption. Some people may have other reasons, or several reasons, for choosing a vegetarian way of life.

Regardless of the reason for choosing vegetarianism, there are a variety of diets that may be followed and still be called vegetarian. The "pure" vegetarian, or vegan (ˈvéj-ən ˈvāǵ-ən) diet consists entirely of foods of the plant origin, including fruits, vegetables, nuts, legumes, and grains. The people following vegan diets are a diversified group. Fruitarians will eat only fruits, vegetables, and nuts that drop from trees; they avoid eating vegetables such as beets and carrots whose harvest causes the destruction of the entire plant. Sproutarians dine on sprouted alfalfa, wheat, beans, and a number of other seeds. Vitarians won't eat seeds, nuts, or grains, but will eat fruits and vegetables. The diet of fruitarians, sproutarians, vitarians, and other such individuals are generally extreme and nutritionally unbalanced. However, a vegan diet (one that includes a wide variety of fruits, vegetables, grains, nuts, seeds, and other plant foods) can be nutritionally balanced and healthful for adults provided it is carefully planned. However, such diets are *not* recommended for young children because it is very difficult for them to get all of the nutrients they need for rapid growth from these diets.

The lacto vegetarian diet consists of all plant foods with the addition of milk and milk products. A lacto vegetarian will drink milk and will eat cheese, yogurt, and other dairy products.

The ovolacto vegetarian diet includes plant foods, milk and milk products, and eggs. This type of diet is the least extreme of the vegetarian diets. It can be followed with ease and with relatively little planning.

The big question in most people's minds is whether or not a vegetarian diet is nutritionally sound. Because of the wide assortment of vegetarian diets, nutritionists are unable to make a blanket generalization about the adequacy of vegetarian diets. It has thus become important to identify the nutrients that *may* be less than adequate in a vegetarian diet and then to evaluate an individual's diet for those nutrients. The following list describes the nutrients that are of concern in a vegetarian diet:

1. **Protein.** Although protein is the one nutrient about which people may be concerned, it is actually one of the easier nutrients to obtain on a vegetarian diet designed for adults. Proteins are made of amino acids, and nearly all foods have some amino acids. The protein in plant foods is called *incomplete protein* because one or more essential amino acids are not present in sufficient amounts to meet human needs. However, if two or more plant foods are eaten simultaneously, they may form a complete protein. For complete protein, the best combinations of plant foods are legumes plus grains or legumes plus seeds. If milk, milk products, and eggs are consumed, an adequate protein content in the diet can be more easily obtained. The foods of animal origin may be combined with plant foods to improve the protein quality of the plant food.

2. **Calcium.** Since milk and milk products are the major sources of calcium, vegetarians who eat only plant foods may lack calcium. Care must be taken to include many other sources of calcium. Good vegetable sources of calcium are the dark-green leafy vegetables (kale, collards, turnip greens, mustard greens, and others), broccoli, and sesame seeds. Blackstrap molasses is another good source of calcium. Nuts and beans are fair sources of calcium.
3. **Vitamin D.** Very few foods contain Vitamin D. These are all of animal origin including liver, egg yolks, butter, and some fish. Milk is often fortified with Vitamin D. If all animal foods are eliminated from the diet, supplemental Vitamin D may be advisable. Although the body can produce Vitamin D in the skin, people who live in colder climates and in cloudy or smog-covered areas may not receive enough sunlight to produce sufficient Vitamin D.
4. **Vitamin $B_{12}$.** Apparently, only foods of animal origin contain naturally occurring Vitamin $B_{12}$. Vitamin $B_{12}$ is actually a by-product of microorganisms and thus is found in meat, eggs, fish, and dairy products. There has been some speculation that microorganisms living on certain seaweeds or other plants produce Vitamin $B_{12}$, but so far no conclusive evidence is available. There is also a conjecture that human intestines may contain the microorganisms that produce Vitamin $B_{12}$. However, for pure vegetarians relying solely on plant foods, supplementation with Vitamin $B_{12}$ is advisable.
5. **Iron.** Iron is found in greatest concentration and availability in red meats. Other foods contain concentrations of iron that may be less available to the body. Generally, the iron in foods of animal origin is more available (absorbable) than foods of plant origin. Good plant sources of iron include prune juice, dry beans, peas, whole grains, spinach, dried fruits, and blackstrap molasses. Nuts and peanut butter have some iron, but they are not the best choice for iron-containing foods.
6. **Zinc.** Zinc also is found in greatest concentration and availability in foods of animal origin including meat, seafood, eggs, milk, and milk products. Whole-grain breads and cereal products contain zinc, but much of this is unavailable to the body. Vegans would be recommended to include plenty of whole-grain foods in their diets in an attempt to meet their bodies' needs for zinc.

The nutritional needs of vegetarians may be met if these nutrients are taken into consideration. In addition to knowing about the nutritional needs of vegetarians, it is important to know how to plan nutritious meals. An adaptation of the "Daily Food Guide" may be useful in planning a vegetarian diet. Included in this lesson is a student sheet describing such an adaptation.

Besides choosing foods according to the adaptation of the "Daily Food Guide," there are several goals to keep in mind while planning a vegetarian diet. They include:

1. Reducing empty-calorie foods, which are foods that provide calories but not essential nutrients.

2. Increasing the intake of bread and cereal products, especially whole-grain products.
3. Using a wide variety of plant foods.
4. Replacing meats with an increased intake of legumes, nuts, seeds, eggs, milk, and milk products.

---

This unit is designed to teach students a more sophisticated way to plan a vegetarian diet. The general rule of thumb for complementing proteins [(1) legumes + grains; (2) legumes + seeds; or (3) grains + milk products] is an easier tool, but it does not allow for the inclusion of various other foods and combinations of foods in the diet. The additional work required to use Sheets 5-7 through 5-8, "Complementing Your Proteins," is especially important for a vegan diet. Vegan diets need to include a wide variety of plant foods that should be eaten in complementary patterns.

## BASIC ACTIVITY

**Time Needed:** Two class periods

**Materials Needed:** Sheets 5-1 through 5-3: "The Vegetarian Diet"
Sheet 5-4: "Vegetarian's Daily Food Guide"
Sheet 5-5: "Complementary Protein Relationships"
Sheet 5-6: "Practice Menu for a Vegetarian Diet"
Chart B: "Daily Food Guide" *(optional)*
Quiz Sheet 5-1

### Class Period 1

1. Conduct an introductory values-voting exercise. Ask the students to respond to the following statements in this manner:

| Thumbs Up–Agree | Both Thumbs Up–Strongly Agree |
|---|---|
| Thumbs Down–Disagree | Both Thumbs Down–Strongly Disagree |

Some of the statements are opinion statements, while others have right or wrong answers. In either case, the students should feel free to express their answers and opinions. Add your own statements if appropriate.

- Americans should cut their meat consumption in half in order to eliminate much of the starvation in the world. *(opinion)*
- Americans eat too much protein. *(opinion)*
- If you eat only plant foods (beans, grains, nuts, seeds, fruits, vegetables) you could get enough protein. *(true)*
- Protein-rich foods are usually high in calories. *(true)*

- Meat has some nutrient in it that no other food has. *(false)*
- Vegetarian diets are more healthful and less expensive than the traditional American diet. *(opinion)*
- I could easily adjust to a vegetarian diet. *(opinion)*
- I could never give up meat altogether. *(opinion)*

2. As time permits, discuss each of these statements by asking for students' reactions to them.
3. Have students read and complete Sheets 5-1 through 5-3, "The Vegetarian Diet."
4. Discuss the final part of the worksheet where they have placed themselves on the continuum. Each student may have a different diet for different reasons. Open up the discussion to these topics.
5. Have students plan a nutritious vegetarian diet by having them complete Sheet 5-5, "Complementary Protein Relationships." Beneath the examples of combination dishes, students should suggest other dishes that include complementary proteins. Additional examples are given in the "Answer Key."
6. Using one or more of their combination dishes, have students plan a well-balanced vegetarian diet for a day. Use Sheet 5-6, "Practice Menu for a Vegetarian Diet," and Sheet 5-4, "Vegetarian's Daily Food Guide," as additional resources.
7. Have students describe their menus and decide as a group which meal they would like to prepare.

**Class Period 2**

1. Have the students prepare the vegetarian meal they chose.
2. Ask the class to evaluate the meal they prepared in terms of eye appeal, taste, and ease of preparation.
3. Proceed with the "Advanced Activity" if you wish; otherwise use the quiz mentioned in step 4.
4. **Evaluation:** Distribute Quiz Sheet 5-1 and have the students complete it independently. (Students can complete the quiz as their meal is cooking.)

## ADVANCED ACTIVITY

**Time Needed:** Two class periods

**Materials Needed:** Sheets 5-1 through 5-3: "The Vegetarian Diet"
Sheet 5-5: "Complementary Protein Relationships"
Sheets 5-7 through 5-8: "Complementing Your Proteins"
Quiz Sheet 5-1

**Class Period 1**

1. Have students review Sheets 5-1 through 5-3, "The Vegetarian Diet."
2. Discuss students' responses to the vegetarian/meat-eater continuum on Sheet 5-3.

3. Have students read and examine Sheets 5-7 through 5-8, "Complementing Your Proteins." Students should list food combinations that complement each other.

4. Have students review Sheet 5-5, "Complementary Protein Relationships," and give additional examples of specific food dishes. If students have difficulty thinking of dishes, have them consult cookbooks containing vegetarian recipes and menus (*see* "References/Resources" at the end of this kit).

### Class Period 2

1. Have students prepare a simple snack that makes use of complementary proteins. One sample snack recipe is given here:

**Peanut Butter Balls**

Ingredients:
1 cup granola *or* 1 cup toasted wheat germ
1 cup nonfat dry milk powder
1/2 cup brown sugar, firmly packed
1/2 cup raisins
*Optional:* chopped dried fruit
toasted sunflower seeds
chopped nuts
1/2 cup *crunchy* peanut butter
1 cup toasted coconut *or* 1 cup toasted sesame seeds, ground

Directions:
a. Mix the cereal, dry milk powder, sugar, raisins, and optional ingredients.
b. Add enough peanut butter to make the mixture stiff but not crumbly.
c. Roll the mixture into balls on waxed paper. Roll the balls in either the coconut or in ground sesame seeds.

2. Elicit from the students the complementary protein relationships in this snack recipe.
*Answers:* legumes + grains (peanuts + granola or wheat germ)
legumes + seeds (peanuts + sesame seeds)
grains + milk product (granola + nonfat dry milk)

3. **Evaluation:** Distribute Quiz Sheet 5-1 and have students complete it independently. Discuss the answers as a class.

## FOLLOW-UP ACTIVITIES

1. Invite someone who is a vegetarian to speak to the class about his or her eating habits.

2. Have students plan and prepare a vegetarian meal for parents.

Name ______________________________________ 

# THE VEGETARIAN DIET

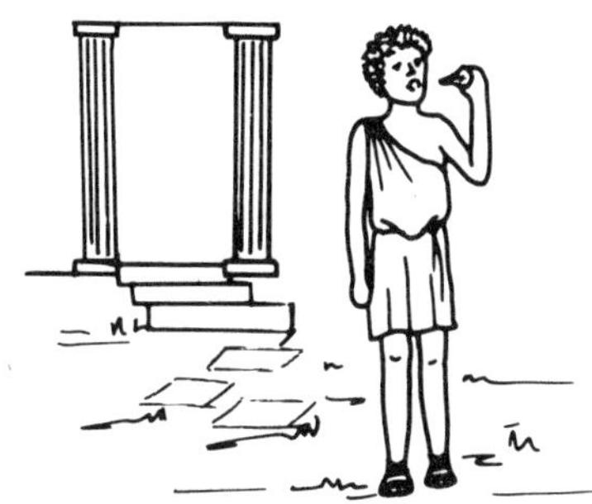

The vegetarian diet has recently become popular in the United States. Some people think that it is a new kind of diet, but it is one of the oldest diets around. In early times, a great emphasis was placed on plant foods in the diet. The early Romans' diet relied mainly on dark breads, thick soups, turnips, beans, olives, and figs.

Many of the world's religious groups throughout history have encouraged a vegetarian diet because of a deep respect for animal life. Today, the Seventh-Day Adventists in this country encourage vegetarian diets.

In the 1800s in this country some people tried to use vegetarian diets for medical purposes. Dr. J. H. Kellogg, director of the Battle Creek Sanitarium in Michigan, tried unsuccessfully to use a vegetarian diet, along with other therapies, to cure diseases such as tuberculosis and arthritis.

No matter what the reason, many people choose to follow vegetarian diets. There are three main types of vegetarian diets and these are illustrated below.

## TYPES OF VEGETARIAN DIETS

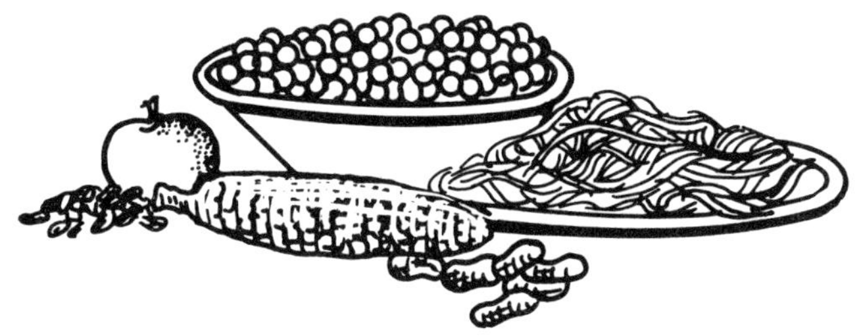

The strictest vegetarian diet is called a *"pure" vegetarian,* or a *vegan* (ˈvéj-ən or ˈvāg-an) *diet.* A vegan diet consists of fruits, vegetables, legumes, grains, nuts, and seeds. There are no animal products included in a vegan diet.

Another type of vegetarian diet is called a *lacto vegetarian diet.* This diet includes foods from a vegan diet plus milk and milk products (*lacto* means "milk").

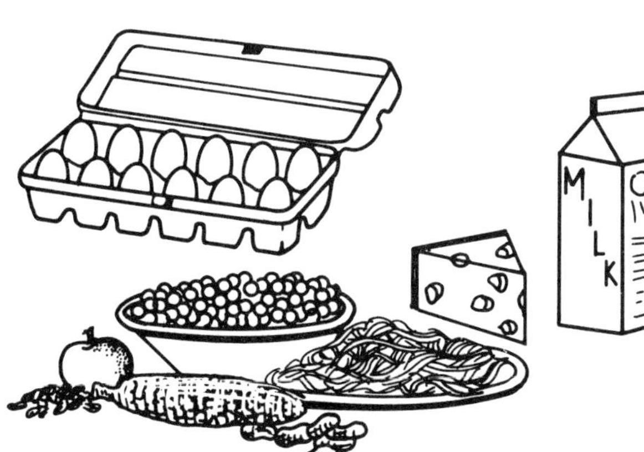


The third type of vegetarian diet is an *ovolacto vegetarian diet.* This diet includes foods from a lacto vegetarian diet, plus eggs (*ovo* means "egg").

## PLANNING A VEGETARIAN DIET

Now let us look at how to plan a vegetarian diet. People who eat meat and people who do not *still* need the same nutrients. People who eat meat can use the "Daily Food Guide" to help plan their diet so that they can get all the nutrients they need. People who do not eat meat can use an adapted version of the "Daily Food Guide" and get all the nutrients they need.

The "Vegetarian's Daily Food Guide" is similar to the regular version. The only difference is that the Meat-Poultry-Fish-Beans group is replaced with the Eggs-Beans-Nuts-Seeds group. This group consists of all the foods that are considered meat alternates. These meat alternates include dried beans, dried peas, lentils, eggs, nuts, seeds, and peanut butter. Since these foods are good sources of protein, iron, and the B vitamins, they can replace meat in the diet. One thing to remember: these protein foods should be eaten along with foods from the Bread-Cereal group. If eaten *together*, these foods meet protein needs better than if eaten alone.

Many people worry that they will not get enough protein if they do not eat meat. But, in reality, most Americans eat more protein than they need because they eat more meat than they need. Protein is found in almost all foods. When you add them all together, you will find that you have eaten a lot of protein without even realizing it!

Protein in plant foods is a little different from protein in animal foods. All protein is made up of amino acids (building blocks). Animal foods have all of the amino acids in the proper amounts in order for you to be able to build body protein. Plant foods have most of the same amino acids, but not in the proper amounts. If you eat certain types of plant foods together, you will have all the amino acids in the proper amounts needed to build protein for your body.

Let us take a look at how plant foods can be put together to provide all the amino acids needed. A vegetarian who eats milk, milk products, and/or eggs consumes complete protein. But, for a vegetarian who does not eat milk, milk products, or eggs, it is very important to eat the correct combination of plant foods for complete protein.

Vegetarians must also make sure they get enough calcium, Vitamin D, Vitamin $B_{12}$, and iron. These nutrients are found mainly in foods of animal origin (meat, poultry, fish, eggs, milk, milk products). A vegan diet may be lacking in these nutrients unless carefully planned or supplemented.

Most grains (wheat, rice, or rye) have all but two amino acids in the proper amounts. Let us call these two amino acids lysine and isoleucine. Beans (kidney, pinto, red, or navy) have all but two *other* amino acids in the right amounts. Let us call these two amino acids methionine and tryptophan. By combining grains plus beans, the four different amino acids are there in the right amounts.



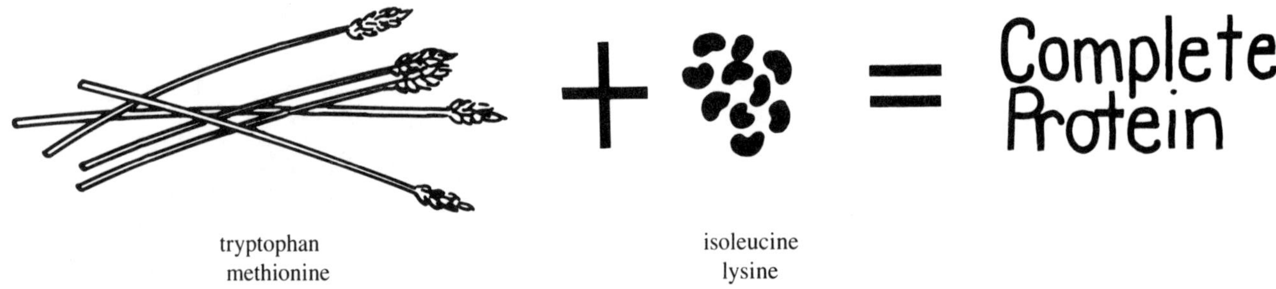

Name ______________________ **Sheet 5-3**

Now try to answer the questions below based on the reading of Sheets 5-1 through 5-2.

1. Vegetarian diets are a modern idea. True False
2. Which religious group in this country today encourages a vegetarian diet?

   ______________________

3. Name the three main types of vegetarian diets and name the foods included in each.

   Diet: ______________ Foods: ______________

   ______________

   Diet: ______________ Foods: ______________

   ______________

   Diet: ______________ Foods: ______________

   ______________

4. Vegetarians need nutrients that are different from those needed by meat-eaters. True False
5. You can get all the nutrients you need without eating meat. True False
6. In the vegetarian version of the "Daily Food Guide," which food group is different from the regular version?

   ______________________

7. For a vegetarian to be sure of getting high-quality protein, he or she must combine these two food groups:

   ______________ and ______________

8. Name four nutrients other than protein that might be in short supply in a vegetarian's diet:

   ______________ ______________ ______________ ______________

Think about your own diet. Place a check mark along the line below to show where you fit into this picture.

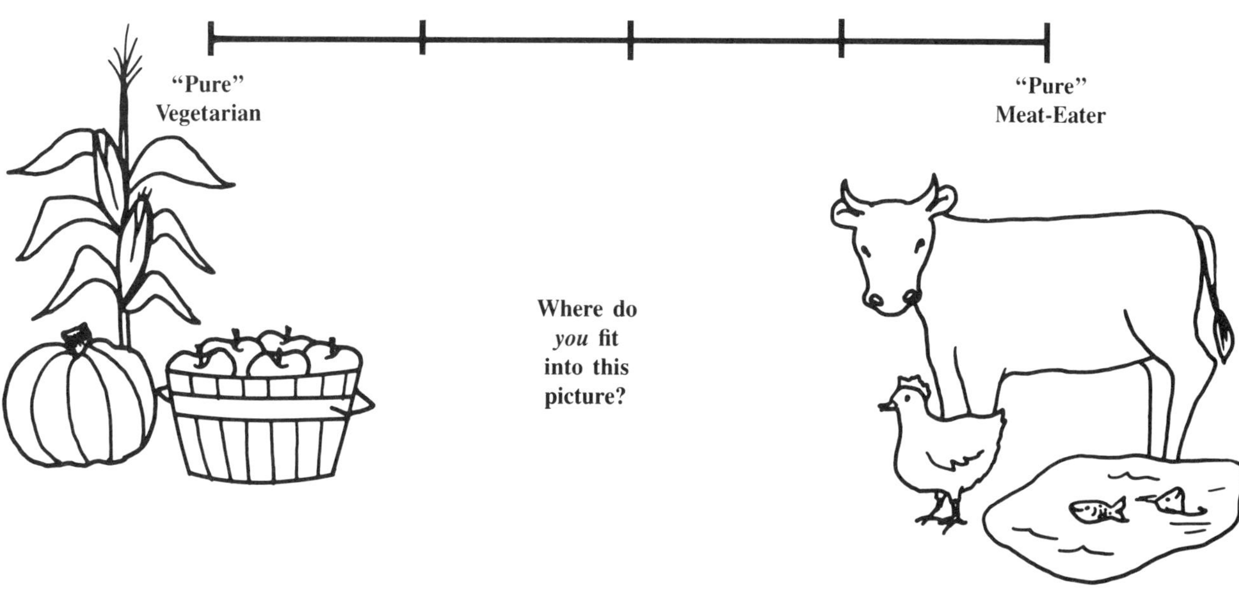

Name ____________________  Sheet 5-4

# VEGETARIAN'S DAILY FOOD GUIDE

| FRUIT-VEGETABLE | BREAD-CEREAL | MILK-CHEESE | EGGS-BEANS-NUTS-SEEDS* | FATS-SWEETS-ALCOHOL |
|---|---|---|---|---|
| **HOW MANY SERVINGS?** | | | | |
| FOUR BASIC SERVINGS DAILY | FOUR BASIC SERVINGS DAILY | BASIC SERVINGS DAILY:<br>*child under 9 2-3 servings<br>*child 9–12 3 servings<br>*teen 4 servings<br>*adult 2 servings<br>*pregnant women 3 servings<br>*nursing women 4 servings | TWO BASIC SERVINGS DAILY | In general, the number of calories you need determines the amount of these "extra" foods you can eat. It's a good idea to concentrate first on the calorie-plus-nutrients foods provided in the other groups. |
| **WHICH FOODS?** | | | | |
| All fruits and vegetables. Include one good Vitamin C source each day. Also frequently use deep-yellow or dark-green vegetables (for Vitamin A) and unpeeled fruits and vegetables and those with edible seeds, such as berries (for fiber). | Select only whole-grain and enriched products. (But include *some* whole-grain bread or cereal, for sure!) Include breads, biscuits, muffins, waffles, pancakes, cereals, pasta, rice, barley, rolled oats, and bulgur. | All types of milk and milk products, including whole, skim, lowfat, evaporated and nonfat dried milks, buttermilk, yogurt, cheese, ice cream, and foods prepared with milk, such as puddings or cream soups. | Includes dried peas, soybeans, lentils, tofu, eggs, sesame seeds, sunflower seeds, nuts, peanuts and peanut butter. Various dried beans and seeds are also in this food group. | Includes butter, margarine, mayonnaise, salad dressings, and other fats and oils; candy, sugar, jams, jellies, and syrups; soft drinks and other highly sugared drinks; alcoholic beverages such as wine, beer, and liquor. Also included are refined but unenriched breads, pastries, and other grain products. |
| **WHAT'S A SERVING?** | | | | |
| Count 1/2 cup as a serving or a typical portion such as one orange, half a grapefruit or cantaloupe, juice of one lemon, a wedge of lettuce, a bowl of salad, or one medium potato. | Count as one serving 1 slice of bread, 1/2 to 3/4 cup of cooked cereal, cornmeal, grits, pasta, or rice; or 1 oz. of ready-to-eat cereal. | Count an 8 oz. cup of milk as a serving. Equivalent amounts of calcium (but different amounts of calories) are found in the following: 1 cup yogurt, 1½ oz. hard cheese, 1½ cups ice milk or ice cream, or 2 cups of cottage cheese. | Two eggs, 1 to 1½ cup cooked dried beans, dried peas, soybeans, or lentils; 4 Tbsp. peanut butter; or 1/2 to 1 cup nuts or seeds count as one serving. | No serving sizes have been defined because a basic number of servings is not suggested for this group. Use these foods in moderation. |
| **WHAT'S IN IT FOR YOU?** | | | | |
| Carbohydrates, fiber, Vitamins A and C. Dark-green vegetables are valued for riboflavin, folacin (B vitamin), iron, and magnesium. Certain greens provide calcium. Nearly all fruits and vegetables are low in fat and none contain cholesterol. | Carbohydrates, proteins, B vitamins, iron. Whole-grain products also provide magnesium, folacin (B vitamin), and fiber. | Calcium riboflavin, protein, vitamins A, $B_6$ and $B_{12}$. Milk products also provide Vitamin D when fortified with this vitamin. Fortified lowfat or skim milk products have the same nutrients as whole milk products but fewer calories. | Protein, carbohydrates, B vitamins, iron, Vitamin E, zinc, magnesium. Nuts and seeds are relatively high in fats. | These foods, with the exception of vegetable oils, provide mainly calories. Vegetable oils generally provide Vitamin E and essential fatty acids. Sweets and alcohol provide mainly calories without other essential nutrients. |

*Eggs provide complete protein. Beans, nuts, and seeds provide incomplete protein. These foods need to be combined with foods from the Bread-Cereal group to form a complete protein.

Name ________________________________ Sheet 5-5

# COMPLEMENTARY PROTEIN RELATIONSHIPS

**Directions:** These sample combinations of nutrients join complementary proteins to form *complete proteins*. Write your own dishes below the examples. Use Sheet 5-4 if you wish.

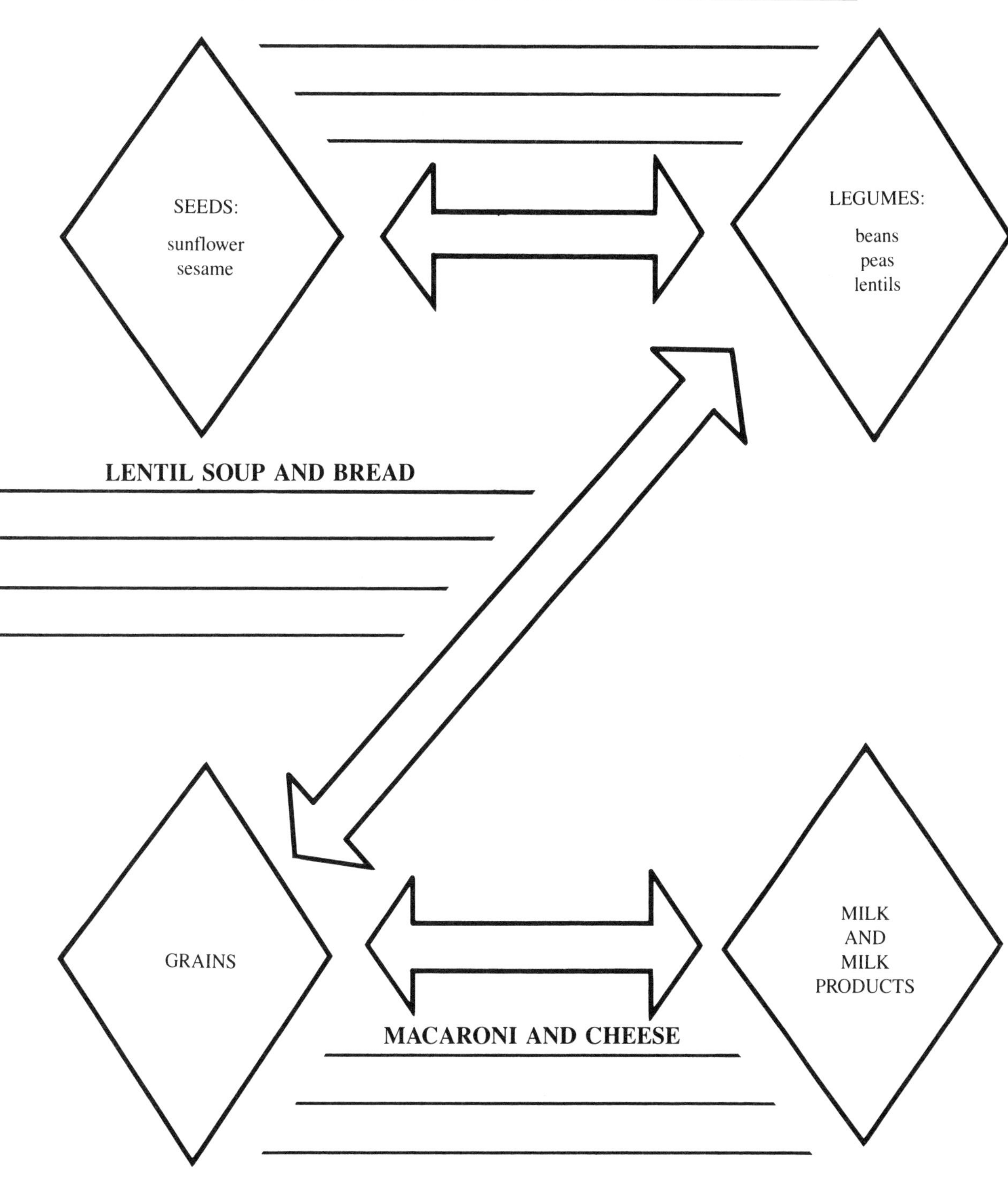

Name ______________________



# PRACTICE MENU FOR A VEGETARIAN DIET

| MEAL/SNACK | FOOD EATEN | AMOUNT | MILK-CHEESE GROUP | EGGS-BEANS-NUTS-SEEDS GROUP | FRUIT-VEGETABLE GROUP | | | BREAD-CEREAL GROUP | FATS-SWEETS-ALCOHOL GROUP |
|---|---|---|---|---|---|---|---|---|---|
| | | | | | Vitamin C-rich | Vitamin A-rich | Other | | |
| | | | | | | | | | |
| TOTAL NUMBER OF SERVINGS: | | | | | | | | | |
| RECOMMENDED NUMBER OF SERVINGS: | | | | | | | | | |

Name ______________________________ Sheet 5-7

# COMPLEMENTING YOUR PROTEINS

**Directions:** Combine two or more foods from the items listed on Sheets 5-7 through 5-8 so that for each of the four amino acids there is an "OK" or " ☺ " in each column.

☺ = good source of amino acid

☹ = not a source of amino acid

OK = fair source of amino acid

**Example:** Combine black beans (tryptophan "OK," isoleucine " ☺ " lysine "OK") with bulgur wheat (methionine "OK")

| FOOD† | AMINO ACIDS | | | |
|---|---|---|---|---|
| | Tryptophan | Isoleucine | Lysine | Methionine |
| <u>Animal Products</u> | | | | |
| eggs | OK | OK | ☺ | OK |
| milk and milk products | OK | OK | ☺ | OK |
| <u>Beans</u> | | | | |
| black beans | OK | ☺ | OK | ☹ |
| chickpeas (garbanzo) | ☹ | OK | ☺ | ☹ |
| common beans (white)* | ☹ | OK | ☺ | ☹ |
| cow peas (black-eyed) | OK | ☹ | ☺ | ☹ |
| kidney beans | ☹ | OK | ☺ | ☹ |
| lentils | ☹ | OK | ☺ | ☹ |
| mung beans | ☹ | ☹ | ☺ | ☹ |
| peas, dried | ☹ | OK | ☺ | ☹ |
| soybeans (soy grits) | OK | OK | OK | ☹ |
| <u>Flours</u> | | | | |
| cornmeal | ☹ | ☹ | ☹ | OK |
| rye flour | ☹ | ☹ | ☹ | OK |
| soy flour | OK | OK | OK | ☹ |
| whole wheat, buckwheat flours | OK | ☹ | ☹ | OK |

*also deficient in valine

†Adapted from *Diet for a Small Planet*. Lappe, F. M., Ballantine Books, New York, 1982.

Name ________________________________________ 

| FOOD‡‡ | AMINO ACIDS | | | |
|---|---|---|---|---|
| | Tryptophan | Isoleucine | Lysine | Methionine |
| Grains | | | | |
| barley | OK | ☹ | ☹ | OK |
| bulgur (cracked wheat) | OK | ☹ | ☹ | OK |
| millet | ☺ | OK | ☹ | OK |
| oatmeal | OK | ☹ | ☹ | OK |
| rice | OK | ☹ | ☹ | OK |
| spaghetti, macaroni, noodles | OK | OK | ☹ | ☹ |
| wheat bran | OK | ☹ | OK | OK |
| wheat germ | ☹ | OK | ☺ | OK |
| Nuts and Seeds | | | | |
| Brazil nuts | ☺ | ☹ | ☹ | ☺ |
| cashews | ☺ | OK | OK | OK |
| peanuts/peanut butter** | OK | ☹ | ☹ | ☹ |
| sesame | OK | ☹ | ☹ | OK |
| sunflower | OK | OK | ☹ | OK |
| **also deficient in threonine | | | | |

‡‡Adapted from *Diet for a Small Planet,* Lappe, F. M. Ballantine Books, New York, 1982.

Write your combinations here:

___________________________________________

___________________________________________

___________________________________________

___________________________________________

___________________________________________

___________________________________________

___________________________________________

___________________________________________

___________________________________________

Name ____________________ Quiz Sheet 5-1

# QUIZ
# THE VEGETARIAN WAY OF LIFE

_____ 1. Which foods would not be included in a vegan diet?

a. Fruits and vegetables c. Nuts and seeds
b. Milk and eggs d. Beans and grains

_____ 2. Which foods would not be included in a lacto vegetarian diet?

a. Milk c. Legumes
b. Cheese d. Eggs

_____ 3. Which diet best describes an ovolacto vegetarian diet?

a. All foods of plant origin
b. All foods of plant origin plus milk, cheese, and eggs
c. All foods of plant origin plus milk, cheese, and yogurt
d. All foods of plant origin plus milk, cheese, yogurt, eggs, fish, and chicken

4. Write a menu plan for one day that represents a well-balanced ovolacto vegetarian diet.

5. On your menu above, label each food from the food groups below:

FV —Fruit-Vegetable group
BC —Bread-Cereal group
MC —Milk-Cheese group
EBNS—Eggs-Beans-Nuts-Seeds group
FSA —Fats-Sweets-Alcohol group

# Unit 6: Nutrition for the Expectant Mother

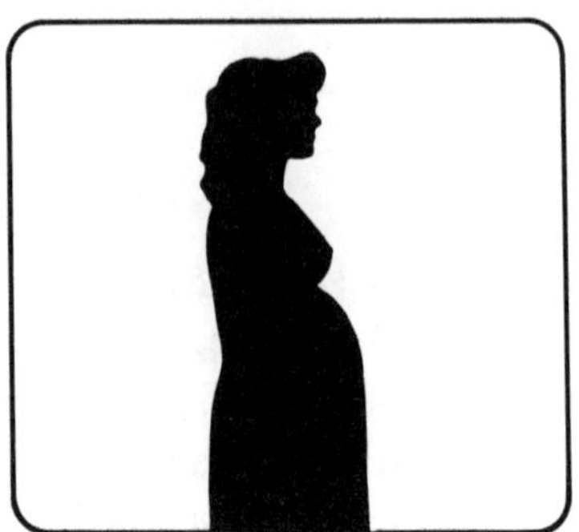

## CONCEPTS

–The "training table" of an expectant mother should include a wide variety of foods.

–The selection of nutrient-dense foods will help to ensure an adequate supply of nutrients during pregnancy without adding unnecessary calories.

–Consumption of alcohol should be curtailed during pregnancy because:

- Consumption of alcohol during pregnancy has been linked to birth defects.
- Alcohol is an empty-calorie food.

## OBJECTIVES

–Students will be able to describe the nutrient needs of a pregnant woman.

–Students will be able to specify how nutritional needs differ for pregnant teenagers.

–Students will be able to select a diet for an expectant mother that meets her calorie and nutrient needs.

–Students will be able to describe the dangers of alcohol consumption during pregnancy.

–Students will be able to describe how consumption of alcohol replaces the more nutrient-dense food choices needed during pregnancy.

## TEACHER'S UNIT INTRODUCTION

Expectant mothers who are asked about their future hopes for either a boy or girl commonly respond, "It doesn't really matter. . . just as long as it's healthy." The growth of a single cell into a baby is an awesome demonstration of the human body's ability to change nutrients from food into a baby. Of course, a successful pregnancy depends on many health-related factors, but an especially important part of good prenatal care is choosing a wide variety of nutritious foods. The anticipation of motherhood provides a strong motivation for many women to become more informed about nutrition and to make more careful food choices for a nutritious diet. A sound understanding of the nutrient needs of pregnancy and of how to select foods to meet those needs is important for every woman, whether she is currently expecting a baby or whether she plans to have a family in the future.

The high school years are an ideal period to gain knowledge about nutrition and pregnancy, particularly when you consider that

(1) One-fifth (20 percent) of all births in the United States involve babies born to teenaged mothers.

(2) One million (10 percent) of all adolescents in the United States become pregnant each year.

(3) 600,000 (60 percent) of the adolescents who become pregnant carry their pregnancy to full term.

(4) One-third of all teenaged mothers are under sixteen years of age.

(5) There is typically no nutrition education offered to young girls who will one day become mothers until the time that they do become pregnant and are under a doctor's care.

Teenaged girls should develop sound food habits for their own benefit *before* they become pregnant. This not only serves them but will also benefit their as-yet-unconceived children. Low nutrient intake of some nutrients prior to conception will reduce the body's nutrient reserves.

Most adolescents lack the physical readiness for pregnancy, although the menstrual cycle may have been established for a few years. Poor dietary intake coupled with this lack of physical maturity are the primary reasons why teenaged pregnancies are considered to be "at risk." This means that teenage pregnancies have a greater than normal chance of having complications. Pregnancy during the teenage years is accompanied by an increased risk of prematurity, low birth-weight infants, toxemia of pregnancy, and maternal anemia.

During pregnancy, the demands of the developing fetus require an increased consumption of all nutrients beyond those levels needed by the teenaged girl's own growing and maturing body.

Chart A, "Recommended Dietary Allowances," lists the nutrient allowances for pregnancy as additions to the nutrient allowances for the nonpregnant woman. You can see that nutrient needs nearly double when a woman is pregnant. The nutrients of particular concern during pregnancy are protein, calcium, iron, and folacin (a B vitamin). In order to achieve adequate levels of these nutrients during pregnancy, a pregnant woman is advised to consume additional servings from the milk group in order to get protein and calcium, and to take a daily supplement of 30-60 milligrams of iron plus 400 micrograms (μg.) of folacin.

The amount of iron and folacin needed during pregnancy is nearly impossible to achieve through diet alone.

The information presented so far has explained how to maximize the health of the mother and the unborn baby through the improvement of her diet. During pregnancy there are other factors that may affect the healthful outcome of pregnancy. Although not strictly "nutrition" issues, these topics cannot be ignored during any discussion of teenage pregnancy.

Consumption of alcohol and caffeine by a pregnant woman may influence the health of her baby. A pattern of mental and physical abnormalities in infants has been linked to heavy consumption of alcohol. Heavy drinking is defined as a daily intake of 3 ounces of pure alcohol, which is the equivalent of four to six drinks per day. This classic pattern of abnormalities is called the Fetal Alcohol Syndrome (FAS) and is described on Sheet 6-3, "For Healthier Babies..."

It is difficult to determine a safe limit of alcohol intake and it is also difficult to assess exactly how alcohol affects the growing fetus. Alcohol's effects depend on the amount the mother drinks and on the length of time between drinks. Small quantities of alcohol, as little as two to three beers or glasses of wine daily, may still affect the child, although the effects may be less pronounced. Symptoms such as short attention span, irritability, restlessness, or hyperactivity may be displayed in the infant of a mother who drinks moderately. "Binge" drinking may also affect the unborn infant, particularly if it occurs early in the pregnancy. In addition to the dangers of alcohol itself, another problem accompanies its use. Many of the daily calories may come from alcohol instead of food. Alcohol has a high calorie content (7 calories/gram of alcohol), but it is very low in nutrients. Beer and wine contain small amounts of several B vitamins, but these amounts are insignificant when compared to the pregnant woman's nutritional needs. Thus, the pregnant woman who drinks alcohol exposes her unborn baby to a double set of risks, that is, to the risks of the alcohol itself as well as to the risk of malnourishment.

Until definite limits are set, complete abstinence from alcohol during pregnancy appears to be the safest route. If a pregnant woman does drink, she should do so in moderation, with no more than one drink per day. Wine and beer seem to be the better choices, since they have the highest nutrient content of all alcoholic beverages and are the lowest in alcohol content.

Another potential hazard to pregnant women is caffeine. Caffeine is found in coffee, tea, cola, and chocolate. This chart lists some common caffeine-containing items and also the level of caffeine that each contains. [Display the following chart on an opaque or overhead projector.]

| FOOD | CAFFEINE (mg.) |
|---|---|
| coffee: | |
| drip | 146/cup |
| brewed | 100/cup |
| instant | 60/cup |
| tea | 46/cup |

| FOOD | CAFFEINE (mg.) |
|---|---|
| cola: | |
| Coke | 64/12 oz. |
| Tab | 45/12 oz. |
| Pepsi Light | 36/12 oz. |
| chocolate: | |
| hot chocolate | 24/cup |
| cocoa (2 tsp.) | 15-25 mg. |
| 1 slice chocolate cake (1/8 cake) | 11-19 mg./slice |

Caffeine is an active central nervous system stimulant. Ingestion of caffeine promotes wakefulness. However, as with any drug, caffeine has other negative side effects including shivering, trembling, irritability, dehydration, diarrhea, and vomiting. Caffeine can also disturb the heart rate and rhythm and can affect coronary circulation, blood pressure, and the secretion of gastric acids. The effects of caffeine on the unborn baby, however, are as yet unclear. Caffeine does cross the placenta easily and can later be found in the newborn infant. Some studies have shown the presence of caffeine-related birth defects in babies born of mothers with high caffeine intakes during early pregnancy (5 or more cups of brewed coffee per day). However, later attempts to duplicate these studies were unsuccessful. Currently, the advice given to pregnant women is to avoid caffeine-containing foods, beverages, and drugs, if possible, or to consume them only sparingly.

---

This unit is designed to concentrate on a very important requirement for a healthy pregnancy, that is, the need to eat a well-balanced diet in order to nourish the mother's body as well as that of her unborn baby. This should be particularly emphasized in the case of the teenaged mother-to-be whose own body is still growing along with that of her unborn child. This unit also encourages you to discuss the adverse effects of other substances, particularly alcohol, in the diet of the mother-to-be. The discussion of caffeine and its relation to pregnancy is left as an optional activity because of the lack of substantive evidence suggesting its harmful effects during pregnancy. The "Follow-Up Activities" in this unit are of particular importance; students should investigate how other nutrition-related topics affect pregnancy (including salt intake, vitamin supplements, drug intake, and smoking). Although this unit is of particular interest to girls, boys can be included by beginning the unit with a careful introduction. The introduction could include a visualization of the growing baby within the mother's body. When you present this imagery exercise to your female students, encourage them to relate the exercise to themselves. In the case of your male students, present the exercise with reference to their mother, sister, or girlfriend. Have the students then imagine this small, growing baby smoking a cigarette, having an alcoholic drink, or eating sugary snacks. The students should then be able to discuss the effects of such actions on the baby.

This unit requires sensitivity and a positive attitude on the part of the teacher in order to instill in the students a sense of importance toward the issue of nutrition during pregnancy.

For the teenager who is pregnant, many critical issues abound. She and her partner are faced with decisions such as whether or not to tell parents, friends, or teachers about their situation and whether or not to have the baby, to keep the baby, to get married, or to run away. To discuss a balanced diet may seem less critical. However, in reality, the chances of a healthy and uncomplicated pregnancy increase with good nutrition. The pregnant teenager will have fewer problems in the long run if she practices good nutrition. To convince the teenager of this idea is the task of the teacher. If a positive attitude toward pregnancy is developed, then a discussion of how to maintain a healthy pregnancy through good nutrition can follow.

## BASIC ACTIVITY

**Time Needed:** Three class periods

**Materials Needed:** Sheets 6-1 through 6-4: "For Healthier Babies . . ."
Chart B: "Daily Food Guide"
Sheet 6-5: "Meal Evaluation"
Sheets 6-6 through 6-7: "Menus for a Pregnant Woman"
Tables 6-1 through 6-2: "Energy and Iron CaPAC Food Composition Table"
Sheet 6-8: "Fizz, Flavor, and Fun!"
Ingredients for drinks on Sheet 6-8
Sheet 6-9: "Booze and Babies Don't Mix!"
Sheet 6-10: "An Ideal Menu for Pregnancy"
Quiz Sheet 6-1

### Class Period 1

1. Distribute Sheets 6-1 through 6-4, "For Healthier Babies . . . ," and have students read them silently. Alternatively, select several students to read the material aloud.

2. On several small slips of paper, write a letter from the word "Baby" and alternate how many times each letter is used. Fold the slips of paper in half and place them in a container.

3. Set up a tournament by dividing the students into groups or by having students compete singly. Read aloud each question below. The first group (or student) to answer the question correctly wins a chance to draw one letter from the container. Students may use the charts or tables in this unit as well as the information on Sheets 6-1 through 6-4 and in Chart B, "Daily Food Guide," to answer the questions. The first group to collect all of the letters to spell the complete word "Baby" wins. If necessary, develop more questions for the tournament using the "Teacher's Unit Introduction" and student worksheets in this unit.

- List three sources of iron. (*Answer:* Iron can be found in red meats, organ meats, poultry, fish, dry peas, beans, and whole-grain or enriched breads and cereals.)
- Name four nutrients that are commonly lacking in the diets of pregnant teens. (*Answer:* Vitamins A and C, iron, and calcium.)

- Name two nutrient-dense foods. (*Answer:* Skim milk, carrots, spinach, tomatoes, cheese, among others.)
- How many extra calories do pregnant women need per day? (*Answer:* 300 calories.)
- List three sources of protein. (*Answer:* Protein can be found in red meats, poultry, fish, eggs, dry peas, beans, milk, and cheese.)
- What is the recommended weight gain during pregnancy? (*Answer:* 24 to 30 pounds.)
- How many pounds of the weight gain during pregnancy account for the development of the baby? (*Answer:* 13-15 pounds).
- Why are pregnant teenagers considered "at risk"? (*Answer:* A pregnant teen is considered "at risk" because her body is growing along with the baby's body. Higher incidences of low birth-weight babies and complications of pregnancy are seen among teenaged girls.)
- List two examples of foods that provide the amount of calcium in one cup of milk. (*Answer:* Either 1½ cups of ice cream, 2 cups of cottage cheese, 1 cup of yogurt, or 2 one-inch cheese cubes equal the amount of calcium in 1 cup of milk.)
- Examine the following statement and if there is an error, state what it is and correct the sentence.

  It is important to gain a lot of weight during the first three months of pregnancy and then to restrict caloric intake to less than 1,200 calories per day for the remainder of the term.

  (*Answer:* Corrected statement: It is important to gain weight slowly throughout pregnancy, and this can be accomplished by adding 300 calories per day to the diet. Restricting calories is unsafe because the mother can deprive her baby of nutrients needed for growth and development.)
- How many alcoholic drinks per day will put a woman at high risk for the development of a baby with Fetal Alcohol Syndrome? (*Answer:* 4 to 6 drinks.)

4. Distribute Sheet 6-5, "Meal Evaluation." Have each student examine each meal and rate them from (1) best to (3) poorest. Have students justify their ratings in a class discussion. Ask the students to describe how they could improve those meals that received a poor rating.

**Class Period 2**

1. Discuss the effects of consuming alcoholic beverages during pregnancy. Emphasize the following points:

- Alcohol intake during pregnancy may cause birth defects.
- High-calorie, low-nutrient beverages that take the place of food and of more nutritious beverage choices do not provide the mother and baby with needed nutrients.
- If an adequate amount of nutritious foods are eaten and large amounts of alcoholic drinks are consumed, the mother may gain excessive weight. The baby may suffer from the effects of the mother's excess weight as well as from the alcohol.

2. Distribute a copy of Sheets 6-6 through 6-7, "Menus for a Pregnant Woman," to each student. Divide the students into groups and have them determine the calories and key nutrients of each diet using Tables 6-1 through 6-2, "Energy and Iron CaPAC Food Composition Table." Have students compare the two diets with respect to calories and nutrients.

3. Have the class brainstorm and list healthful alternatives to alcoholic beverages. Distribute Sheet 6-8, "Fizz, Flavor, and Fun!" to each student. Select the beverage recipes that are the most appealing to the students. Plan the preparation of them for Class Period 3.

**Class Period 3**

1. Divide the class into four groups and have each group prepare one of the beverage recipes on Sheet 6-8.

2. Have students sample each beverage.

3. Have students describe the nutrient contribution of each of the beverages. Knowledge of the key nutrient contributions of the food groups is helpful here. Students should consult Chart C, "Key Nutrients in Food," as they analyze the beverages. The specific key nutrient compositions of the beverages are given below.

**Nutrient Composition of "Fizz, Flavor, and Fun!" Recipes**

| ONE SERVING | Calories | Protein (gm.) | Vitamin A (IUs) | Vitamin C (mg.) | Calcium (mg.) |
|---|---|---|---|---|---|
| Orange Smoothee | 115 | 2 | 302 | 50 | 60 |
| Orange Buttermilk Shake | 220 | 6 | 345 | 26 | 219 |
| Pineapple Cooler | 150 | 2 | 281 | 57 | 38 |
| Peanut Butter Eggnog | 245 | 10 | 536 | 2 | 198 |

4. Distribute Sheet 6-9, "Booze and Babies Don't Mix!" Have students complete the worksheet and then review the correct answers with them. Discuss any questions that arise.

5. Proceed with the "Advanced Activity" if you wish; otherwise use the quiz mentioned in step 6.

6. **Evaluation:** Distribute Quiz Sheet 6-1 and have students complete it independently. Discuss the answers as a class.

## ADVANCED ACTIVITY

**Time Needed:** One class period

**Materials Needed:** Tables 6-1 through 6-2: "Energy and Iron CaPAC Food Composition Table"

Chart A: "Recommended Dietary Allowances"
Chart E: "Dietary Calculation Chart"
Sheet 6-10: "An Ideal Menu for Pregnancy"
Quiz Sheet 6-1

1. Distribute Chart A, Chart E, and Sheet 6-10, "An Ideal Menu for Pregnancy," and Tables 6-1 through 6-2, "Energy and Iron CaPAC Food Composition Table."

2. Have the students construct a one-day "ideal" menu for a pregnant girl between 15 and 18 years of age.

3. Have students calculate the amounts of selected nutrients in the menu they created on Sheet 6-10 on Chart E, "Dietary Calculation Chart." Although students should realize the importance of consuming all nutrients during pregnancy, only the daily iron, calcium, protein, vitamins A and C, and caloric needs should be calculated in this activity. (Calculations of all nutrients require additional time, but do not improve the students' understanding of the concepts.)

4. Have the students compare their calculations to the RDAs for a 15- to 18-year-old pregnant girl.

5. Discuss student findings as a class.

6. **Evaluation:** Distribute Quiz Sheet 6-1 and have students complete it independently. Discuss the answers as a class.

## FOLLOW-UP ACTIVITIES

1. Because teenage pregnancy is a sensitive issue, it is important to encourage the students to talk about their own concerns, fears, anxieties, or simply attitudes toward pregnancy. Have students suggest nutrition-related topics of importance in pregnancy such as: salt intake, drug intake (prescription and nonprescription drugs), vitamin supplements, vegetarianism, cravings, smoking (which robs the body of nutrients), or similar topics of interest. If appropriate, have students also suggest nonnutrition-related topics to discuss such as: teenage marriage, family conflicts, body image during pregnancy, or similar topics. Have students research these topics through library research and interviews. Ask students to present their findings to the class in whatever format they wish (report, demonstration, role-play, speaker, debate, roundtable discussion, advertising, etc.).

2. Have students talk to their mothers or other mothers about how their diets changed while they were pregnant. Compare these changes in diet with the changes in diet suggested at the present time.

3. Display the following table, "Progressive Effects of Alcohol," on an overhead or opaque projector. Discuss how these effects could endanger both the mother and her unborn child. For example, a very small amount of alcohol may be enough to make a pregnant woman unsteady and prone to falls or to other accidents due to carelessness. At the other extreme, a state of unconsciousness due to heavy alcohol consumption could lead to a situation where the baby would not get enough oxygen and, as a result, would suffer brain damage.

**Progressive Effects of Alcohol**

| Physical or Mental Changes Due to Alcohol | Number of Drinks Needed to Induce Changes |
|---|---|
| RELEASE OF TENSION<br>carefree sensation<br>tensions and inhibitions lessened | 1–2 |
| LOSS OF INTELLIGENT BEHAVIOR<br>decreased judgment<br>decreased self-control<br>increased emotional responses | 2 |
| DECREASED MUSCULAR CONTROL<br>decreased reaction time<br>slurred speech<br>tremors | 4–6 |
| INFLUENCE ON SENSE ORGANS<br>double vision<br>blurred vision<br>loss of ability to judge distances<br>impaired hearing<br>dizziness | 8 |
| UNCONSCIOUSNESS<br>decreased breathing rate<br>decreased heart action and blood pressure<br>decreased body temperature<br>coma<br>death | 12 or more |

Name ____________________ Sheet 6-1

# FOR HEALTHIER BABIES...

## FIGHT BOREDOM—EAT A VARIETY OF FOODS

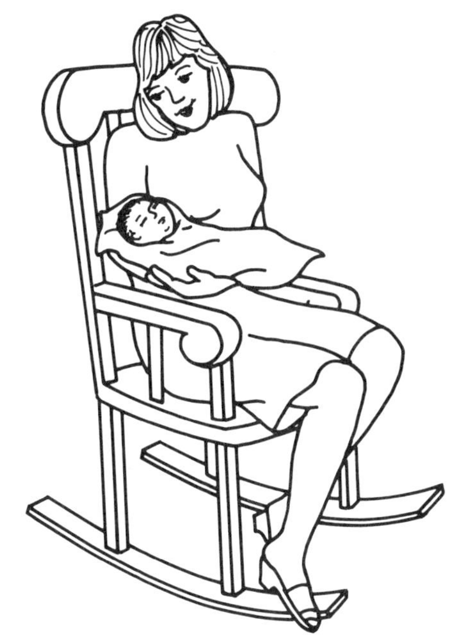

Poor food habits are common among pregnant women, and especially among pregnant teens. Teens often use fad diets to control weight, and they frequently skip breakfast as well. A large portion of the total calories in a teenager's diet comes from empty-calorie snack foods such as soft drinks, potato chips, and candy. Poor snack food choices appear to be made at the expense of vegetables, milk, and milk products. This results in diets that are low in calcium, iron, Vitamin A, and Vitamin C—all of which are very important for the health of both the growing fetus and of the mother-to-be herself.

The best way for a pregnant woman to get all of the foods she needs is to eat a variety of wholesome nutrient-dense foods. By using the "Daily Food Guide," her choices of foods become clear. The following chart shows the recommended foods to eat for a healthier baby.

**DAILY FOOD GUIDE***
for a Young Mother-to-Be

| | |
|---|---|
| Fruit-Vegetable | 4 basic servings daily |
| Bread-Cereal | 4–6 basic servings daily |
| Milk-Cheese | 5 basic servings daily |
| Meat-Poultry-Fish-Beans | 2–3 basic servings daily |

## GAIN THE RIGHT AMOUNT OF WEIGHT

Many women are concerned about their weight and about staying thin. During pregnancy, a woman may not want to gain a lot of weight, so she refuses to eat enough to provide for both herself and for her unborn baby. More complications of pregnancy are seen in underweight mothers and in mothers who don't gain enough weight. Women who are underweight at conception need to gain more weight than women who are not underweight when they become pregnant. For the underweight, pregnant teen, weight gain above the recommended level may be especially desirable because her body is still growing along with that of her unborn baby.

While gaining too little weight during pregnancy is not good for either the mother or the infant, gaining too much weight has risks as well. Being overweight at conception and gaining too much weight during pregnancy increase the risk of complications. However, pregnancy is not the time to diet! Women who are overweight at the time of conception should be expected to gain at least 18 pounds during pregnancy. This weight gain is due to the development of the baby as well as to the growth of the mother's tissues (breasts, uterus, blood). This development requires many nutrients such as iron, calcium, and protein. These nutrients should be supplied from the foods in her diet. Remember that obesity is a condition that involves the storage of excess fat and that this excess can be used for energy (calories) during pregnancy. However, this stored fat will not provide the important nutrients needed for growth.

*Refer to Chart B, "Daily Food Guide," for more details.

The recommended weight gain during pregnancy is 24 to 30 pounds. The rate at which weight is gained is as important as the total weight gained. It is recommended that weight be gained slowly at first, with three pounds gained by the end of the first three months. In the last six months, there should be a steady increase of about one pound per week. Why should a woman gain so much total weight during pregnancy when she expects to give birth to a baby weighing only about seven pounds? The following illustration shows the distribution of weight in pregnancy.

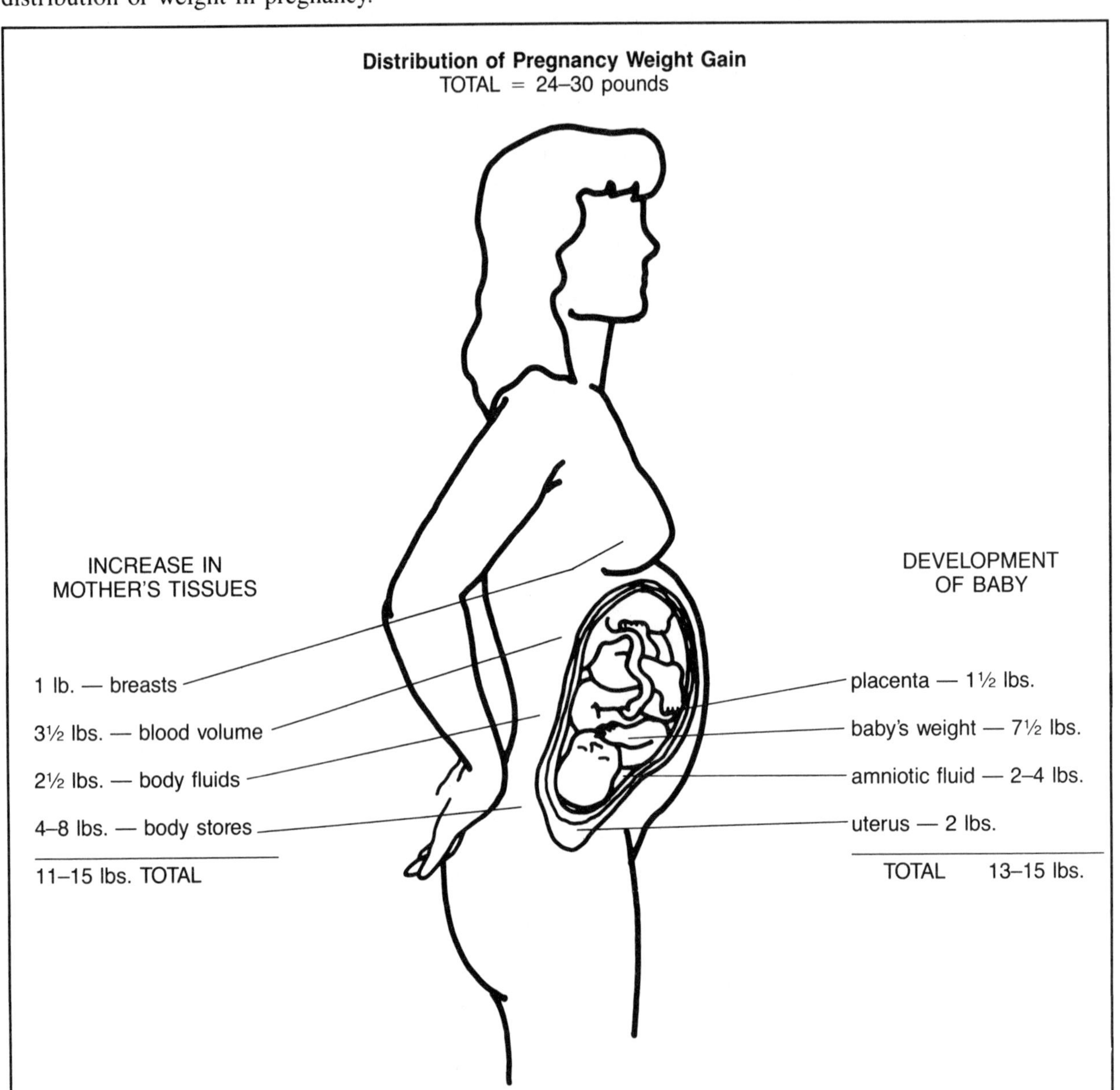


Notice that a normal pregnancy requires an increase in the mother's tissues of 11-15 pounds, which is about the same as that represented by the weight of the baby's tissues. The 13-15 pounds required strictly by the baby is lost within one week of delivery.

The gradual increase in weight during pregnancy can be achieved by consuming about 300 calories more than normal each day. Because other nutrient needs increase at this time, foods should be chosen that are high in nutrients compared to their calorie content. The table on Sheet 6-3 lists examples of combinations of foods that are about 300 calories per serving and that are good sources of one or more nutrients. Through the selection of nutrient-dense foods, the expectant mother is more likely to have a healthy baby without gaining unneeded weight.

Name ______________________________ Sheet 6-3

| Nutrient-Dense Foods to Meet Pregnancy Needs | |
|---|---|
| Food | Calories |
| 1 cup skim milk | 85 |
| 1 carrot | 35 |
| 1 slice raisin bread | 70 |
| 1 banana | 100 |
| Total | 290 |
| 1 slice whole wheat bread | 55 |
| 2 Tbsp. peanut butter | 180 |
| 1 small apple | 80 |
| Total | 315 |
| 1 cup creamed cottage cheese | 235 |
| 1 cup canned peaches, packed in water | 75 |
| Total | 310 |

## AVOID ALCOHOL DURING PREGNANCY

Beverages containing alcohol are consumed daily by many people and are a part of social life for many teens. Although a moderate consumption of alcohol may not have permanent, serious effects on an individual, there are many unanswered questions about the effects of alcohol on the unborn child. An expectant mother may want to reduce, or completely eliminate, alcohol in her diet.

Numerous mental and physical defects are seen in some infants whose mothers drank heavily during the pregnancy. This condition, called Fetal Alcohol Syndrome (or FAS), is associated with a number of birth defects. The chart on Sheet 6-4 shows the wide range of effects of Fetal Alcohol Syndrome.

A high risk of Fetal Alcohol Syndrome is observed when pregnant women drink at least three ounces of pure alcohol per day (equivalent to four to six drinks). One drink is usually considered to be twelve ounces of beer, four ounces of wine, or one mixed drink. However, it is uncertain if a safe level of alcohol intake during pregnancy exists. The wisest course for the pregnant woman is to stay away from alcoholic beverages.

A woman does not need to be considered an alcoholic for her child to be affected by alcohol. Irritability, reduced attention span, restlessness, and hyperactivity have been shown to appear in later childhood in some children whose mothers either drank moderately (two drinks per day) throughout pregnancy or had episodes of "binge" drinking.

Consumption of alcoholic beverages may not only expose the unborn baby to a high-risk substance, but alcohol also contributes little (if any) nutrients to the pregnant woman. Alcoholic beverages have a high calorie content but few nutrients. (*See* Tables 6-1 through 6-2, "Energy and Iron CaPAC Food Composition Table.")

**Physical and Mental Defects Associated with FAS**

Physical Defects:

- Growth deficiency: low birth-weight
  small head circumference
  reduction in weight and height for age
  throughout childhood
- Facial abnormalities: low nasal bridge
  narrow eyes with folds over inner corners
  short, upturned nose
  cleft lip
  underdeveloped groove in center of upper lip
- Defective organs, including heart and genitals
- Malformed arms and legs

Mental Defects:

- Brain impairment: poor coordination
  restlessness, irritable temperament, and hyperactivity
  learning difficulties and poor attention span
  lower IQ
  mental retardation

It is recommended that pregnant women consume 300 calories above their caloric needs during pregnancy. Consuming two 12-ounce beers or two mixed drinks adds about 300 calories to the diet but contributes few nutrients. If these beverages are consumed with an adequate diet, the extra calories are stored as fat and the mother may gain excess weight. More nutritious choices are needed during pregnancy.

Name ______________________________ Sheet 6-5

# MEAL EVALUATION

**Directions:** Three examples each are given for breakfast, lunch, dinner, and snacks on the menus below. For each meal or snack, rate the examples as best (1) to poorest (3) by writing 1,2, or 3 in the box in the lower right-hand corner. Be prepared to justify your choices in a class discussion and to tell how the best choices contribute nutrients to a pregnant woman's diet. Use Chart B, "Daily Food Guide," to help justify your answers.

| BREAKFAST A | B | C |
|---|---|---|
| 1 oz. sugar-coated cereal with ½ cup whole milk<br>1 cup hot tea | ½ cup orange juice<br>1 cup skim milk<br>1½ oz. cheddar cheese cube<br>1 slice bread | 1 cinnamon doughnut<br>1 cup hot coffee with sugar |
| **LUNCH A** | **B** | **C** |
| 4 carrot sticks<br>1 hamburger with bun<br>1 banana<br>1 cup skim milk | 1 cup vegetable soup<br>1 apple<br>1 cup skim milk<br>4 chocolate cookies | 1 piece fried fish<br>10 potato chips<br>12 oz. diet cola<br>1 piece apple pie |
| **DINNER A** | **B** | **C** |
| 1 hot dog with bun<br>12 oz. orange soda<br>1 scoop chocolate ice cream<br>1 vanilla cupcake<br>12 oz. beer | 1 baked chicken breast<br>1 cup spinach salad with salad dressing<br>1 dinner roll<br>1 corn on the cob<br>1 cup chocolate pudding<br>8 oz. water | 1 broiled pork chop<br>10 french fries<br>1 dinner roll and margarine<br>1 piece German chocolate cake |
| **SNACK A** | **B** | **C** |
| 1 cup pineapple chunks<br>4 saltine crackers<br>1 cup whole milk | 1 bag potato chips<br>12 oz. beer | 1 chocolate candy bar<br>¼ cup raisins |

Name ________________________________ Table 6-1

# ENERGY AND IRON CaPAC FOOD COMPOSITION TABLE

| Food and Serving Size | Weight | Energy | Iron | Ca | P | A | C |
|---|---|---|---|---|---|---|---|
| | g. | cal. | mg. | mg. | g. | IUs[1] | mg. |
| Alcoholic cocktail, highball–8 ounces | 240 | 165 | – | – | – | – | – |
| Apple, fresh–1 medium | 138 | 80 | 0.1 | 10 | * | 125 | 6 |
| Apple pie–1/7 of 9″ diameter | 135 | 400 | 1.0 | 11 | 3 | 175 | 3 |
| Applesauce, sweetened–½ cup | 128 | 115 | 1.3 | 10 | * | 51 | 1 |
| Apricots, fresh–3 | 108 | 55 | 0.6 | 5 | * | 2,890 | 11 |
| Avocado–½ | 114 | 190 | 0.6 | 11 | 2 | 330 | 16 |
| Banana–1 | 119 | 100 | 0.7 | 12 | 1 | 230 | 12 |
| Beef pot pie–4¼″ diameter | 227 | 560 | 4.1 | 32 | 23 | 1,860 | 7 |
| Beer–12 ounce | 360 | 150 | T | 18 | 1 | 0 | 0 |
| Beet greens, cooked–½ cup | 73 | 15 | 1.4 | 72 | 1 | 3,697 | 11 |
| Beets, cooked–½ cup | 85 | 30 | 0.4 | 12 | 1 | 20 | 5 |
| Biscuit–1, 2½″ diameter | 40 | 155 | 0.7 | 47 | 3 | T | T |
| Blueberries, fresh–½ cup | 73 | 45 | 0.7 | 11 | * | 72 | 10 |
| Bologna–1 slice, 1 ounce | 28 | 85 | 0.5 | T | 3 | 0 | 0 |
| Bread, enriched: | | | | | | | |
| cracked wheat–1 slice | 25 | 65 | 0.3 | 22 | 2 | T | T |
| rye (light)–1 slice | 25 | 60 | 0.4 | 19 | 2 | 0 | 0 |
| white–1 slice | 25 | 70 | 0.6 | 21 | 2 | T | T |
| whole wheat–1 slice | 23 | 55 | 0.5 | 23 | 3 | T | T |
| Broccoli, cooked–½ cup | 78 | 20 | 0.6 | 68 | 2 | 1,937 | 70 |
| Cabbage, cooked–½ cup | 73 | 15 | 0.2 | 32 | 1 | 94 | 24 |
| Cantaloupe–¼, 5″ diameter | 133 | 40 | 0.5 | 19 | 1 | 4,505 | 44 |
| Carrot, raw–1 medium | 81 | 35 | 0.6 | 30 | 1 | 8,910 | 6 |
| Cauliflower, cooked–½ cup | 68 | 15 | 0.5 | 14 | 2 | 40 | 37 |
| Cheese, American–1 slice, 1 ounce | 28 | 95 | 0.2 | 163 | 6 | 260 | 0 |
| Chicken[a]–½ breast | 98 | 195 | 1.0 | 10 | 29 | 100 | 0 |
| Chili con carne, w/beans–1 cup | 230 | 305 | 4.3 | 82 | 19 | 150 | 0 |
| Chocolate bar–1 ounce | 28 | 150 | 0.3 | 65 | 2 | 80 | T |
| Chocolate chip cookie–1 medium | 12 | 60 | 0.2 | 4 | * | T | 0 |
| Coffee, black– 6 ounce | 173 | 5 | 0.2 | T | 0 | 0 | 0 |
| Corn, canned–½ cup | 83 | 70 | 0.4 | 4 | 3 | 290 | 3 |
| Corn grits, enriched–½ ounce dry (½ cup prepared) | 123 | 60 | 0.4 | 1 | 2 | 73 | 0 |
| Cupcake, yellow w/chocolate icing–1 average | 46 | 185 | 0.4 | 20 | 2 | 209 | T |
| Doughnut, cake, plain–1 | 42 | 165 | 0.6 | 17 | 2 | 30 | T |
| Egg, plain–1 | 51 | 80 | 1.1 | 29 | 6 | 265 | 0 |
| Fruit cocktail–½ cup | 128 | 100 | 0.5 | 11 | 1 | 178 | 3 |
| Gelatin (Jell-O)–½ cup | 120 | 70 | 0 | 0 | 2 | 0 | 0 |
| Gingerbread, homemade–1 piece | 76 | 275 | 4.1 | 134 | 3 | 28 | 2 |
| Grapefruit–½ | 98 | 40 | 0.4 | 16 | * | 78 | 37 |
| Grapes, fresh–½ cup | 80 | 55 | 0.3 | 10 | * | 80 | 3 |
| Hamburger, no roll–1 | 85 | 245 | 2.7 | 10 | 21 | 34 | 0 |
| Ice cream, regular–⅔ cup | 89 | 180 | 0.1 | 117 | 3 | 363 | 0 |
| Lamb chop–2½ ounce | 71 | 255 | 0.9 | 6 | 16 | 0 | 0 |
| Lettuce, iceberg–½ cup | 28 | 5 | 0.1 | 5 | * | 90 | 2 |
| Liver, beef–3 ounce | 85 | 195 | 7.5 | 9 | 22 | 45,390 | 23 |

[1]To convert RDA for Vitamin A to IUs, multiply μgRE by 5.

[a]Values for these foods are averages of several varieties, brands, cuts of meat, or methods of preparation.

*Less than one gram protein.

**Fortified with Vitamin A.

[T]Means food contains only trace amount of this nutrient.

# ENERGY AND IRON CaPAC FOOD COMPOSITION TABLE

| Food and Serving Size | Weight | Energy | Iron | Ca | P | A | C |
|---|---|---|---|---|---|---|---|
| | g. | cal. | mg. | mg. | g. | IUs[1] | mg. |
| Macaroni, cooked–½ cup | 70 | 80 | 0.7 | 10 | 3 | 0 | 0 |
| Macaroni and cheese, prepared from mix–¾ cup | 156 | 290 | 1.6 | 114 | 9 | 560 | 0 |
| Milk, fluid: | | | | | | | |
| chocolate, 2% butterfat–8 ounce | 250 | 180 | 0.6 | 285 | 8 | 500** | 2 |
| skim–8 ounce | 245 | 85 | 0.1 | 300 | 8 | 500** | 2 |
| whole–8 ounce | 244 | 160 | 0.1 | 290 | 8 | 340 | 4 |
| Oatmeal, cooked–½ cup | 123 | 67 | 1.2 | 10 | 3 | 0 | 0 |
| Ocean perch, breaded, fried–2½ ounce | 70 | 160 | 0.9 | 23 | 13 | T | T |
| Orange, fresh–1 | 131 | 65 | 0.5 | 54 | 1 | 260 | 65 |
| Oysters, raw–6 | 90 | 60 | 4.8 | 84 | 8 | 276 | 0 |
| Peach, fresh–1 | 100 | 40 | 0.5 | 9 | * | 1,330 | 7 |
| Peanut butter–1 tablespoon | 15 | 90 | 0.3 | 9 | 4 | 0 | 0 |
| Pepper, green, raw–1 | 164 | 35 | 1.1 | 15 | 2 | 689 | 210 |
| Pizza, with cheese–⅐ of 10″ diameter | 57 | 140 | 1.0 | 89 | 5 | 251 | 3 |
| Plum, fresh–1 | 28 | 20 | 0.1 | 3 | * | 85 | 1 |
| Popcorn, plain–1 cup | 12 | 45 | 0.2 | 1 | * | 2 | 0 |
| Pork chop–3 ounce | 85 | 330 | 3.3 | 11 | 26 | 0 | 0 |
| Potato: | | | | | | | |
| baked–1 | 165 | 145 | 1.1 | 14 | 4 | T | 31 |
| chips–14 | 28 | 160 | 0.5 | 11 | 2 | 0 | 4 |
| french fries–½ cup | 55 | 150 | 0.7 | 8 | 2 | T | 12 |
| Prunes–10 medium | 96 | 240 | 4.0 | 50 | 2 | 1,540 | T |
| Pumpkin pie–⅐ of 9″ diameter | 135 | 290 | 1.2 | 106 | 6 | 2,467 | 3 |
| Raisins–¼ cup | 42 | 125 | 0.9 | 23 | 1 | 7 | T |
| Strawberries, whole–½ cup | 75 | 30 | 0.7 | 16 | 1 | 45 | 44 |
| Sweet potato, baked–1 | 146 | 205 | 1.3 | 58 | 3 | 11,826 | 32 |
| Tapioca pudding–½ cup | 116 | 150 | 1.2 | 77 | 2 | 19 | 1 |
| Tomato, fresh–1 medium | 123 | 30 | 0.6 | 16 | 1 | 1,107 | 28 |
| Tuna, canned in oil, drained–½ cup | 80 | 160 | 1.5 | 6 | 23 | 65 | 0 |
| Turnip greens, cooked–½ cup | 73 | 15 | 0.8 | 133 | 2 | 4,567 | 50 |
| Turnips, cooked–½ cup | 78 | 20 | 0.3 | 27 | * | T | 17 |
| Veal roast–3 ounce | 85 | 200 | 2.7 | 10 | 22 | 0 | 0 |
| Watermelon, fresh–1 piece | 426 | 140 | 0.8 | 84 | 3 | 1,596 | 42 |
| Wine, red–3½ ounce | 104 | 90 | 0.4 | 9 | * | 0 | 0 |
| Yogurt: | | | | | | | |
| skim milk–1 cup | 227 | 125 | 0.2 | 452 | 13 | 16 | 2 |
| whole milk–1 cup | 227 | 140 | 0.1 | 216 | 8 | 280 | 1 |

[1]To convert RDA for Vitamin A to IUs, multiply μgRE by 5.

[a]Values for these foods are averages of several varieties, brands, cuts of meat, or methods of preparation.

*Less than one gram protein.

**Fortified with Vitamin A.

[T]Means food contains only trace amount of this nutrient.

Name ____________________ Sheet 6-6

# MENUS FOR A PREGNANT WOMAN—A

**Directions:** Use Table 6-1 through 6-2, "Energy and Iron CaPAC Food Composition Table," to determine the calories and key nutrients in each food below. Then compare Diets A and B. Use T for "trace" and * for "less than 1 gram."

| | Calories | Iron (mg.) | Calcium (mg.) | Protein (gm.) | Vitamin A (IUs) | Vitamin C (gm.) |
|---|---|---|---|---|---|---|
| BREAKFAST | | | | | | |
| 1 cup black coffee | | | | | | |
| 1 slice white toast | | | | | | |
| 1 Tbsp. peanut butter | | | | | | |
| MIDMORNING | | | | | | |
| 3 chocolate chip cookies | | | | | | |
| LUNCH | | | | | | |
| 2 slices cheese pizza | | | | | | |
| 1 glass (3½ oz.) red wine | | | | | | |
| MIDAFTERNOON | | | | | | |
| 28 potato chips | | | | | | |
| 1 12-oz. beer | | | | | | |
| DINNER | | | | | | |
| 1 alcoholic cocktail | | | | | | |
| 1/2 chicken breast | | | | | | |
| 1/2 cup corn, canned | | | | | | |
| EVENING | | | | | | |
| 1 12-oz. beer | | | | | | |
| 1 cup popcorn, plain | | | | | | |
| TOTAL | | | | | | |

Name ______________________________ Sheet 6-7

# MENUS FOR A PREGNANT WOMAN—B

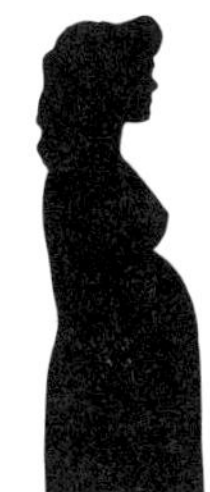

**Directions:** Use Table 6-1 through 6-2, "Energy and Iron CaPAC Food Composition Table," to determine the calories and key nutrients in each food below. Then compare Diets A and B. Use T for "trace" and * for "less than 1 gram."

| | Calories | Iron (mg.) | Calcium (mg.) | Protein (gm.) | Vitamin A (IUs) | Vitamin C (gm.) |
|---|---|---|---|---|---|---|
| BREAKFAST | | | | | | |
| 1/2 cup oatmeal | | | | | | |
| 1 orange | | | | | | |
| 1 cup skim milk | | | | | | |
| 1 slice whole wheat toast | | | | | | |
| MIDMORNING | | | | | | |
| 1/2 cup grapes | | | | | | |
| 1/2 cup tapioca | | | | | | |
| LUNCH | | | | | | |
| 2 Tbsp. peanut butter | | | | | | |
| 2 slices whole wheat bread | | | | | | |
| 1 cup skim milk | | | | | | |
| 1 plum | | | | | | |
| MIDAFTERNOON | | | | | | |
| 1-oz. slice, American cheese | | | | | | |
| 1 apple | | | | | | |
| DINNER | | | | | | |
| 1 pork chop | | | | | | |
| 1/2 cup broccoli | | | | | | |
| 1/2 cup french fries | | | | | | |
| 1 cup skim milk | | | | | | |
| 1 slice pumpkin pie | | | | | | |
| EVENING | | | | | | |
| 1 medium carrot | | | | | | |
| 1 package (1/4 cup) raisins | | | | | | |
| TOTAL | | | | | | |

Name ________________________________________ 

# FIZZ, FLAVOR, AND FUN!

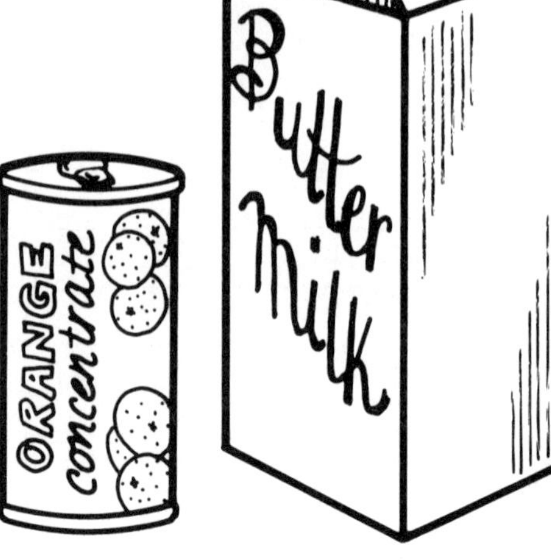


### Orange Smoothee

6-ounce can frozen orange juice concentrate
1 cup milk
1 cup water
1/4 cup sugar
1/2 teaspoon vanilla
10 ice cubes

Place all ingredients in a blender. Blend until smooth and serve. Makes 6 servings, 115 calories each.

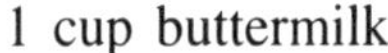

### Orange Buttermilk Shake

1 cup buttermilk
1 scoop vanilla ice cream
1/2 cup orange juice
2 tablespoons brown sugar

Beat ingredients with a spoon or mixer until smooth; then serve. Makes 2 servings, 220 calories each.

### Pineapple Cooler

46-ounce can unsweetened pineapple juice
2 tablespoons lemon juice
6-ounce can frozen orange juice concentrate
10-ounce bottle club soda

Mix the juices and frozen concentrate. Add club soda before serving and pour over ice. Makes 8 servings, 150 calories each.

### Peanut Butter Eggnog

3-1/2 cups milk
2 egg yolks
1/4 cup creamy peanut butter
1 teaspoon vanilla
2 egg whites
1/2 cup whipped cream

In a blender, blend the egg yolks, peanut butter, vanilla, and *half* of the milk until frothy. Pour into a punch bowl and stir in the remaining milk. With a mixer, beat the egg whites until stiff peaks form. Fold the egg whites into the milk mixture. Then fold whipped cream into the mixture and serve. Makes 6 servings, 245 calories each.

Name ______________________________ Sheet 6-9

# BOOZE AND BABIES DON'T MIX!

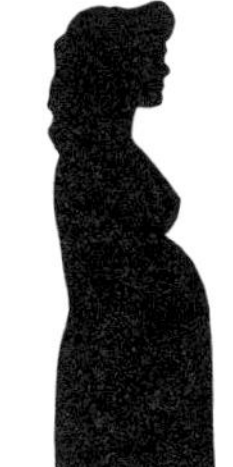

**Directions:** Read each statement. If it is true, circle "T." If it is false, circle "F."

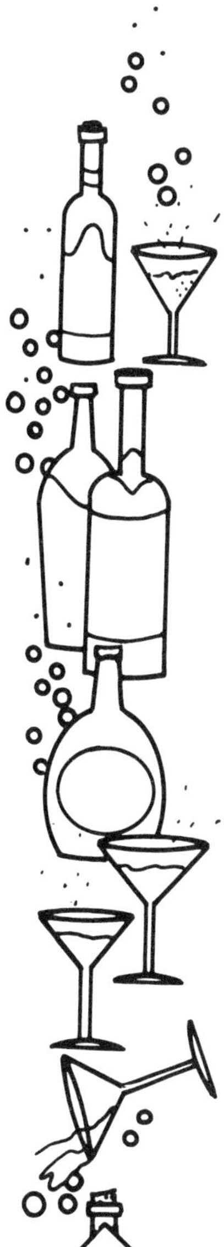

1. In Fetal Alcohol Syndrome, children have a calm, peaceful temperament. T F
2. In Fetal Alcohol Syndrome, there is an increased chance of having a high birth-weight baby. T F
3. In Fetal Alcohol Syndrome, there is a greater chance of having a child with a lower IQ. T F
4. Alcohol is diluted as it crosses the placenta to the fetus. T F
5. Alcohol affects all cells in the body. T F
6. The most critical period for development of the baby's brain and central nervous system is during the last three months of pregnancy. T F
7. An after-dinner drink every day will definitely not harm an unborn child. T F
8. The surest way to avoid FAS is not to drink any alcohol while pregnant. T F
9. If a child is hyperactive or a slow learner, it is undoubtedly because the mother drank during pregnancy. T F
10. A one-night drinking binge during pregnancy may be just as harmful to the fetus as consuming lesser amounts of alcoholic beverages daily. T F
11. The number of alcoholic women of childbearing age has steadily been decreasing. T F
12. Pure alcohol contains very few calories. T F

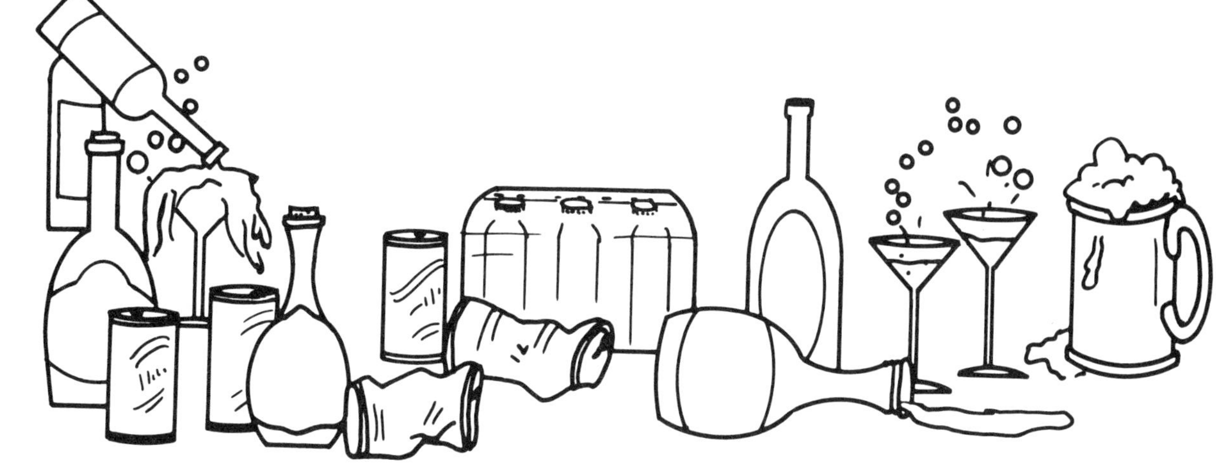

Name ______________________________ Sheet 6-10

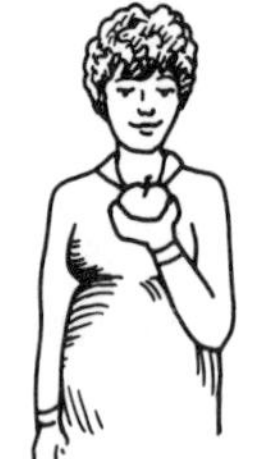

# AN IDEAL MENU FOR PREGNANCY

**Directions:** Use Tables 6-1 through 6-2, "Energy and Iron CaPAC Food Composition Table," and Chart A, "Recommended Dietary Allowances," to create a one-day "ideal" menu for a pregnant girl between 15 and 18 years of age.

| **Breakfast:** |
|---|
| **Snack:** |
| **Lunch:** |
| **Snack:** |
| **Dinner:** |
| **Snack:** |

Name ______________________________ Quiz Sheet 6-1

# QUIZ
# NUTRITION FOR THE EXPECTANT MOTHER

_____ 1. Which of these should the expectant mother cut down on during pregnancy?

a. Pastries
b. Nonfat milk
c. Pasta
d. Fruits

_____ 2. A pregnant woman needs to eat more foods from:

a. The Milk-Cheese group
b. The Meat-Poultry-Fish-Beans group
c. The Fats-Sweets-Alcohol group
d. Answers a and b

_____ 3. Karen is pregnant. Which of the following menus would be her best dinner choice?

a. Fried chicken
Corn-on-the-cob
Mashed potatoes and margarine
Nonfat milk
Apple pie

b. Hot dog and bun
Potato salad
Wedge of watermelon
12 ounces of cola

c. Meat enchiladas
Spinach salad
Cornbread and margarine
Fresh peach
Ice Cream

d. Broiled pork chop
French fries
Buttered corn
Chocolate chip cookies
Whole milk

4. Name several nutrient-dense foods. On the back of this sheet, discuss the importance of nutrient-dense foods in the pregnant woman's diet with respect to both meeting the RDAs and gaining weight.

______________________________________________

______________________________________________

_____ 5. Debbie has just found out she is pregnant. She weighs 120 pounds. About how much should she weigh right before the baby is born?

a. 124–130 pounds
b. 134–140 pounds
c. 144–150 pounds
d. 152–160 pounds

6. Although safe limits for alcohol consumption are not known, explain what has been recommended for pregnant women and why.

______________________________________________

______________________________________________

_____ 7. Which of the following is a major characteristic of Fetal Alcohol Syndrome:

a. Calm, peaceful temperament
b. Mental retardation
c. Large head circumference
d. All of the above

# Unit 7: Nutrition for Infants and Children

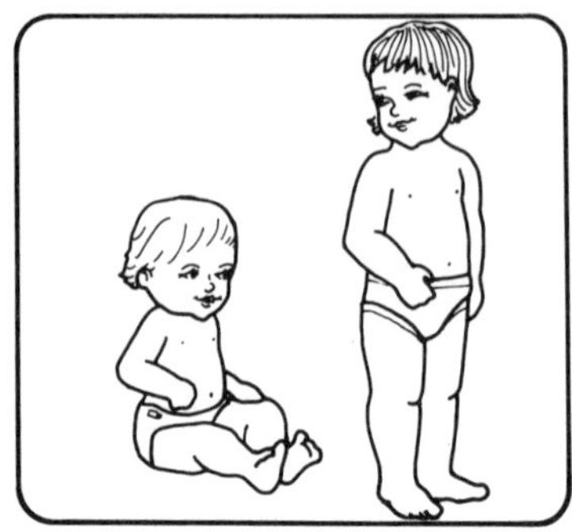

## CONCEPTS

–Nutrition affects the health of people of all ages and at all stages of the life cycle, including infancy and childhood.

–People at each stage of the life cycle possess different nutritional needs.

## OBJECTIVES

–Students will be able to judge nutritional appropriateness of a menu for infants and for children.

–Students will be able to describe nutritional needs during infancy and will be able to plan nutritional meals for infants.

–Students will be able to describe nutritional needs during childhood and will be able to plan nutritional meals for children.

## TEACHER'S UNIT INTRODUCTION

Nutritional needs change during a person's lifetime. The needs of an infant are obviously different from the needs of an adult. Each stage of the life cycle needs special nutritional attention.

**Infancy.** If we consider nutritional needs on the basis of body weight, the nutrient needs during infancy are higher than during any other stage of life. The infant grows at a rapid rate. By four to six months of age, most babies double their birth-weight. Body length increases by 50 percent during the first year. If infants continued to grow at this rate, they might weigh 1,823 pounds and stand 19 feet tall by the time they were five years old! Luckily, the growth spurt during infancy gradually slows down and only comes back for a shorter time during adolescence.

The rapid rate of growth during infancy demands large quantities of the nutrients important for cell and tissue growth. Nearly all of the nutrients are involved, but especially important are protein, calcium, and iron. The energy needs of an infant are also high. More calories per pound of body weight are required during infancy than during any other time of life.

Keeping this information in mind, let's look at the practical side of nutrition for infants. First, we need to know what types of food a baby needs to supply all of the nutrients required. Second, we need to know how much food to feed.

The first food infants receive is milk, either breast milk or formula. The question of which type of milk to feed the infant is the individual mother's decision. A look at the advantages and disadvantages of each method can help during decision-making. This chart presents both the positive and negative sides of each method. [Display the following chart using either an opaque or overhead projector.]

| | **Breast** | **Formula** |
|---|---|---|
| ADVANTAGES | *The nutrients in breast milk match exactly the needs of the infant. | *People other than the mother can feed the infant. |
| | *The breast milk present directly after birth (colostrum) possesses anti-infective properties for the baby. | *Bottle-feeding allows the mother the freedom to do other things, such as hold a full-time job. |
| | *Breast milk is always available. | *Some mothers may be either ill or taking medication and for health reasons should not breast-feed. |
| | *There is no need for bottles, equipment, or preparation skills. | *The mother can measure the amount of milk the infant consumes and thus control weight gain if necessary. |
| | *If the mother eats inexpensive foods while breast-feeding, breast milk is cheaper to feed than formula. | *The composition of formulas may be altered to suit the infant's needs. |
| | *Babies rarely have any allergic reactions to breast milk. | |
| | *Breast-feeding often helps the mother return to her prepregnancy weight and physical condition more quickly. | |

| | Breast | Formula |
|---|---|---|
| DISADVANTAGES | *Other people cannot feed the baby, except for giving the baby water.<br>*Some women feel uncomfortable with breast-feeding for physical or psychological reasons.<br>*Breast-feeding restricts the mother's freedom to leave the baby for more than a few hours at a time. | *Formulas do not exactly match breast milk.<br>*Bottle-feeding involves more preparation time and skill.<br>*The water supply must be safe.<br>*Many formulas are expensive, especially the ready-to-feed type.<br>*Cow's milk can produce allergies. |

The next question to consider is: When should solid foods be introduced? Breast milk or iron-fortified formula, alone, is an excellent diet for an infant during the first several months of life. For some infants, breast milk may need to be supplemented with flouride and/or iron. Formula usually supplies these nutrients. There are no nutritional reasons to add solid foods until at least four months of age, and probably not until six months. By the age of six months, the iron that had been stored in the infant from birth has been drained and the infant is in need of a dietary supply. Iron supplements or iron-fortified cereals should be started at this time. In addition, at six months breast milk or formula alone is not sufficient to meet most infants' calorie needs. The chart on Sheet 7-2, "What Is Good for the Baby to Eat?," describes the sequence for introducing solid foods to infants.

Homemade or commercially prepared baby foods can be fed to the infant. Commercially prepared baby foods are sometimes a more expensive source of nutrients because starch, sugar, fat, water, and other "fillers" may be added to the food. This type of baby food can thus contain more empty calories than the variety made at home. However, commercially prepared baby foods offer a convenience value not provided when making them at home. Homemade baby foods should be prepared carefully to make sure that the nutritional value is high and that the food is free from contamination. A simple description of homemade baby foods is presented on Sheet 7-3, "What Is Good for the Baby to Eat?"

**Childhood.** After about one year of age, an infant is considered to be a child and will be eating most foods from the family table. However, children's nutrient needs are slightly different from those of the rest of the family. Children need nearly the same quantity of nutrients as their parents do, but they need fewer calories. The foods children eat must be nutrient-dense in relation to calories. Children cannot afford to eat empty calories.

Snacking is an activity commonly engaged in by children. Young children's stomachs cannot hold enough food to last the five or six hours between regular meals. Snacking is a necessary way to provide extra nutrients and calories between meals. As long as they are well chosen, snacks can make a valuable contribution to children's diets.

---

Unit 7 is designed as two learning centers. In order to economize on expenses and space, you may want to use cupboards and cabinets to display the centers instead of using elaborate backdrops. The following are step-by-step directions for creating each learning center.

### Nutrition in Infancy Learning Center

1. Construct a backdrop to stimulate interest. Attach pictures of infants or breast-feeding women to the posterboard and display them in front of the backdrop with jars or boxes of baby food and/or baby dolls.
2. Construct a flipchart to parallel Sheets 7-1 through 7-3, "What Is Good for the Baby to Eat?," by attaching Sheets 7-1, 7-2, and 7-3 to the posterboard with rings holding the tops together. Make a tape recording of the script on Sheets 7-4 through 7-5, "More About Good Food for the Baby," to play along with the flipchart. The mounted information sheets and tape recordings are designed to complement one another: Sheet 7-1 goes with Sheet 7-4; Sheets 7-2 and 7-3 go with Sheet 7-5. On the tape recording announce the appropriate sheets to use. (Alternatively, use the complete package of Sheets 7-1 through 7-5 as a single handout for students to read silently at the learning center.
3. Sheet 7-6, "Review of What Is Good for the Baby to Eat," provides a short-answer self-quiz to review learning center information.
4. Set up the backdrop, flipchart, tape, tape recorder, and copies of Sheets 7-1 through 7-6 for the learning center.
5. Include additional resource materials if desired (*see* "References/Resources" at the end of this kit). Provide additional topics for students to research in these references. (*see* the "Follow-Up Activities" for this unit).

### Nutrition in Childhood Learning Center

1. Construct a backdrop to stimulate interest. Use photos of young children eating and mount them on a posterboard; include a display of small bowls, plates, cups, utensils, and children's cookbooks in front of the backdrop.

2. Construct a pocketboard as illustrated here and label it "Nutrition for Children." In appropriate pockets, place cards with pictures of single foods. In the pocket labeled "Combinations" include pictures of mixed dishes such as soups and casseroles. Include at least six different food choices in each pocket.

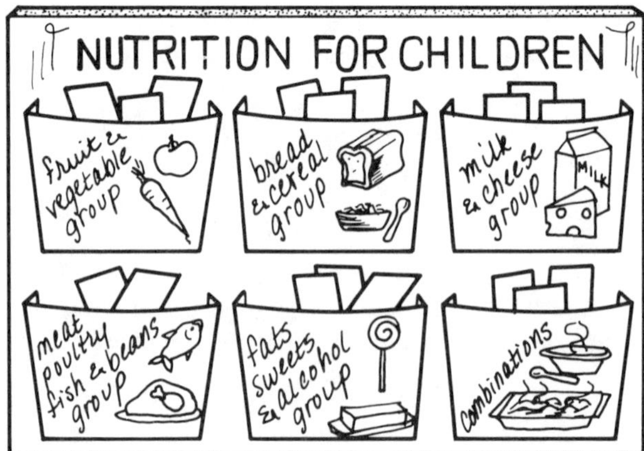


3. For the learning center, set up the backdrop, pocketboard, and copies of Sheet 7-7, "Nutrition for Children"; Sheet 7-8, "Special Nutritional Needs at Different Life Stages"; and Chart B, "Daily Food Guide."
4. Include additional resources if desired (*see* "References/Resources" at the end of this kit).

This unit requires familiarity with menu planning. If students are not familiar with menu planning, it may be wise to spend some time discussing the principles of menu planning introduced in Units 13, 14, and 15. Unit 7 also acts as an introduction to Unit 8 in which nutrition for progressive life stages is discussed.

## BASIC ACTIVITY

**Time Needed:** One class period

**Materials Needed:** Sheets 7-1 through 7-3: "What Is Good for the Baby to Eat?"
Sheets 7-4 through 7-5: "More About Good Food for the Baby"
Sheet 7-6: "Review of What Is Good for the Baby to Eat?"
Sheet 7-7: "Nutrition for Children"
Sheet 7-8: "Special Nutritional Needs at Different Life Stages"
Chart A: "Recommended Dietary Allowances"
Chart B: "Daily Food Guide"
*Optional:* tape recorder(s)
*Optional:* cassette tape(s)
Backdrops for learning centers (*see* Teacher's Unit Introduction)
*Optional:* additional resource materials (*see* "References/Resources" at the end of this kit)
Quiz Sheet 7-1

1. Introduce this activity by conducting a brainstorming session about why students need to have information concerning nutrition during infancy and childhood. Encourage them, as potential parents and adults, to discuss the importance of knowing about each phase of the life cycle *before* it begins. Teenagers may be interested in infants and children, but

they might not see this activity as being personally relevant. The introductory discussion is designed to promote the idea that these topics are important.

2. Have students visit each learning center and complete the appropriate worksheets. You may have them work individually or in pairs. To ease the movement of students through the centers, you may want to make several sets of tapes and flipcharts for the "Nutrition in Infancy Learning Center."

3. To close the activity, bring the students together for a large-group discussion that compares and contrasts the differences in individual nutritional needs at different life stages. At this point, you may also want to distribute copies of Chart A, "Recommended Dietary Allowances," to demonstrate the varying levels of the many different nutrients needed by each life-stage group.

4. **Evaluation:** Distribute Quiz Sheet 7-1 and have students complete it independently. Discuss the answers as a class.

## FOLLOW-UP ACTIVITIES

1. Have students interview children or guardians of children at different stages of the life cycle: a mother of an infant, a young child, and an older child. They should ask questions about the diet habits and activity patterns of the children. In addition, have the students ask the mothers what kind of nutrition information that they wish they had learned in school and that they believe would have helped them with diet planning for pregnancy and for feeding infants and children.

2. Assign readings from the selected materials in the "References/Resources" at the end of this kit. Have students write summary reports or present the information in another format such as a demonstration or display.

3. Arrange a visit to a preschool or day-care center where young children eat at least one meal. Have students observe the children's eating behavior. Discuss the feeding program with the director. Then have several students design a nutrition or food activity for the children and carry it out with the director's permission. Their findings should then be presented to the class in whatever format they wish.

4. Have students visit the baby food section of a grocery store and do a label-reading activity. For example, have them select a group of foods that meet the U.S. RDAs for a baby for one day.

Name ____________________ 

# WHAT IS GOOD FOR THE BABY TO EAT?

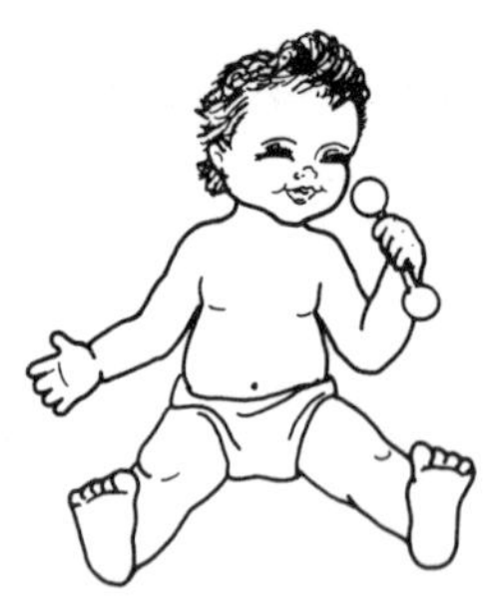

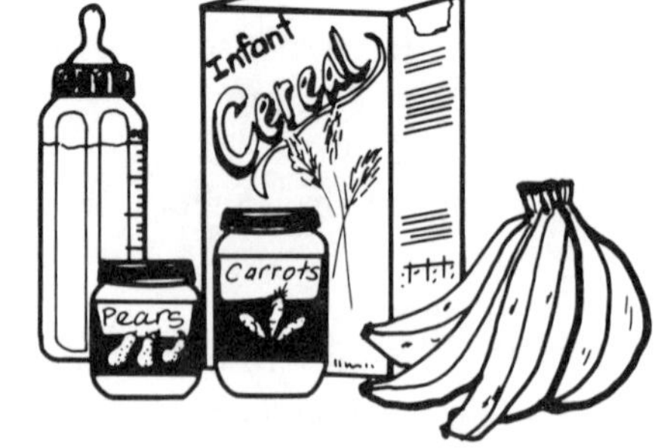


## BREAST-FEEDING

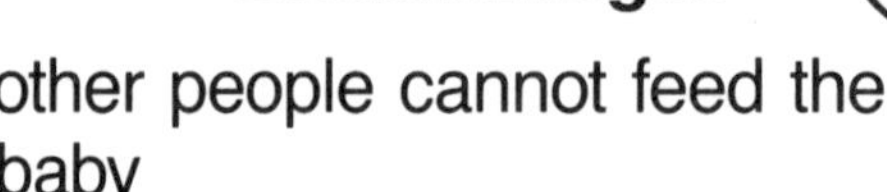

### Advantages

+ designed for baby's special nutritional needs
+ protects from infections
+ can be less expensive
+ always available and safe
+ fewer allergies

### Disadvantages

– other people cannot feed the baby
– some women are uncomfortable or embarrassed about breast-feeding
– some women may be unwilling or unable physically to breast-feed

## BOTTLE-FEEDING

### Advantages

+ other people can feed the baby
+ mother is free to do other things

### Disadvantages

– can be more expensive
– must sterilize equipment and prepare formula
– must have safe water supply
– cow's milk in some formulas can cause allergies
– formulas imitate breast milk but not exactly
– formulas do not provide immunities

# WHEN DO BABIES NEED SOLID FOODS?

4–6 months

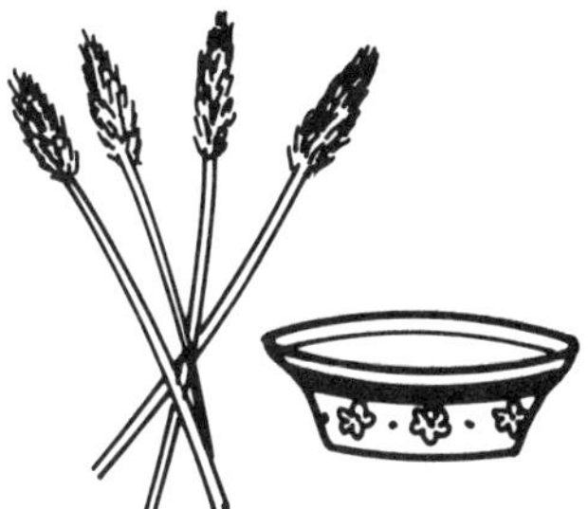

**Cereals Are Usually the First Food**

♡ use iron-fortified cereals

♡ use rice first, then oatmeal, and next barley

4–6 months

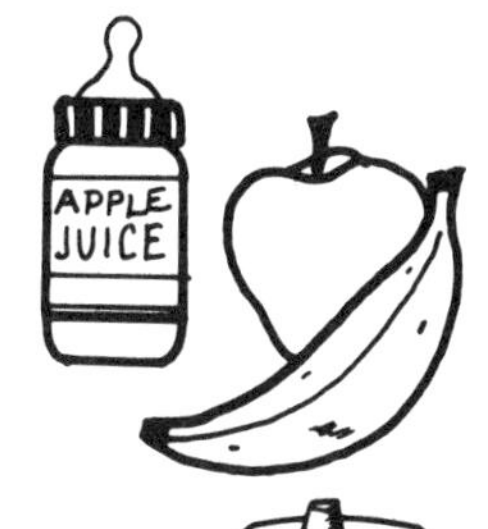


**Fruits, Vegetables, and Juices Next**

♡ use real fruit juices, not fruit drinks

♡ feed a single fruit or vegetable at one time

♡ start with bananas or applesauce (no sugar, please)

6–8 months

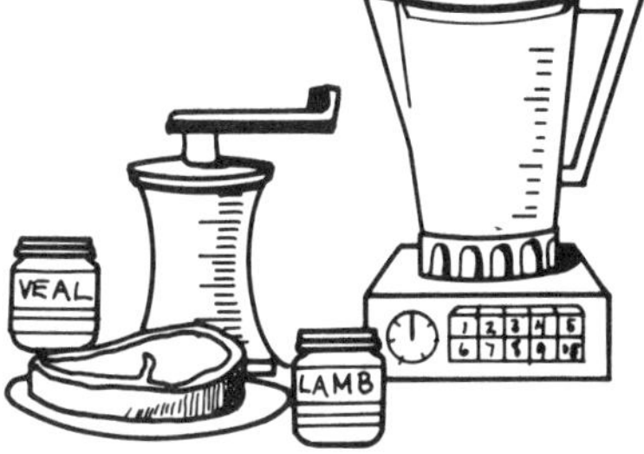


**Strained Meats Are Next**

♡ avoid combination dinners—they have less protein and iron

8–10 months

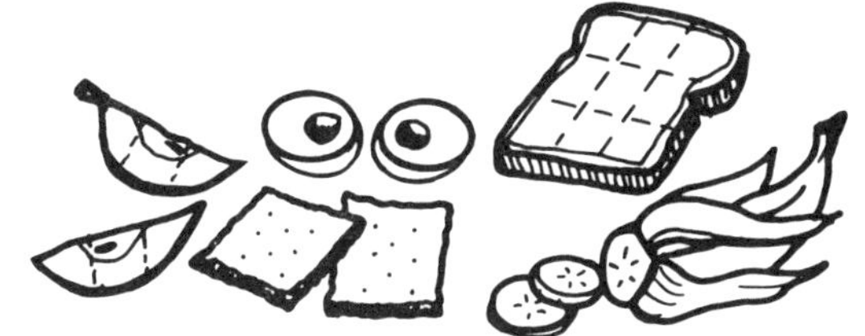

**Serve Finger Foods**

♡ foods baby can pick up

♡ serve small portions

♡ avoid chewy or hard foods

♡ eggs, crackers, soft fruit chunks

10–12 months

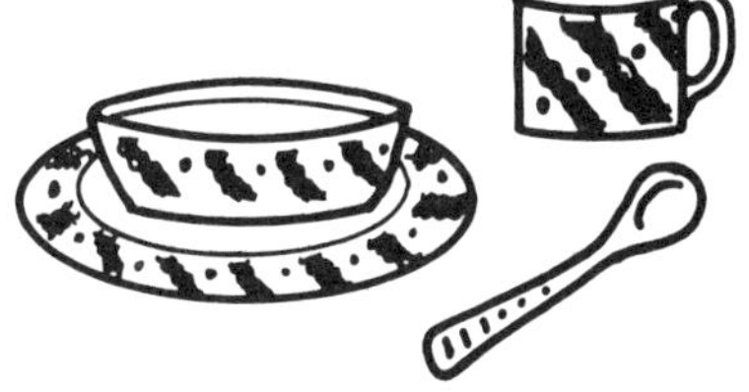

**Foods From the Table—Like Everyone Else**

♡ use small plates and utensils made for children

♡ avoid exotic seasonings

♡ serve small portions

♡ avoid heavy use of seasonings including salt

## HOW TO MAKE BABY FOOD:

1. Select fresh, wholesome foods.
2. Wash all equipment and food thoroughly.
3. Prepare food by removing peel, excess fat, seeds, bones, or other hard, indigestible parts.
4. Bake, broil, or steam food until tender. Do not fry foods for baby.
5. Use fork and strainer, food mill, or blender. Mash food with liquid (milk, formula, juice, or water) until very smooth. Do not add sugar or salt.
6. Serve at room temperature.

**CAN YOU TELL WHAT BABY IS EATING FROM THE FOOD LABEL?**

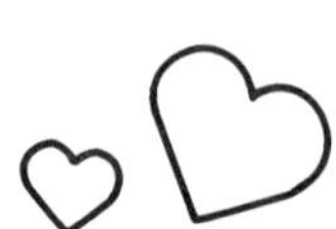

The baby needs love, plenty of rest, and good nutrition to grow healthy and happy!

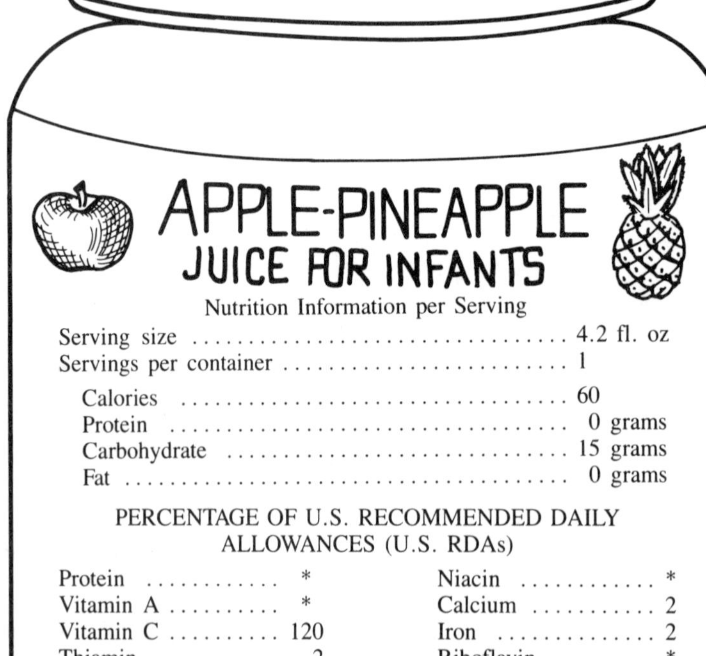

APPLE-PINEAPPLE
JUICE FOR INFANTS
Nutrition Information per Serving
Serving size ........ 4.2 fl. oz
Servings per container ........ 1
Calories ........ 60
Protein ........ 0 grams
Carbohydrate ........ 15 grams
Fat ........ 0 grams
PERCENTAGE OF U.S. RECOMMENDED DAILY ALLOWANCES (U.S. RDAs)
Protein ........ *
Vitamin A ........ *
Vitamin C ........ 120
Thiamin ........ 2
Niacin ........ *
Calcium ........ 2
Iron ........ 2
Riboflavin ........ *
*Contains less than 2% of the U.S. RDAs of these nutrients.

# MORE ABOUT GOOD FOOD FOR THE BABY

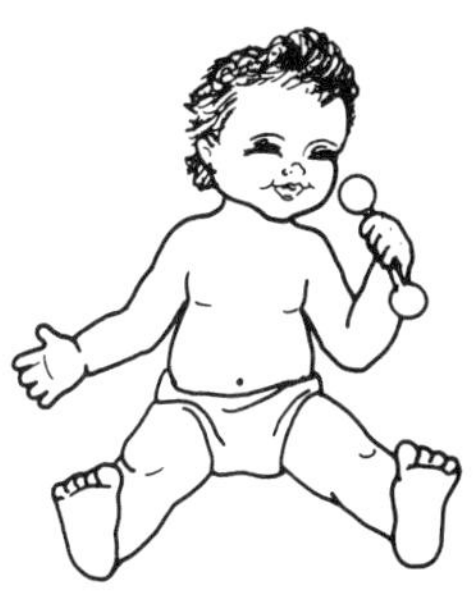

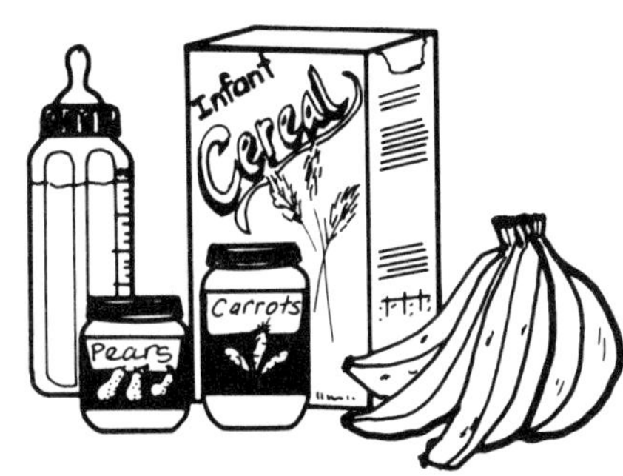


Babies need special care. Everyone knows that! But did you know that babies have special nutritional needs? The kinds and amounts of food babies eat are very important for their health. When babies are first born, they need only breast milk or milk formula to grow and be healthy. Later, they need other foods. First, let us talk about milk.

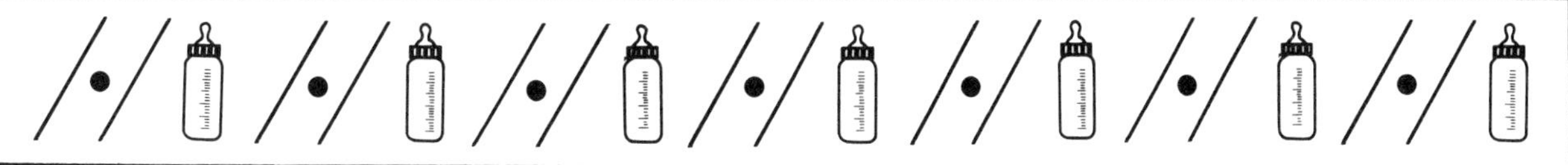

Babies can get their milk in two ways. They can either be breast-fed or they can be bottle-fed. We will talk about breast-feeding first, and later we will talk about bottle-feeding.

There are five reasons why breast-feeding is a good idea. First, breast milk is designed by nature to be just right for the baby's nutritional needs. Second, breast milk contains special substances that help babies fight infections. Third, breast milk is always available from the mother, and it is safe, too. Fourth, breast milk can be less expensive than store-bought milk. It depends partly on what the mother eats. The mother must eat more food when she breast-feeds, but if she eats inexpensive foods, the breast milk will cost less than store-bought milk. Fifth, breast milk is good for the baby because most babies are not allergic to it. Some infants are allergic to the cow's milk used in most formulas.

Breast-feeding is not perfect, though. There are three reasons why breast-feeding is not always a good idea. First, other people, such as the father, are not able to feed the baby. Second, some mothers are uncomfortable or embarrassed about breast-feeding. Third, some women are unable or unwilling to breast-feed because of an illness, a job, or family responsibilities.

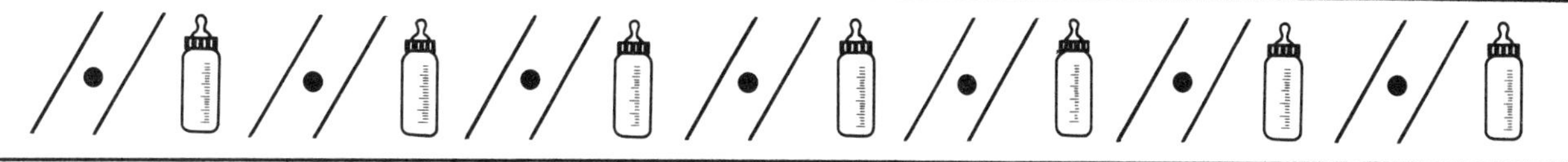

Bottle-feeding began in the early 1900s when people realized they could change cow's milk to make it similar to human milk. At first, mothers used cow's milk formulas only in an emergency. Gradually, many women began using formulas for feeding their babies. Today more women use formula than breast milk. However, there is a trend toward breast-feeding once again.

Bottle-feeding does have some advantages. Bottle-feeding allows other people to feed the baby. It also allows the mother the freedom to do other things, such as holding a full-time job. There are some problems with bottle-feeding, though. Formulas can be expensive, especially the ready-to-feed kind. Bottles and equipment must be sterilized and the formula must be prepared; this takes time and some skill. To prepare a formula, there must be a safe, clean supply of water. Cow's milk, the kind of milk used in most formulas, can cause allergies in some babies. Formulas do not have the exact makeup of nutrients that human milk has. Formulas also do not have the special substances that protect the baby against infections.

A mother has the choice of which kind of milk to feed her baby: breast milk or formula. It is important for her to know all about both kinds before she makes her decision.

Foods other than milk should be introduced into a baby's diet gradually. Four to six months of age is the earliest time at which most babies need solid foods. Cereals are the easiest foods for a baby to digest. Cereals fortified with iron are usually introduced first. Fruits, vegetables, and juices are introduced into a baby's diet next. Finally, strained meats or meat alternates are introduced. By the time infants reach their first birthday, they may be eating most of the foods their family is eating. Exotic spices and rich foods should not be offered to the infant.

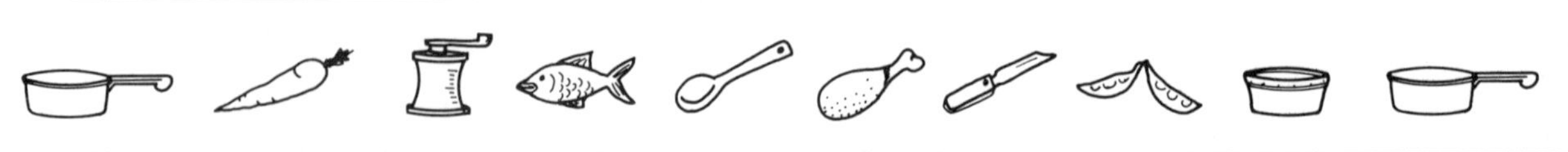

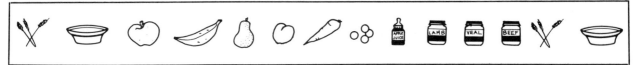

Homemade baby food can be just as nutritious as store-bought baby food. If it is prepared carefully, homemade baby food may be more nutritious than the store-bought varieties. Commercial baby food may have extra water, sugar, starch, fat, or other "fillers." It may contain more calories and fewer nutrients.

When making baby food at home, it is important to prepare and store the food carefully. The nutrients may be lost or destroyed if the food is overcooked or stored too long.

Look at the general recipe for making baby food at home. Doesn't it look easy?

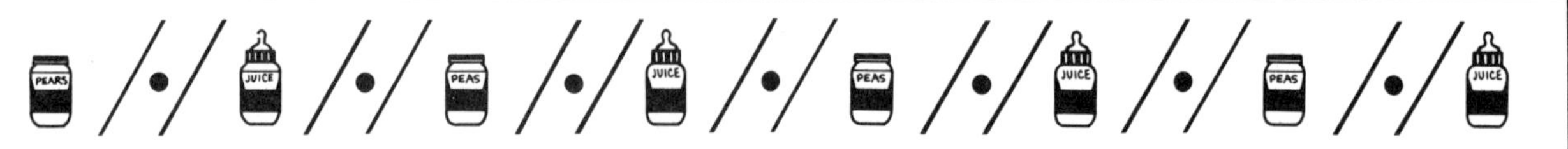


Nutrition labeling tells you what is in the food you buy. On baby food jars and boxes, the label tells many things. The illustrated label tells you that in one serving of apple-pineapple juice for infants there are 60 calories, 0 grams of protein, 15 grams of carbohydrate, and 0 grams of fat. It also tells you what percentage of the U.S. RDA for each nutrient is provided by the serving. On baby food labels, the U.S. RDAs are a set of standards made especially for infants under the age of twelve months. For example, one serving of the juice provides 120 percent of the U.S. RDA for Vitamin C and 2 percent for thiamin.

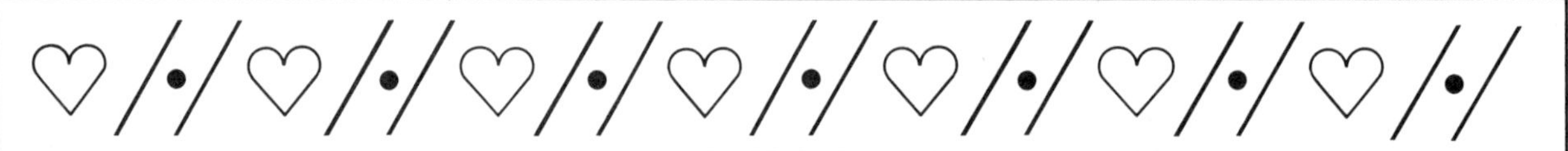

Babies need good nutrition to grow strong and healthy! They also need plenty of love and rest to stay healthy and happy.

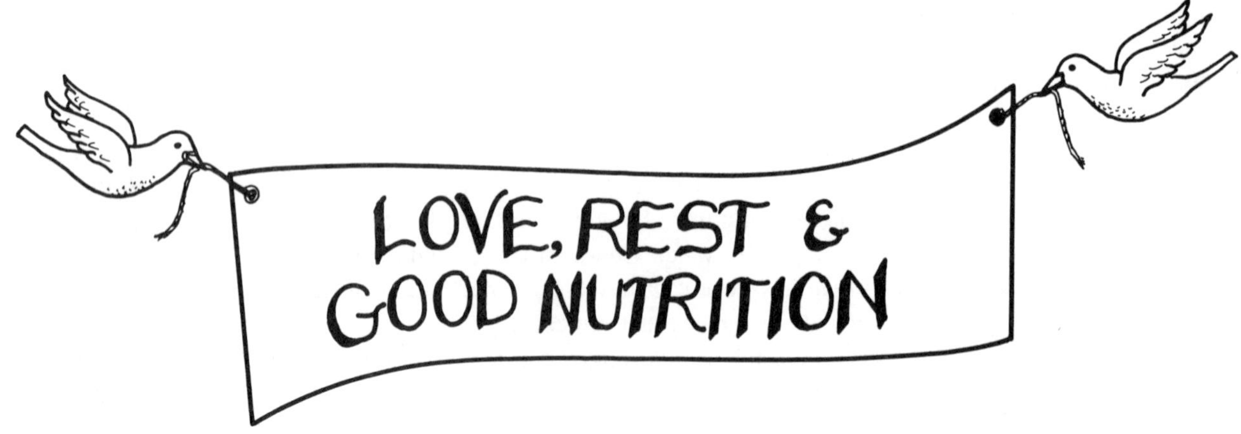

# REVIEW OF "WHAT IS GOOD FOR THE BABY TO EAT?"

**Directions:** Review the information on Sheets 7-1 through 7-5 by answering the questions below.

1. When babies are first born, the only food they need is
   ______________ or ______________.
2. Babies can get their milk in two ways:
   ______________ or ______________.
3. Name one reason why breast-feeding is a good idea: ______________.
   ______________.
4. Name one problem with breast-feeding: ______________.
   ______________.
5. Name one reason why bottle-feeding is a good idea: ______________.
   ______________.
6. Name one problem with bottle-feeding: ______________.
   ______________.
7. Which type of feeding is usually more expensive? ______________
8. Which type of feeding causes fewer allergies? ______________
9. List the order in which these foods should be introduced to the infant:
   _____ finger foods _____ cereal _____ fruits/vegetables _____ table foods _____ meats
10. Commercial baby food sometimes contains extra ______________, ______________, ______________, ______________, or other ______________. It may contain more ______________ and fewer ______________.
11. These two things destroy nutrients in the process of making homemade baby foods:
    ______________ and ______________.
12. What three things do babies need to grow strong and healthy?
    ______________, ______________ and ______________.

# NUTRITION FOR CHILDREN

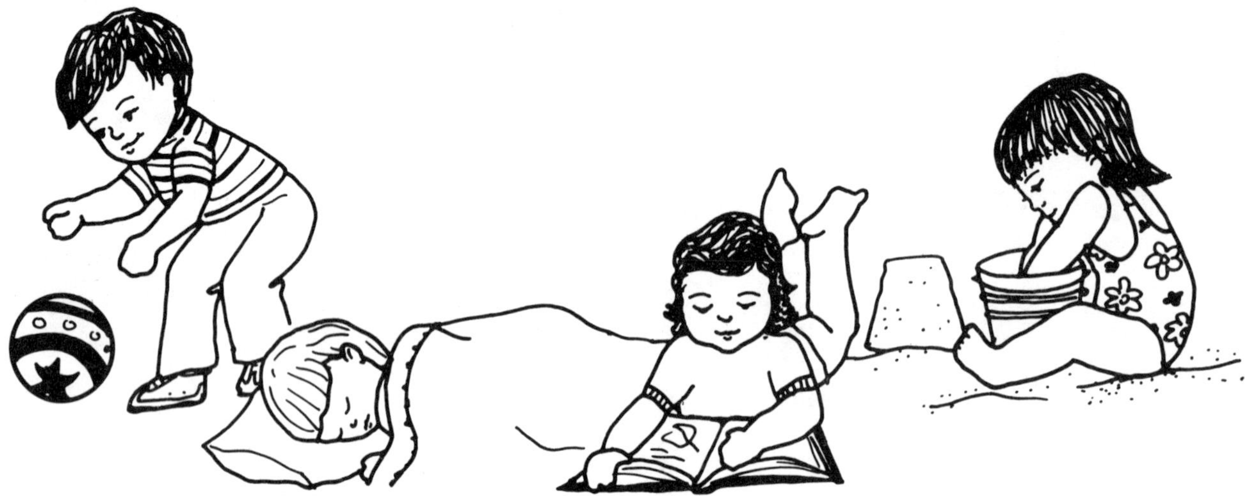

Children are special people. Their nutritional needs depend on many things—on how fast they are growing . . . on how much they sleep . . . on how much they run and play.

Children need the same *kinds* of foods everyone else needs. But children need different *amounts* of these foods. For example, children who are still growing need plenty of calcium for growing bones (two to three servings of milk a day). They need to eat and drink foods from the Milk-Cheese group in order to supply themselves with the extra calcium.

See the chart on Sheet 7-8, "Special Nutritional Needs at Different Life Stages." Other than the Milk-Cheese group, children need almost, but not quite, the same amount of foods that other people of different ages need. Some children might not be able to eat adult-sized servings, however. At lunch time, for example, small children may only want to eat half a slice of bread and one or two tablespoons of peanut butter. Their stomachs may not be big enough to hold more. Later in the day, they may need a snack of one or two crackers with cheese, or half a banana with half a glass of milk. On the other hand, some children who are very active and who are growing at full-speed may want to eat as much or more than many adults. Do not be too surprised if a seven year old can "out-eat" you someday!

The two keys to understanding children's nutritional needs are *individuality* and *variety.* Each child is unique and has different nutritional needs at different times. Besides individuality, children need variety. Variety in the diet ensures that each child will get what he or she needs nutritionally. Variety means eating a lot of different kinds of foods.

---

## SPECIAL NEEDS

Every child likes certain foods and dislikes others. Yet, every child has similar nutritional needs. How can you provide enough calcium for a child who does not like to drink milk? Or, how can you provide enough protein for a child who will not eat meat? Every problem has a solution!

**Directions:** Solve the nutritional problems of Kim and Angela, below. Use Chart B, "Daily Food Guide," and Sheet 7-8 as references. To solve the problems, select foods found in the "Nutrition for Children" pocketboard and write them on the back of this sheet.

1. Kim is six years old. She likes to eat and drink almost anything . . . anything except milk, that is. Fluid milk of any kind makes her turn up her nose in disgust. Plan a nutritious day's diet for Kim.
2. Angela is just starting first grade. Her mother needs some interesting ideas for nutritious meals to pack for lunch so that Angela will be motivated to eat. Plan three menus for Angela's school lunch. Remember that lunch should provide about 1/3 of her daily nutritional needs.

# SPECIAL NUTRITIONAL NEEDS AT DIFFERENT LIFE STAGES

| | MILK-CHEESE GROUP (# Servings) | MEAT-POULTRY-FISH-BEANS GROUP (# Servings) | FRUIT-VEGETABLE GROUP (# Servings) | BREAD-CEREAL GROUP (# Servings) |
|---|---|---|---|---|
| **Pregnant Women**<br>Pregnant women need about 300 extra calories per day. The extra food should be high in calcium, iron, and protein. These nutrients are found in the Milk-Cheese group and in the Meat-Poultry-Fish-Beans group. | 3–5 | 3 | 4 | 4 |
| **Infants**<br>Infants need only breast milk or milk formula when they are born. As they grow, they begin to need different foods. By 4 to 6 months of age, they need a variety of foods beginning with cereals, then fruits/vegetables, and meat or meat alternates in addition to milk. By one year of age, infants may eat most of the foods children and adults eat. Serving sizes are proportionately smaller for infants. | * | * | * | * |
| **Children**<br>Children's needs vary from day to day and from child to child. Serving sizes are about ½ of adult portions. | 2–3 | 1–2 | 3–4 | 3–4 |
| **Teenagers**<br>Teenagers are growing at a rapid rate and need lots of nutrients. They especially need plenty of calcium for bone growth. Calcium is found in the Milk-Cheese group. | 4 | 2 | 4 | 4 |
| **Adults**<br>Depending upon activity level, adults need fewer calories to maintain desirable weight. Especially important is a steady dietary supply of calcium to prevent osteoporosis (a condition of weakened, brittle bones) because the body cannot absorb and store calcium as it once did. | 2 | 2 | 4 | 4 |
| **Elderly**<br>The elderly need fewer and fewer calories as they age. They need the same or more nutrients, however. Choosing foods high in nutrients and low in calories is important. Especially important is a steady dietary supply of calcium to prevent osteoporosis. Brittle bones in the elderly result both in increased bone breakage in minor accidents and in slow recuperation. | 2 | 2 | 4 | 4 |

Name ______________________________ Quiz Sheet 7-1

# QUIZ
# NUTRITION FOR INFANTS AND CHILDREN

1. The following foods may be fed to an infant. Next to each food, write the age at which the food may be introduced into the infant's diet. Remember there is a range of ages for each food.

| Age Range | Food |
|---|---|
| ______________________ | Strained meats |
| ______________________ | Cereals |
| ______________________ | Table foods |
| ______________________ | Fruits, vegetables, and juices |
| ______________________ | Finger foods |

2. Plan one day's menu for a six-year-old child using the recommended serving sizes.

| Meal (M) Snack (S) | Food | Amount | Fruit-Vegetable group 3–4 serv. | Bread-Cereal group 3–4 serv. | Milk-Cheese group 2–3 serv. | Meat-Poultry-Fish-Beans group 1–2 serv. | Fats-Sweets-Alcohol group |
|---|---|---|---|---|---|---|---|
| | | | | | | | |
| TOTAL NO. OF SERVINGS: | | | | | | | |
| RECOMMENDED NO. OF SERVINGS: | | | | | | | |

_____ 3. Which group of foods would you feed a six-month-old baby for lunch?

a. Ice cream, applesauce, peaches
b. Cereal, applesauce, peaches
c. Cheese and crackers, Jell-O, mashed banana
d. Whatever my family eats

_____ 4. Which of the following would make the best lunch for a three-year-old child?

a. Milk, egg salad sandwich, apple
b. Hot dog, potato chips, Coke
c. Peanut butter toast, banana, Kool-Aid
d. Juice, vegetable soup, banana

# Unit 8: Nutrition for Adolescents, Adults, and the Aged

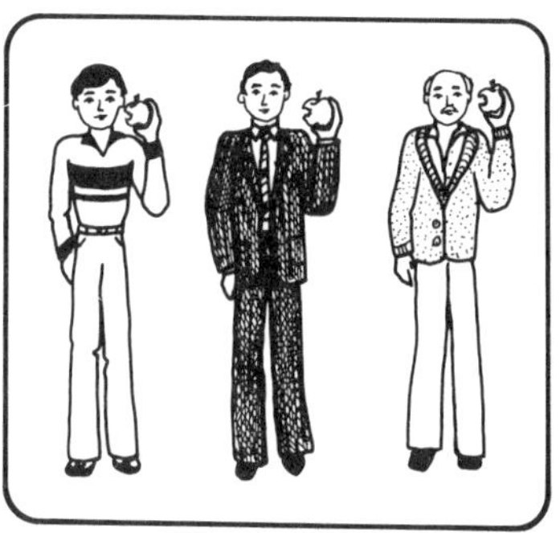

## CONCEPTS

_Nutrition affects the health of people of all ages and at all stages of the life cycle, including adolescence, adulthood, and the later years.

–People at each stage of the life cycle possess different nutritional needs.

## OBJECTIVES

–Students will be able to name at least one unique nutritional need at each stage of the life cycle, including adolescence, adulthood, and the later years.

–Students will be able to discuss how nutritional needs change with age.

–Students will be able to analyze the nutritional needs, problems, and issues of different age groups.

## TEACHER'S UNIT INTRODUCTION

**Adolescence.** The period of adolescence, ranging from late childhood to early adulthood, is a time not only of rapid physical growth and development, but also of significant psychological and social changes. Physical, psychological, and social factors affect the nutritional status of any individual. Let us look at each one of these aspects as they affect teenagers.

**Physical Factors.** Adolescence begins with changes in hormone activity and ends with the last stage of sexual and physical maturation. The time at which the greatest amount of change occurs is from 10 to 14 years of age. With girls this generally occurs earlier than in boys. This period of rapid growth is called puberty.

The most obvious changes teenagers experience is their growth spurt. Youngsters can add inches to their height in a year's time. Because this growth is so rapid, nutrient needs increase sharply during this time as well. The nutrients associated with bone growth, that is, calcium, phosphorus, Vitamin D, and protein, are needed in amounts that are greater than at any other life stage except for a woman who is pregnant or breast-feeding.

In addition to growing taller, teenagers are also adding to their body size in terms of weight. Both boys and girls are adding lean body mass (muscle), although boys generally add more muscle than girls do. This rapid growth in muscle increases the need for protein.

In addition to bone and muscle, blood is also growing at a rapid rate, and requires additional nutrients. Blood volume increases during adolescence and requires the production of extra hemoglobin. Hemoglobin is the oxygen-carrying molecule that relies on iron to do its work. For girls, adolescence marks the beginning of the menses, which also demands the production of extra hemoglobin. Thus, the increased blood volume and the beginning of menstruation increase the need for the blood-forming nutrients. These nutrients include primarily iron and protein.

The final area of concern is caloric needs. Because of their rapid growth rate, most adolescents experience an increased caloric need. Girls and boys differ in their caloric needs and in the timing of their growth spurt. Girls' growth spurt peaks at about age 13 when their need for calories reaches about 2,200 per day. In contrast, boys' growth spurt peaks later, at about age 15, when their daily caloric need approaches 2,800 calories. Teenagers who are involved in athletics or who are otherwise exceptionally active may have caloric needs well above these amounts.

Although for the most part teenagers' caloric needs are high, there seems to be a growing proportion of the adolescent population who are overweight. In teenagers, this is often expressed not as increased consumption of foods, but rather as a more sedentary life style. Most teenagers lead active and energetic lives, but there are those who do not. These teenagers' caloric needs may be lower than normal. The problem with overweight in the teenage years is in trying to restrict calories while at the same time providing additional nutrients needed for normal bone, muscle, and blood growth.

**Psychological Factors.** Many psychological factors influence the eating habits of teenagers. These influences, in turn, affect their nutritional status. The effects may be positive or negative, but are more often negative.

Teenagers' diets may be inadequate in several nutrients. Iron, calcium, Vitamin A, and Vitamin C are the ones most often lacking. In general, teenagers who have poor diets are those who skip meals, eat smaller quantities of food at meals, and eat fewer snacks. The inadequacies in teenagers' diets may be due to several different psychological states that teenagers experience.

Teenagers are often preoccupied with their own body image. Girls desire extreme slenderness while boys wish to be tall and muscular. The desire to look a certain way or to fit a certain image, and the distorted body image that many teenagers possess, oftentimes lead them to adopt eating habits that are nutritionally unsafe.

The struggle for independence often exhibited during adolescence may also affect eating habits. Teenagers may want to eat more meals away from home with their friends. They want to be in charge of their own food intake. In addition, their search for independence may lead them to a life style of always being "on the go." The consequences of these practices may lead to nutritionally unbalanced eating habits.

**Social Factors.** Perhaps more than at any other time, adolescence is a time when friends and social relationships are of top priority. Teenagers begin to feel the importance of being accepted into peer groups. This intense need for social acceptance affects nearly every aspect of a teenager's life. Amidst the turmoil, the eating habits of the teenager emerge. Oftentimes, the peer groups say, "I'll eat what *I* want, not what my mother (or father, or teacher) says is good for me!" Thus, eating habits may become nutritionally unbalanced.

Finally, two areas of special concern for teenagers' nutritional health deserve special attention. These areas are athletics and eating disorders. Both of these issues have profound effects on the nutritional status of adolescents.

Athletics in the schools has become a big business. Competition is stiff. Often, special diets are encouraged because of the belief that certain foods will help give someone "the edge" in a contest. Fasting and dehydration are promoted as acceptable ways to shed pounds. Vitamin, mineral, or protein supplements are espoused. These practices are unnecessary and potentially dangerous from a nutritional point of view. The best nutritional guidelines for athletes are the same as those for nonathletes, with the addition of extra calories and water as needed to meet the demands of training and competition. Emphasis, as with nonathletes, should be placed on avoiding "empty-calorie" foods and on eating a variety of nutritious foods.

The second area of concern in teenage nutrition is eating disorders. Although it is by no means a common disorder, the disease called anorexia nervosa affects nearly one out of a hundred teenaged girls. Teenaged boys, children, and adults rarely exhibit this disorder. Generally the disorder is characterized by a distorted body image, extreme thinness, self-starvation followed by gorging, self-induced vomiting, excessive use of laxatives, and a preoccupation with food and nutrition. Unless anorexia nervosa is treated in its early stages, it may lead to death by starvation. Its victims simply refuse to eat. Although extreme cases may be fatal, it is thought that many other teens are affected by it to a certain extent because of a preoccupation with slimness that has been exacerbated by the constant exhortations of the advertising industry that in order to be attractive, an individual has to be slender.

Bulimia is another eating disorder that has also been described as a "binge-purge" disorder. It has been estimated that from 10 to 50 percent of teenaged girls experience the binge-purge cycle, although probably fewer are truly bulimic. The binge behavior consists of secretively consuming large amounts of high-calorie foods (from 3,000 to 20,000 calories) in a short period of time, usually in less than two hours. Purging allows the bulimic to control his or her weight through self-induced vomiting, diuretic and laxative abuse, and rigorous exercise. Bulimics are rarely more than 15 percent underweight or overweight.

This chart lists the warning signs of anorexia and bulimia. [Display the chart on an opaque or overhead projector.] You should become familiar with these disorders and with their symptoms so that you can recognize a problem in yourself, your friends, or your family. Recognizing the problem is one step toward seeking professional help. [Associations and resources that help persons correct eating disorders are listed in "References/Resources" at the end of this kit.]

| WARNING SIGNS | |
|---|---|
| **Anorexia Nervosa** | **Bulimia** |
| • Abnormal weight loss of 25% or more with no known medical illness accounting for the loss. | • Concern about weight and attempts to control weight by diet, vomiting, or laxative and diuretic abuse. |
| • Reduction in food intake, denial of hunger, and decrease in consumption of fat-containing foods. | • Eating pattern that alternates between binges and fasts. |
| • Prolonged exercise despite fatigue and weakness. | • Secretive about binges and vomiting. |
| • Intense fear of weight gain. | • Consumption of high-calorie foods during binges. |
| • Peculiar patterns of handling food. | • In most cases, individuals are within a normal weight range; some may be slightly underweight or overweight. |
| • Amenorrhea in women. | • Occurrence of depressive moods. |
| • In some cases, bulimic episodes of binge eating followed by vomiting or laxative abuse. | |

**Adulthood.** The period of life between adolescence and the later years is generally regarded as a time relatively free from physical stress and change. Growth and development have, for the most part, ceased. Critical aspects of the aging process have not yet begun, so life appears stable and problem-free.

However, adults do have unique nutritional needs that are important and worthwhile subjects for discussion. One of the most important nutritional issues during adulthood is the maintenance of ideal body weight. As the body ages, the basal metabolic rate progressively decreases. In addition, activity levels generally decline. These two major events occur over a long period of time so that they may seem subtle or even nonexistent. However, a lower basal metabolic rate plus a lower activity level lead to decreased calorie use. Weight gain will result if the number of calories consumed remains the same. Thus, throughout adulthood, calorie needs decrease. Because the calorie needs of adults decrease so gradually, many adults do not notice a gradual increase in body weight until it becomes a problem.

Overweight is one of the most common problems of adults. Overweight, in turn, may be an aggravating factor in many of the chronic and degenerative diseases that affect adults in their later years. Those diseases that may be affected by diet (in ways other than by excessive weight) include heart disease, high blood pressure, stroke, diabetes, and liver disorders. The U.S. government has recently published a series of Dietary Guidelines for Americans aimed at reducing these diet-related diseases. The Dietary Guidelines are described in Unit 19.

The second unique nutritional need of adults is related to young adult women in their childbearing years. During this time, diet is vitally important as a preparatory step for pregnancy and breast-feeding. These issues were discussed in Unit 6. In addition, young women taking birth control pills appear to have an increased need for certain nutrients, particularly for some of the B vitamins. Although vitamin supplements may not be advisable because of the complicated interactions of these nutrients, it may be wise to suggest that users of oral contraceptive pills increase their intake of foods rich in folacin and pyridoxine (two of the B vitamins.) Foods rich in folacin include dark-green, leafy vegetables such as spinach; other green vegetables such as asparagus, cabbage, and peas; dry beans and peas; whole-grain breads and cereals; and orange juice. Food sources of pyridoxine include many meats such as beef, ham, lamb, liver, pork, and veal; whole-grain breads and cereals; and some fruits and vegetables such as bananas, cabbage, lima beans, potatoes, spinach, and strawberries.

**The Later Years.** Nutrition plays a role in many of the aging processes. Although many older adults believe food and nutrition to have miraculous powers, there are no magical foods or special vitamin/mineral supplements that can act as an elixir. However, a nutritous diet throughout life and during the later years may lead to the retention of good health and to the maintenance of an active life.

One of the major nutrition-related problems afflicting older adults is osteoporosis. *Osteoporosis* is a disorder of the bones characterized by a decrease in bone mass. This decrease often results in decreased height and in an increased susceptibility to bone fractures and lower back pain. The cause of osteoporosis is not known, but diet, hormonal changes, and the level of physical activity are believed to be implicated. Although methods for prevention and cure have not been established, most experts currently agree that a calcium intake of 800–1200 milligrams per day and maintenance of a physical exercise program throughout adulthood may be beneficial. The calcium-to-phosphorus ratio also appears to be significant in the development of osteoporosis. Calcium should be in a 1:1 relationship with phosphorus in the diet. But, because the American diet is high in phosphorus, the ratio is often skewed. Foods high in phosphorus include protein-rich foods, soft drinks, and many processed foods.

In addition to maintaining adequate calcium in the body, it is important for older adults to maintain adequate levels of all of the other nutrients, while at the same time decreasing the amount of calories they consume. Thus, avoidance of empty-calorie foods during the later years is of particular concern. The elderly need to make the most of their calories by consuming foods with a relatively high nutrient-to-calorie ratio.

The physical needs of adults in their later years are not the only factors affecting their nutritional status. As with teenagers, older adults are subjected to psychological and social changes that may affect nutrient intake. Although it is impossible to discuss all of these changes in detail, several of them are:

- singleness and loneliness
- apathy and lack of motivation

- poverty
- physical disabilities (arthritis, loss of teeth, etc.)
- poor appetite

There are several governmental programs designed to alleviate some of these problems. The Meals-on-Wheels program and the Congregate Meals Program attempt to provide food and social stimulus for the elderly. The former program delivers hot meals to the homes of senior citizens who have difficulty shopping, preparing, or serving meals, or who cannot leave their home. The Congregate Meals Program, on the other hand, provides meals in a location central to many older adults. There the participants are able to obtain a nutritious meal as well as to enjoy a social outlet with their peers.

---

In presenting Unit 8, it is important to mention eating disorders among teenagers in order to warn them about the dangers involved and also to alert them to the warning signs in themselves, in their friends, and in their family. However, discretion should be exercised when discussing the disorders in case there are students in the class afflicted with them. For more information about eating disorders and how to handle them, contact a local nutritionist, your state department of health, or a physician. Or, you can write to the organizations listed in "References/Resources" to obtain more information.

This unit should be presented as a topics-oriented unit. A person in each stage of the life cycle requires the same nutrients but in varying amounts. The concerns at each stage, however, vary. Students are most likely to be interested in their own nutritional concerns; however, they should be encouraged to look closely at the other topics. At this age, they should be encouraged to consider the needs of others.

## BASIC ACTIVITY

**Time Needed:** One class period

**Materials Needed:** Sheet 8-1: "Trivial Truths... The Facts of Life" (gameboard)
Sheets 8-2 through 8-3: "Trivial Truths" (playing cards)
Chart A: "Recommended Dietary Allowances"
Chart F: "Height/Weight and Recommended Energy Intake"
Quiz Sheet 8-1

1. Introduce this activity with a short discussion of nutritional needs during each stage of the life cycle. Several of these issues will be covered in more detail in later units. Emphasize the following points:

- Nutritional needs change as a person matures and grows older.
- Nutritional needs during the teenage years are high because of growth and activity levels.
  - –Teenagers need more calcium and adequate phosphorus for bone growth.
  - –Teenagers need more iron for blood and tissue growth. Additional blood and oxygen are needed to help organs and other tissues grow. Without adequate iron, teenagers

may develop iron-deficiency anemia, a disease characterized by lack of energy, pale complexion, and increased susceptibility to infection. It can be cured by eating iron-rich foods and/or by taking iron supplements.

–Teenagers' calorie needs vary. If they are active in sports and other activities, their requirements are high. However, there are some sedentary teenagers who fall into an overweight or obese state during the teenage years. These teenagers need fewer calories and more exercise.

–Teenagers' diets are often low in iron, calcium, Vitamin A, and Vitamin C.

- Anorexia nervosa is a disorder that usually affects teenaged girls and that is characterized by a distorted body image, extreme thinness, self-starvation, self-induced vomiting, excessive use of laxatives, and a preoccupation with food and nutrition. Bulimia is another eating disorder that follows a binge-purge cycle. Bulimics, however, usually maintain normal weight and appearance.
- Use of any drugs, including alcohol and birth control pills, can alter nutrient needs. Both of these drugs increase the need for B vitamins.
- Nutritional needs change with advancing age.

  –Calorie needs decrease. Basal metabolism, and often the activity level of the individual, decrease with age.

  –Nutrient needs other than calories remain the same.

  –Adults need to avoid empty-calorie foods in order to maintain weight.
- Adults may be able to reduce the risk of heart disease by avoiding foods high in fat, particularly saturated fats and cholesterol. Saturated fats are any oils or fats that are solid at room temperature, such as nuts, margerine, solid shortening, avocado, butter, fat marbling in meats, and lard. Cholesterol is found in animal foods such as eggs, shrimp, shellfish, organ meats, beef, butter, cheese, and cream.
- Adults can also reduce the risk of hypertension (high blood pressure) by avoiding excess salt in their diet.
- Maintaining ideal weight may reduce the risk of heart disease, high blood pressure, diabetes, stroke, and liver disorders.
- The elderly have similar concerns as adults in needing to avoid empty-calorie foods.
- Osteoporosis is a disease of aging. It can often be prevented by maintenance of an adequate calcium status, by moderate exercise, and by avoidance of excessive amounts of phosphorus. It is more likely to develop in women than in men.
- Cancer is also a disease of aging. Several types of cancer have been related to diet. A high-fat, low-fiber diet has been associated with colon and breast cancer.
- Constipation is a common complaint of the elderly. It can often be relieved by an increased consumption of fiber. Good food sources of fiber include bran, whole-grain breads and cereals, fruits, vegetables, and seeds.
- The government is interested in assisting the elderly in maintaining their nutritional health. Two programs, Meals-on-Wheels and Congregate Meals, are designed to improve the nutrient intake and overall health of the elderly by providing nutritious meals and by reducing depression and loneliness.

In addition to these points for discussion include any others from the "Teacher's Unit Introduction" that you feel are appropriate.

2. Distribute Chart A, "Recommended Dietary Allowances," and Chart F, "Height/Weight and Recommended Energy Intake," and have students make comparisons between the various age groups.

3. During the discussion, encourage students to share personal remarks about themselves, friends, or family who may have a nutritional need similar to that being discussed. Ask them to notice the difference between themselves, their parents, and their grandparents in terms of activity level and related dietary habits.

4. Have students play the game "Trivial Truths . . . The Facts of Life" by following these rules. You may adapt the game to your class size by preparing one set of cards for every four students and distributing one gameboard (Sheet 8-1) to each student.

a. Four players can participate in each game.
b. Each player receives a copy of the gameboard and each group receives a complete (copied) set of playing cards (Sheets 8-2 through 8-3), which they cut apart and place face down.
c. Each player selects three markers to use as playing pieces. Markers can be coins, pieces of paper or cardboard, or plastic pieces.
d. The game starts by having each player place his markers on his gameboard, with one marker on the triangle, square, and circle below the large arrows. Each arrow represents a different stage in the life cycle—adolescence, adulthood, and the later years.
e. Each group decides who goes first and the game continues to that player's left. The first player is asked a question from a "Trivial Truths" card selected by the player to his or her left. The answering player can choose the category of the question by shape (triangle for adolescence, square for adulthood, circle for the later years).
f. If the question is answered correctly, the player takes another turn. If the question is answered incorrectly, the game passes to the player to the left. After two correct answers on a turn, the game passes to the next player.
g. The object of the game is to move each marker to the top of each of the three arrows by answering questions correctly. Once a player has all three markers at the top spots, he or she must answer all three questions on the "Trivial Truths" card on a single turn in order to reach the star. The winner is the first player to move all three markers onto the star.
h. The teacher arbitrates any disputes regarding answers. Note that the answers are provided on the playing cards in boldface type.

5. Proceed with the "Advanced Activity" if you wish; otherwise use the quiz mentioned in step 6.

6. **Evaluation:** When students have completed the game, distribute the Quiz Sheet 8-1 and have students complete it independently. Following completion of the quiz, conduct a summary discussion of the unit.

## ADVANCED ACTIVITY

**Time Needed:** Two class periods

**Materials Needed:** Chart A: "Recommended Dietary Allowances"
Additional resource materials (*see* "References/Resources" at the end of this kit)
Chart F: "Height/Weight and Recommended Energy Intake"

### Class Period 1

1. Briefly present the idea that each of the stages of the life cycle poses particular problems or concerns. The following list summarizes possible topics to be investigated by students in each category:

**Adolescence:** athletics, eating disorders (anorexia nervosa, bulimia), fad diets, alcohol, nutrient/drug interactions

**Adulthood:** weight control, Dietary Guidelines for Americans, birth control pills and diet, pregnancy, breast-feeding

**The Later Years:** osteoporosis, heart disease, diabetes, obesity, arthritis, high blood pressure, Congregate Meals, Meals-on-Wheels

2. Have each students choose a topic of interest, conduct an investigation, and prepare a report on the topic. Students should use the materials listed in "References/Resources" to conduct their research.

### Class Period 2

1. Have each student summarize his or her findings in a presentation or report to the rest of the class. Encourage students to be creative in their presentation formats (demonstration, role-play, commercial, etc.).

2. **Evaluation:** Distribute Quiz Sheet 8-1 and have students complete it independently. Following the quiz, conduct a summary discussion of changing nutritional needs during the life cycle.

## FOLLOW-UP ACTIVITIES

1. Have students interview or survey people from each stage of the life cycle, including other adolescents in school; adults at home, in school, or in the community; and the elderly at home or in the community. Have them ask questions about the person's activity level and dietary habits. Students should write about their findings in a report and accompany it with graphs summarizing their data.

2. Conduct a discussion revolving around the social and ethical issues of the elderly and their nutritional needs.

3.Invite a senior citizen to talk to the class about foods, dietary habits, and exercise habits from the past.

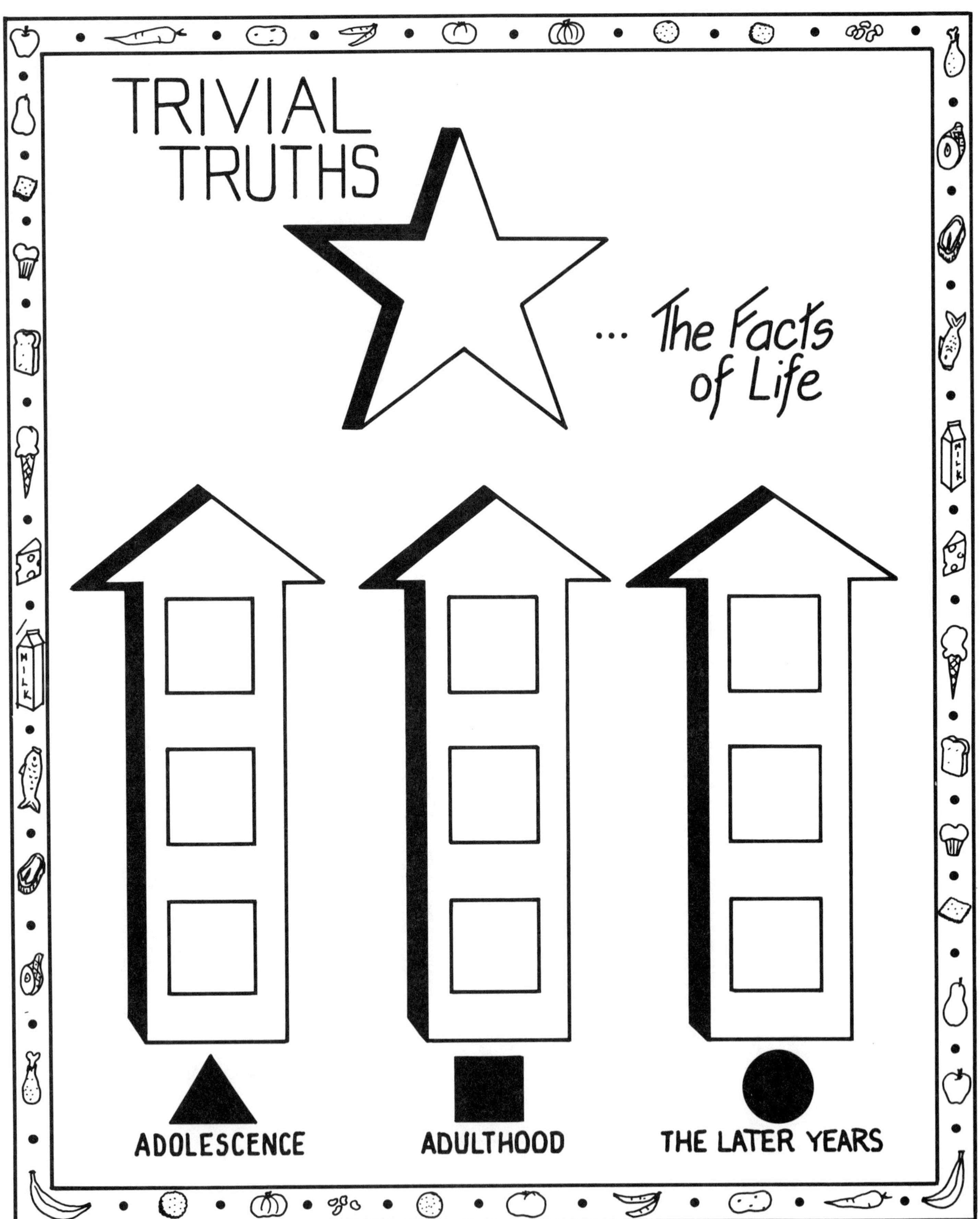
TRIVIAL
TRUTHS
... The Facts of Life
MILK
ADOLESCENCE
ADULTHOOD
THE LATER YEARS

# TRIVIAL TRUTHS PLAYING CARDS

▲ What vitamin is associated with bone growth? **(Vitamin D)**

■ Truth or Baloney! As the body ages, basal metabolism increases. **(Baloney)**

● Osteoporosis can be related to a low intake of what mineral? **(Calcium)**

▲ What two minerals are associated with bone growth? **(Calcium, phosphorus)**

■ What condition results when more calories are eaten than are needed? **(Overweight or obesity)**

● Do the elderly need a high or low nutrient-to-calorie ratio? **(High)**

▲ What is the name of the oxygen-carrying molecule in the blood (without it you are anemic)? **(Hemoglobin)**

■ Truth or Baloney! You will gain weight by age 40 if you maintain the same diet and exercise habits you had at age 20 **(Truth)**

● What is the name of a government program designed to provide food for the elderly? **(Congregate Meals or Meals-on-Wheels)**

▲ What mineral is needed for blood production? **(Iron)**

■ What vitamin is needed in larger amounts by women using birth control pills? **(B vitamins)**

● What physical problem causes the elderly to eat soft foods? **(Dentures or loss of teeth)**

▲ What two minerals are often lacking in teenagers' diets? **(Iron, calcium)**

■ Name two diseases that can be triggered by obesity. **(Any 2: heart disease, high blood pressure, diabetes, stroke, liver disorders)**

● What emotional problem of the elderly causes them to lose interest in foods? **(Depression or loneliness)**

▲ What vitamins are often lacking in teenagers' diets? **(Vitamins A and C)**

■ If 2 peanuts have 10 calories, and you ate 2 peanuts more than your calorie needs require every day for a year, how much weight would you gain? **(1 pound)**

● The life expectancy of a child born today is about how many years? **(70–75 years)**

▲ Truth or Baloney! Athletes need more protein than nonathletes. **(Baloney)**

■ How many calories per gram does alcohol contain? **(7 calories/gram)**

● Excess of what nutrient aggravates high blood pressure? **(Sodium)**

▲ What is the name of an eating disorder associated with self-starvation? **(Anorexia nervosa)**

■ What form of cancer is associated with a low-fiber diet? **(Colon cancer)**

● The lack of what dietary substance can be the cause of constipation? **(Fiber)**

# TRIVIAL TRUTHS PLAYING CARDS

| | |
|---|---|
| ▲ What is the name of the eating disorder associated with binging and purging? **(Bulimia)**<br>■ What form of cancer has been associated with a high-fat diet? **(Breast or colon cancer)**<br>● Name two good sources of fiber. **(Any 2: bran, whole grains, fruits, vegetables, seeds)** | ▲ Who needs more calories: a 15-year-old boy or a 15-year-old girl? **(The boy)**<br>■ Name three rich food sources of cholesterol. **(Any 3 of these: egg, shrimp, shellfish, organ meats, beef, butter, cheese, cream)**<br>● A low-calcium, high-phosphorus diet is associated with what disease? **(Osteoporosis)** |
| ▲ Who needs more calcium: a 16 year old or a 25 year old? **(The 16 year old)**<br>■ Name one plant source of cholesterol. **(None)**<br>● Who is more likely to develop osteoporosis: men or women? **(Women)** | ▲ Which has more calories: a 12-ounce beer or two slices of bread? **(Beer)**<br>■ Name one plant source of saturated fat. **(Any of these: nuts, margarine, solid shortening, avocado)**<br>● Name one nondairy food high in calcium. **(Any of these: sardines, salmon, leafy greens, sesame seeds, molasses)** |
| ▲ What nutrients are needed for the body to handle alcohol? **(The B vitamins)**<br>■ Truth or Baloney! Adults need more Vitamin $B_{15}$ than teenagers. **(Baloney: Vitamin $B_{15}$ isn't even a vitamin!)**<br>● Truth or Baloney! Vitamin E can prevent aging. **(Baloney)** | ▲ What nutrition-related disease is marked by lack of energy, pale complexion, and increased susceptibility to infection? **(Iron-deficiency anemia)**<br>■ How many pounds of sugar does the average American adult eat each year? **(100–300 pounds)**<br>● Truth or Baloney! The elderly need fewer vitamins than the young. **(Baloney: They need about the same.)** |
| ▲ If you ate this meal at a fast-food restaurant, what food group would be missing: hamburger on a roll, french fries, soft drink? **(Milk-Cheese group)**<br>■ Who needs more protein: a 25 year old or a 50 year old? **(They both need the same amount of protein.)**<br>● Who needs more calories: a 50 year old woman or a 75 year old man? **(The 50 year old, because of age alone)** | ▲ If you ate a slice of sausage pizza, what food group would be missing? **(None)**<br>■ Who needs more calories: a 16-year-old boy or a 25-year-old man? **(The 16 year old)**<br>● An elderly man should drink whole milk, drink skim milk, or not drink milk at all. **(Drink skim milk)** |

# QUIZ
# NUTRITION FOR ADOLESCENTS, ADULTS, AND THE AGED

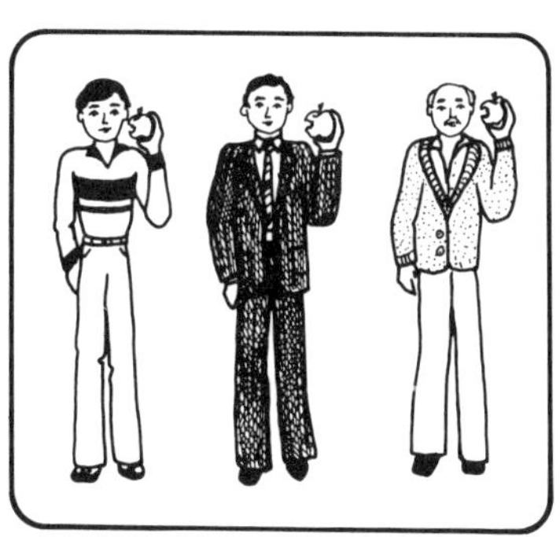

____ 1. Teenagers who have poor dietary habits often:
- a. Skip meals
- b. Eat large amounts of simple carbohydrates
- c. Eat few fruits and vegetables
- d. All of the above

____ 2. Teenagers' diets are often lacking in:
- a. Protein
- b. Calcium
- c. Vitamin E
- d. Fat

3. Cathy Candy is a young teenager who does not care about the food she eats. She thinks good nutrition is not all that important. Sara Spinach, on the other hand, thinks good nutrition is of the utmost importance. She tries as hard as she can to learn more about nutrition and how to eat well. Sara thinks this is important to her health now and in the future.

**Directions:** Write a short paragraph about each teenager's viewpoint. Defend each as well as you can. Then place yourself on the line somewhere between them, and write about how *you* feel about nutrition. Use the back of this sheet for your answers.

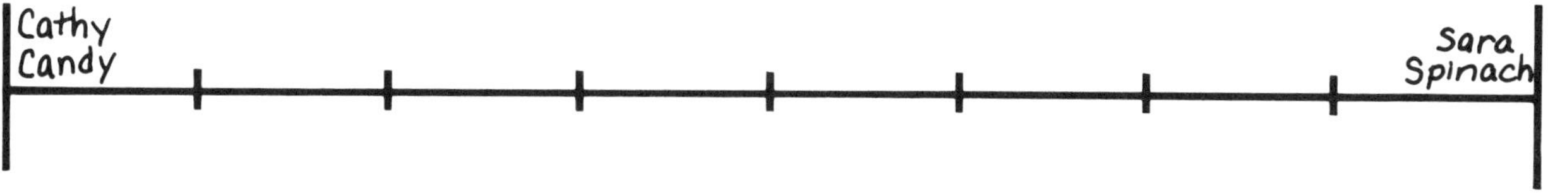


____ 4. Which is true for adults as they grow older?
- a. Calorie needs go up.
- b. Nutrient needs stay the same.
- c. Empty-calorie foods should be eaten.
- d. Calcium is no longer needed.

____ 5. Which of the following is a nutritional strategy for the elderly?
- a. Balancing calorie intake with calorie output
- b. Eating low-fiber foods to keep the intestines healthy
- c. Choosing empty-calorie foods to maintain preferred weight
- d. Choosing high-phosphorus foods to prevent osteoporosis

# Section IV

# Meal Planning and Preparation

# Unit 9 Interpreting Ingredient Labels: Nutritive Food Additives

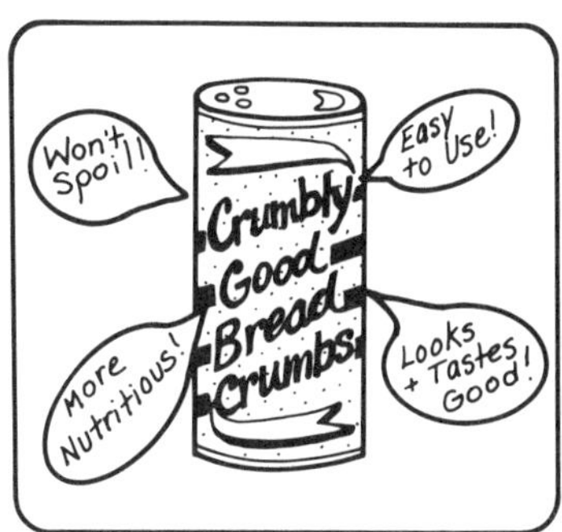
Won't Spoil!
Easy to Use!
Crumbly Good Bread Crumbs
More Nutritious!
Looks + Tastes Good!

## CONCEPTS

–Nutritive food additives are any vitamins, minerals, or protein added to food products.

–"Enrichment" or "fortification" are two terms used to describe the process of adding nutritive food additives to food.

–"Superfortification" of food products is not necessary and may give consumers a false sense of nutrition security.

–Food additives serve many functions and can be categorized according to function. These categories include: (a) nutritive food additives (to make food more nutritious); (b) preservatives (to keep food safe); (c) quality-giving additives (to make food preparation easier); (d) cosmetic additives (to make food look and taste good).

## OBJECTIVES

–Students will be able to name four general functions of food additives.

–Students will be able to differentiate between enrichment and fortification.

–Students will be able to evaluate fortified foods based on their total contribution to the diet.

## TEACHER'S UNIT INTRODUCTION

Nutritive additives encompass all vitamins, minerals, and protein added to food to increase its nutritional quality. The addition of nutritive food additives to foods is termed "enrichment" or "fortification." In the past, enrichment and fortification were intended to have distinct and different definitions under the food-labeling laws. "Enrichment" was defined as the replacement of vitamins and minerals lost in the processing of the food. In contrast, "fortification" was used to describe the addition to foods of nutrients that may be lacking in the diet. Because the FDA found that the majority of consumers were confused by this terminology, the most current FDA policy statement (1980) allows the terms to be used interchangeably to indicate the addition of one or more vitamins, minerals, or protein to food.

The addition of nutrients to food started in the 1920s and 1930s when iodine was added to salt to prevent goiter (an enlargement of the thyroid gland due to an iodine deficiency) and Vitamin D was added to milk to protect against rickets (a Vitamin D deficiency disease in which bones are poorly mineralized). These two examples illustrate that the reason for adding nutrients during this time period was to prevent the occurrence of deficiency diseases. As the food supply changed, and consumers began to rely on food manufacturers for their foods instead of growing and processing food at home, nutritive additives were put in foods to restore nutrients that were destroyed during processing and storage. The addition of thiamin, riboflavin, niacin, and iron to white flour began during this time period. These four nutrients as well as many others are normally lost during the processing of wheat for flour production. However, only these four nutrients have been replaced. Today the food supply has evolved to the point where substitute foods (for example, textured vegetable protein products and fruit-flavored drinks) and many convenience, highly processed foods dominate the marketplace. New technology has made it very easy to add nutrients to foods. Numerous foods now have vitamins, minerals, or protein added to them. Contrary to the original reasons for the enrichment or fortification of foods, today food manufacturers add nutrients to foods for a variety of reasons.

The largest segment of food products hit by the fortification wave are breakfast foods, particularly cereals and breakfast substitutes. One justification for the fortification of cereals is that young children do not eat large quantities or varieties of foods. Fortifying cereals contributes to the nutrient intake of these children. Also, people who do not plan time for breakfast can receive some nutrition through fortified substitutes.

These justifications do not satisfy the Consumers Union. Members of this organization charge the cereal companies with "superfortifying" their products simply to increase selling power. Further, they charge that a person who eats such a fortified product might think he or she is protected from a nutrient imbalance for the remainder of the day. Food intake may then become haphazard and poor in nutritional quality.

There is a misconception among consumers that the addition of vitamins and minerals to foods always makes the product superior to comparable unfortified products. It must be realized that the addition of nutrients that are already received in adequate quantities through a normal diet has no benefit. The body uses what it needs and either excretes the excess or stores it. Storage of some nutrients (vitamins A and D, for example) can have serious consequences because they are toxic when levels stored in the body exceed a certain limit. Many of the vitamins and minerals that are added to foods are not normally contained in these foods. For instance, Vitamin A is added to numerous fortified breakfast cereals. Normally, vitamin A is found in fruits and vegetables. This might give consumers a distorted view of the natural sources of nutrients. Worse yet, a consumer may develop a false sense of security; that is, he or she may feel that there is no need to eat fruits and vegetables because he or she received Vitamin A in the fortified breakfast cereal. However, fruits and vegetables provide other nutrients (like trace minerals) and fiber which may not have been added to the cereal.

Regular consumption of highly processed, fortified foods to the exclusion of their more natural counterparts has generated some concern among nutritionists. Essential trace minerals and fiber may be present in lower amounts of highly processed foods than in foods in their more natural state. Conversely, the highly processed foods may supply quite a bit of sugar and/or fat. The fortification of fabricated foods, that is, the addition of nutrients in significant amounts, give these foods the appearance of being nutrient-dense. These fabricated, fortified foods in reality belong in the "other" food group because of their high sugar and/or fat content, but are considered nutrient-dense because of the fortification with some vitamins and minerals. The ingredient labels on some instant breakfast powders, some presweetened breakfast cereals, breakfast bars, and fortified drink mixes substantiate these points.

---

The information and activities on food additives have been divided between Units 9 and 10 of this kit. Unit 9 deals exclusively with the category of additives labeled nutritive food additives. The category of additives labeled quality-giving additives has not been included in the main body of these units because of a need to limit the amount of time devoted to this issue. Quality-giving additives are not unimportant, but they have less bearing on the nutritional content and safety of foods, which are the issues of utmost importance to nutritionists. Cosmetic additives are discussed because of their extremely controversial nature. This unit and Unit 10 do not propose the elimination of cosmetic additives nor of highly processed, highly fortified foods from the diet. Rather, the intent is to enable the student to make informed choices about the use of certain additives in his or her diet. Another purpose is to acquaint the student with the roles enrichment and fortification play in increasing the nutritional quality of today's food supply.

During the "Basic Activity," students are asked to investigate the nutrient contributions of fortified, ready-to-eat cereals. The U.S. RDA amounts given for the ready-to-eat cereal in Chart D, "Food Composition Table for Selected Nutrients," are based on about 60 varieties of cereals. Since vitamin and mineral values will vary somewhat among fortified cereals, students may find somewhat higher or lower values on cereals they eat at home. During one of the activities, you will be assigning students to compare the values given in their food composition table with one or more of the cereals they eat at home. The name of each cereal and of the U.S. RDA values could be copied on notebook paper and posted in a designated area in the room. Product comparison could then be made between cereals.

## BASIC ACTIVITY

**Time Needed:** Three class periods

**Materials Needed:** Sheet 9-1: "Look at the Chemicals Mother Nature Puts in Whole Milk!"
Sheets 9-2 through 9-3: "Chemicals You Eat"

Sheets 9-4 through 9-5: "Food Label Table"
Sheets 9-6 through 9-7: "To Add or Not to Add"
Sheet 9-8: "E•N•R•I•C•H"
Chart B: "Daily Food Guide"
Chart D: "Food Composition Table for Selected Nutrients"
Several fortified food containers: breakfast bars, instant breakfast, ready-to-eat cereals, canned fruit drink or mix, whole milk, skim milk, or nonfat dry milk, margarine, iodized salt
Quiz Sheet 9-1

**Class Period 1**

1. This activity should be used as an introduction to the concept of chemicals in food and food additives. It will demonstrate that even completely natural foods are composed of complex chemicals, many of which can be used by our own bodies. Distribute Sheet 9-1, "Look at the Chemicals Mother Nature Puts in Whole Milk!," and discuss the following questions:

- Did you ever think of milk as containing all of the chemical substitutes you see here? No one added them. They all occur naturally. Does this surprise you?
- Do you recognize any of the nutrients listed on the milk carton on Sheet 9-1? Which ones? *(Possible answers:* Ascorbic acid or Vitamin C, riboflavin, thiamin, amino acids, fatty acids, calcium, phosphorus, water, carbohydrates).
- A child may define milk as something that comes from a cow. How might a food chemist define milk? *(Answer:* A liquid produced from a mammal that is made of many chemicals, some of which are nutrients.)
- Do you suppose that some of the chemicals naturally occurring in milk are added to certain processed foods? Which ones and why? *(Answer:* Yes. Examples include adding thiamin and riboflavin to improve the nutritional quality of flour, bread, and cereals; adding lecithin to salad dressings and ice cream so that the fat will remain evenly distributed; adding citrates and ascorbic acid (Vitamin C) to canned and frozen fruits to help preserve them; and using carotene as the coloring agent in margarine and cheese. Thus, several chemicals that are added to processed foods to preserve them, color them, make them of better quality, and make them more nutritious can be found naturally in milk!)

2. Distribute Sheets 9-2 through 9-3, "Chemicals You Eat." Also distribute Sheets 9-4 through 9-5, "Food Label Table," so the students may refer to examples of preservative, nutritive, cosmetic, and quality-giving additives.

3. Have students silently read Sheets 9-2 through 9-3, "Chemicals You Eat."

4. Elicit from students the functions of food additives and write them on a transparency or on the chalkboard. The four additive functions are described on Sheet 9-3. Have students give examples of each from Sheets 9-4 through 9-5. Discuss the controversy surrounding food additives. Elicit students' concerns, written on Sheet 9-3, and also emphasize these points:

- Some people say food additives are good for you for the following reasons:
  - –Additives allow for a longer shelf life, for wider availability, and for distribution of a variety of foods.
  - –Some additives have been used for years.
  - –Some additives are naturally occurring compounds, so they must be safe.
  - –Additives can improve the texture, flavor, and appeal of food.
- Other people say food additives are harmful because of the following reasons:
  - –No one can prove that any additive is completely safe.
  - –Some additives that have been used for years have recently been shown to be unsafe or to be of questionable safety (Red color #2, #3, and #40; Carbon Black, cyclamates, saccharin, sodium nitrite, and others).
  - –Many additives are used for appeal purposes only and therefore are unnecessary from a nutritional or safety point of view. Food manufacturers attempt to sell products by making them more colorful or superflavorful.

5. Discuss the following information on Sheets 9-2 through 9-5 by conducting a values-voting exercise. Ask the following (and other) questions about food additives:

- Do you trust the government to keep your food safe?
- Do you think food additives should be controlled by the government?
- Should food additives that are possibly dangerous be allowed in foods?
- Should the food industry be responsible for testing the safety of food additives? Should the government? Should consumers?

**Class Period 2**

1. Distribute Sheet 9-6 through 9-7, "To Add or Not to Add," and Sheet 9-8, "E•N•R•I•C•H." Have students complete the worksheets individually or in pairs. Students will make decisions as to whether certain food additives should or should not be given in various situations. The concept of "enrichment" is introduced. In order to complete the activity, students will need to refer to Sheet 9-8, which provides a comparison of the thiamin, riboflavin, niacin, and iron content of enriched, unenriched, and whole-grain products.

2. Lead a discussion about the concept of "enrichment." Discuss students' answers to questions on the worksheets.

3. Discuss "fortification" by accepting input from students in an attempt to define the word "fortify." Ask students how foods might be fortified. Discussion should lead to a definition of fortification that includes the following:

- Fortification is a process which, like enrichment, is an example of nutritive food additives in use.
- Unlike enrichment, fortification adds larger amounts of one or more nutrients to certain foods.
- Fortification results in making certain foods rich sources of nutrients they do not contain in their natural state.

4. To illustrate these three points, students should compare one slice (one ounce serving) of enriched white bread with one ounce of a ready-to-eat fortified cereal using Chart D, "Food Composition Table for Selected Nutrients." One ounce of cereal is usually between one-half and one cup of cereal, depending on the kind. For each of the nutrients listed, students should identify which food has the highest U.S. RDA value; they should also determine mathematically how much higher the U.S. RDA value is in one food relative to the other. The students should arrive at answers similar to the ones below.

| Food | Protein | Vitamin A | Vitamin C | Thiamin | Riboflavin | Niacin | Calcium | Iron |
|---|---|---|---|---|---|---|---|---|
| Enriched Bread (1 oz.) | Same | – | – | – | – | – | – | – |
| Fortified Cereal (1 oz.) | Same | 5,000 times more | 60 times more | 30 times more | 30 times more | 30 times more | 2 times* more | 30 times more |

*However, both bread and cereal are considered to be poor sources.

Students may point out that the bread has fewer calories. However, the calorie difference is small (only 40 calories) and thus, even from a nutrient-density standpoint, the fortified cereal is a significantly better source of Vitamin A, Vitamin C, thiamin, riboflavin, niacin, and iron.

5. Students should recall which food group the cereals should be categorized under as well as which nutrients the food group is recognized for contributing. If necessary, students can refer to Chart B, "Daily Food Guide." Students should conclude that the Bread-Cereal group is not recognized as being a good source of vitamins A and C. However, many fortified cereals are rich sources of these two nutrients. Thus, fortification can make a food a rich source of one or more nutrients not generally found in the food in its natural state.

6. Assign students to look for fortified foods in their homes. Magazine advertisements could also be a source. Students should bring to class the actual containers or magazine pictures of fortified foods from which they can construct a resource center or a collage of fortified foods. Students should compile a list of the fortified foods and should identify the nutrients added to each food.

**Class Period 3**

1. Using their fortified food lists along with the containers or pictures of fortified foods, students should volunteer examples of fortified foods and should be able to name the respective nutrients added to the foods. Familiarize the students with each of the following fortified foods and with the key nutrients each food provides:

breakfast bars
instant breakfast
ready-to-eat cereals
canned fruit drink or mix
whole milk
skim milk or nonfat dry milk
margarine
iodized salt

2. Proceed with the "Advanced Activity" if you wish; otherwise use the quiz mentioned in step 3.

3. **Evaluation:** Distribute Quiz Sheet 9-1 and have students complete it independently. Conduct a summary discussion about nutritive food additives using the quiz answers as a springboard.

## ADVANCED ACTIVITY

**Time Needed:** One to two class periods

**Materials Needed:** Sheet 9-9: "Fortified Foods"
Chart E: "Dietary Calculation Chart" (two copies per student)
Table 9-1: "Mini Food Composition Table"
Chart A: "Recommended Dietary Allowances"
Quiz Sheet 9-1

1. Distribute Sheet 9-9, "Fortified Foods," and Chart E, "Dietary Calculation Chart."

2. Have students review the menus for Hardly Fortified Helen and Fortified Frances. Students should then calculate the intake of the nutrients in the menus using Chart E. Table 9-1 contains all of the information students will need. Note that this source does not contain all of the nutrients found on food labels, but it does contain a number of the major nutrients. Table 9-1 may be copied and distributed to each student or placed in the library as a reference.

3. After totaling all of the nutrients consumed by each fictional character, students should compare the intake to the Recommended Dietary Allowances (RDAs) for a female aged 15 to 18 years. These RDA figures are found in Chart A, "Recommended Dietary Allowances." On the chalkboard or on a transparency, list the RDA values for each of the nutrients on Chart E. Have students convert actual values to the percentage of the RDA consumed and then have them record these calculations on their copies of Chart E. For example, Frances consumed 374 milligrams of Vitamin C. The RDA for Vitamin C for females aged 15–18 years is 60 milligrams. Therefore, the percent consumed was:

$$\frac{374}{60} \times 100 = 623\%$$

Completion of the worksheets may take two class periods or could be assigned as homework. After students finish them, conduct a class discussion on their findings. Use the following questions to lead the discussion:

- Which menu did not reach ⅔ (67 percent)* or more of the RDA for any of the nutrients? *(Answer:* Fortified Frances. She had 64 percent of the RDA for calcium.)

---

*An intake that is at least ⅔ (67 percent) of each nutrient is considered to be an adequate intake since the RDA for each nutrient includes a wide safety margin. Diets that contain less than 67 percent of the RDA for any nutrient may be inadequate.

- Which menu had the highest values for any single nutrient? *(Answer:* Fortified Frances. She had 623 percent of the RDA for Vitamin C.)
- What are the dangers of consuming vitamins and minerals in excess of those provided by a normal diet? *(Answer:* Vitamins and minerals may accumulate in the body and become toxic.)
- What happens to water-soluble vitamins when consumed in excess of bodily needs? *Answer:* They are eliminated through the kidneys.)
- What benefits do fortified foods have in the diet? *(Answer:* They may provide nutrients that are lacking in your diet.)
- What problems do you think fortified foods cause? *(Answer:* Nutrient excess, reliance on convenience foods, deficiency of fiber and trace minerals, excess sugar and fat.)
- After this exercise, how do you feel about fortified foods? *(Answers will vary.)*

4. **Evaluation:** Distribute Quiz Sheet 9-1 and have students complete it independently. Discuss the answers as a class.

## FOLLOW-UP ACTIVITIES

1. Have students keep a food diary to check the frequency with which fortified foods are consumed.
2. Have students conduct a debate on the pros and cons of iron fortification.
3. Have students select one food additive and do an investigative report including: safety testing, history, limits for use, foods in which it is found, and functions.
4. Set up a hypothetical situation in which consumers are in conflict with the government (FDA) and/or food industry regarding food additives. Set up a debate in which half of the students support the consumers and half of the students support the government and/or food industry. An example of one situation might be as follows:

Timmy Miller is allergic to the protein found in corn. Whenever he eats a food containing corn or a corn product, such as corn syrup or cornstarch, he gets a headache and has stomach cramps. Timmy's mother tries to keep him away from all foods containing corn. Since many products do not contain ingredient lists, she is never sure if a food contains corn or a corn product. At the school cafeteria, she has no way of controlling what he eats.

As the debate moderator, you might want to pose some questions such as: Should the food industry be forced to fully disclose their ingredients? Is the consumer responsible for seeking out the desired information? Should the food industry be forced to discontinue using some food substances or additives because a few people are adversely affected? Would a fair approach be to put all ingredient information on the label and let each consumer take the responsibility for deciding whether or not to purchase the product?

5. Have students write an essay describing what should be done in the future concerning food additives. Should there be stricter regulations? Fewer regulations? Should all additives be eliminated? Should more additives be used?

6. Have students play "The Additive Game." Before the day of the activity, gather labels from various food products that list ingredients. You may want to bring the actual food containers to class, but do not let the students see them. With the students' abilities in mind, try to find foods with fairly long ingredient lists. You may also ask each student to bring in one food label or container, but tell them not to let the other students see them.

To play the game, read the list of ingredients to the students. Alternatively, list the ingredients on the chalkboard or on a transparency. Have students try to guess what food product you are describing. If students have difficulty, you may want to list all of the food products on the board so that they can guess the food from a limited selection.

# LOOK AT THE CHEMICALS MOTHER NATURE PUTS IN WHOLE MILK!

The ingredients on this milk carton are a partial listing of the chemical ingredients found in whole milk.

None of the chemicals listed has been "added" to the milk.

Natural foods are very complex chemical substances used by our bodies!

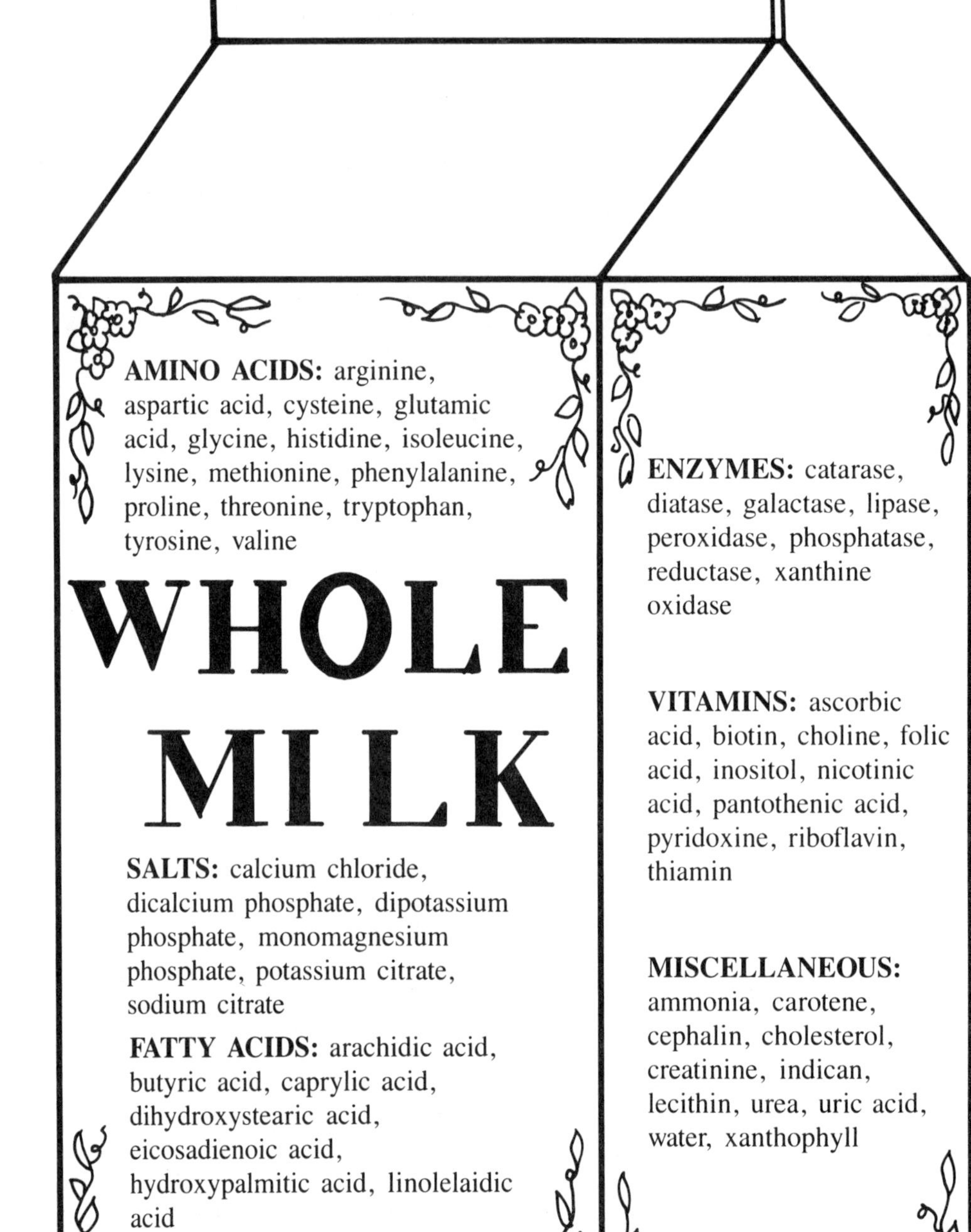
**AMINO ACIDS:** arginine, aspartic acid, cysteine, glutamic acid, glycine, histidine, isoleucine, lysine, methionine, phenylalanine, proline, threonine, tryptophan, tyrosine, valine
WHOLE
MILK
**SALTS:** calcium chloride, dicalcium phosphate, dipotassium phosphate, monomagnesium phosphate, potassium citrate, sodium citrate
**FATTY ACIDS:** arachidic acid, butyric acid, caprylic acid, dihydroxystearic acid, eicosadienoic acid, hydroxypalmitic acid, linolelaidic acid
**CARBOHYDRATES:** lactose
**ENZYMES:** catarase, diatase, galactase, lipase, peroxidase, phosphatase, reductase, xanthine oxidase
**VITAMINS:** ascorbic acid, biotin, choline, folic acid, inositol, nicotinic acid, pantothenic acid, pyridoxine, riboflavin, thiamin
**MISCELLANEOUS:** ammonia, carotene, cephalin, cholesterol, creatinine, indican, lecithin, urea, uric acid, water, xanthophyll

# CHEMICALS YOU EAT

Did you know that you eat lots of chemicals every day of your life? All foods, and everything in nature too, are made of chemicals. Chemicals are the basis of life.

Food additives are chemicals, too. Some food additives are made by people in laboratories; other food additives are found in nature. They are all chemicals.

Why is there so much fuss lately about food additives? One reason is that some people think that food additives are dangerous to our health, and other people think that food additives are completely safe. Even the experts cannot agree! Today there are over 10,000 different food additives used in the foods we eat. With so many additives on the market, it is very confusing to figure out if they are all safe for us to eat.

The Food and Drug Administration (FDA) is the government agency that helps keep our food safe. Since 1958, it has required all new food additives to be tested for safety. These tests are done on laboratory animals. The FDA decides, from the results of the tests, whether the additive is safe to use. The FDA also decides how much of the food additive may be added to a particular food to maintain a safe level for consumption.

Some consumers say that the FDA is not the only one responsible for deciding the safety of food additives. Consumers say that they, too, can decide if they think a food additive is safe enough to eat. They can decide to avoid a particular food if they think it is unsafe. Consumers are teaching themselves about food additives so that they can choose which foods (and which food additives) they will buy when they go to the grocery store. If all consumers stopped buying certain foods, then the food companies would stop making these foods. Consumer advocacy (or consumer groups taking action) is a way for *you* to protect your food supply.

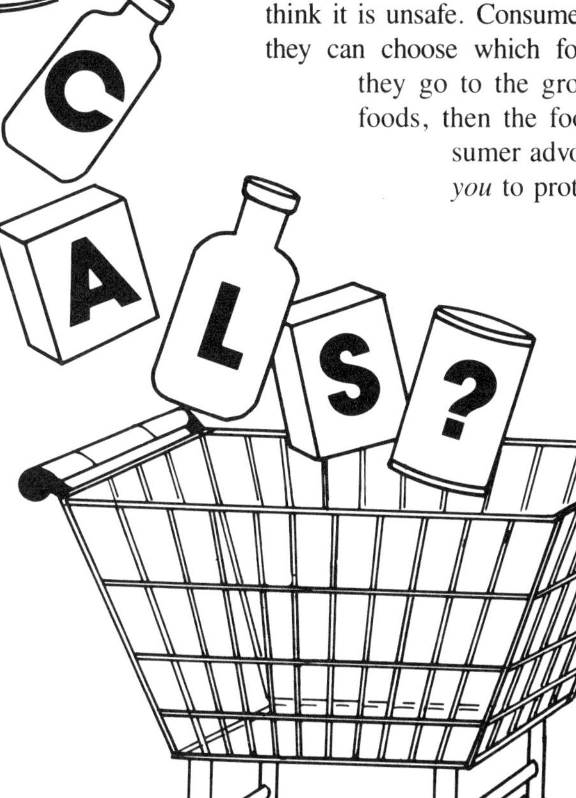


Let us look at what consumers are saying about food additives. Some consumers say that no food additive can be guaranteed to be completely safe for everyone. Some of their questions about food additives are listed here:

1. Just because the additive does not harm test animals, does that guarantee that it is safe for humans?

2. The additives are tested on healthy animals. How might certain additives affect animals (and humans) who have health problems?

3. Many people eat foods containing several different food additives. Is it possible that food additives could combine and be harmful in that way?

4. Today we have better ways to test food additives than we did 10 or 20 years ago. Is it possible that the food additives we tested years ago would be found unsafe today?

You are a consumer, too. What questions do you have about food additives? Write them on the back of this sheet.

---

You have the responsibility to yourself, your family, and your friends to learn about food additives and to make wise decisions about which ones you will eat.

Let us look at food additives a little more closely. There are so many different food additives on the market that it becomes difficult to remember all of them. To make things easier, we can classify food additives according to their function in foods. The four major functions of food additives are:

1. **To make food more nutritious.** Sometimes nutrients will be added to food. They may be replacing nutrients that were lost during processing. For example, thiamin and niacin are two nutrients put back into white flour because these nutrients are removed during milling. Nutrients are also added to food just to make it more nutritious. For instance, ascorbic acid (Vitamin C) is added to apple juice because it has only a little Vitamin C occurring naturally in the juice.
2. **To keep food safe.** Certain food additives slow down the spoiling or aging of food. They are used as preservatives. These additives allow you to keep food on the shelf longer. If food is less perishable, its cost is usually reduced. This allows you to buy food that may be grown far away or stored for long periods of time.
3. **To help in food preparation.** Some food additives are useful in the preparation and processing of food. For example, many of the gum additives are used to hold together food products such as puddings and salad dressings so that they do not separate.
4. **To make food look and taste good.** Some food additives increase the color or flavor of the food. Colors are often used for cosmetic purposes. They are used to make the food look more appealing to the consumer. Flavors and flavor enhancers are used to make the food taste better.

So, you can see that there are many reasons why people use food additives. But what was it like before we knew all about these chemicals? Believe it or not, food additives have been around since the earliest recorded histories. Salt was used in ancient Rome to preserve meats and vegetables. Food colors from beets, berries, and insects were used in ancient civilizations and are still used in some areas of the world. Marco Polo traveled thousands of miles to purchase exotic spices to add flavor to European diets. The recipe for pemmican, a dried meat dish prepared by native Americans and also eaten by American colonists, called for salt, sugar, and vinegar as preservatives. People used chemicals that occurred in nature as food additives before they knew about chemistry. Today people still use these naturally occurring chemicals. They also use chemicals made in laboratories.

The "Food Label Table" on Sheets 9-4 through 9-5 identifies the different food additives, the functions they perform, and the foods in which they are found. The table also tells you which additives are safe in the amounts allowed. Check the food additives on this table with the listings of ingredients on food packages. Keep it handy in the kitchen or take it with you to the grocery store so that you can become a wise consumer.

# FOOD LABEL TABLE

**Directions:** This table lists nutritive, preservative, quality-giving, and cosmetic food additives. Use the key below to check the food additives on Sheets 9-4 and 9-5 with the listings of ingredients on food packages.

KEY: ▲ Safe in quantities allowed
○ Caution

| NUTRITIVE ADDITIVES ...MAKE FOOD MORE NUTRITIOUS | COMMONLY APPEAR IN THESE FOODS: |
|---|---|
| ▲ ascorbic acid (Vitamin C) | instant potatoes, cereals, beverage mixes, soft drinks |
| ▲ beta carotene (pre-Vitamin A) | margarine, butter, shortening, nondairy creamers |
| ▲ ferrous gluconate (iron) | black olives, baked goods, cereals |
| ▲ niacinamide (niacin) | baked good, cereals, other grain products |
| ▲ potassium iodide (iodine) | salt, baked goods |
| ▲ riboflavin (Vitamin $B_2$) | baked goods, cereals, other grain products |
| ▲ thiamin (Vitamin $B_1$) | baked goods, cereals, other grain products |
| ▲ tocopherol (Vitamin E) | cereals, other grain products |

| PRESERVATIVE ADDITIVES ...KEEP FOOD FROM SPOILING | COMMONLY APPEAR IN THESE FOODS: |
|---|---|
| ▲ ascorbic acid (Vitamin C) | bologna, other cured meats, oily foods |
| ○ BHA and BHT (Butylated Hydroxyanisole, -toluene) | convenience foods, cereals, chewing gum, candy, potato chips, oils |
| ▲ calcium (or sodium) propionate | baked goods |
| ▲ citric acid, sodium citrate | instant potatoes, ice cream, fruit drinks, canned fruits and vegetables, candy, soft drinks |
| ▲ EDTA | canned fruits and vegetables, canned shellfish, salad dressings, mayonnaise, sandwich spreads, margarine, soft drinks |
| ▲ heptyl paraben | beer, other beverages, pastries, salad dressings, relishes |
| ▲ lactic acid | cheeses, soft drinks, frozen desserts, Spanish olives |
| ▲ propyl gallate | chewing gum, oils, meat products, chicken soup base |
| ▲ sodium benzoate | fruit juices, soft drinks, pickles, salad dressings, preserves |
| ▲ sodium bisulfite | soft drinks, wine, grape juice, canned fruits, powdered soup mixes |
| ○ sodium nitrite, sodium nitrate | cured meats, fish and poultry including hot dogs, bologna, ham, smoked fish, bacon |
| ▲ sorbic acid, potassium sorbate | cheese, syrup, jelly, mayonnaise, soft drinks, wine, dried fruits, margarine, canned frostings |
| ▲ sulfur dioxide | dried fruits |
| ▲ tocopherol | oils |

| QUALITY-GIVING ADDITIVES ...HELP IN FOOD PREPARATION | COMMONLY APPEAR IN THESE FOODS: |
|---|---|
| ▲ acetic acid | candy, sauces, salad dressings |
| ▲ alginate | ice cream, whipped cream, yogurt, canned frostings, candy |
| ○ brominated vegetable oil (BVO) | soft drinks, fruit drinks |
| ▲ calcium (or potassium) bromate | flour, baked goods |
| ▲ calcium (or sodium) stearolyl lactylates | baked goods, cake fillings, whipped cream, processed egg whites |
| ▲ carboxymethyl cellulose | ice cream, beer, pie fillings, jellies, canned frostings, diet foods, bread, candy |
| ▲ carrageenan | sour cream, syrup, gelatin products, milk drinks, soft drinks, ice cream, infant formula |
| ▲ casein, sodium caseinate | ice cream, ice milk, frozen desserts, nondairy creamers |
| ▲ citric acid, sodium citrate | gelatin products, jams, jellies candy, instant potatoes, soft drinks, fruit drinks |
| ▲ glycerine, glycerol | marshmallows, candy, baked goods |
| ▲ gums: Arabic, carob bean, ghatti, karaya, locust bean | chewing gum, sauces, desserts, salad dressings, syrup, soft drinks, cheese, baked goods, candy |
| ▲ lactic acid | cheese, soft drinks, frozen desserts |
| ▲ lecithin | margarine, chocolate, ice cream, baked goods |
| ▲ modified food starch | sauces, soups, pie fillings, canned meats |
| ▲ mono- and diglycerides | baked goods, peanut butter, cereals, candy, margarine |
| ▲ pectin | jellies, sauces, canned frostings, yogurt |
| ▲ phosphoric acid, phosphates | candy, shortening, soft drinks, cereals, cured meats, cheese |
| ▲ polysorbates | frozen desserts, baked goods, nondairy creamers, candy |
| ▲ propylene glycol | candy, canned frostings, baked goods |
| ▲ silicon dioxide | salt, nondairy creamers, baking powder, seasonings |
| ▲ sodium bicarbonate | baked goods, baking soda |

| COSMETIC ADDITIVES ...MAKE FOOD LOOK AND TASTE GOOD | COMMONLY APPEAR IN THESE FOODS: |
|---|---|
| ○ artificial colors | soft drinks, fruit drinks, ice cream, cured meats, baked goods, cereal, candy, gelatin products |
| ○ artificial flavors | baked goods, ice cream, gelatin products, soft drinks, candy, cereal |
| ○ aspartame (NutraSweet) | some diet soft drinks, diet beverages, diet foods |
| ○ caffeine | coffee, tea, cocoa (naturally occurring), soft drinks (added) |
| ▲ caramel | soft drinks, baked goods |
| ▲ ferrous gluconate | black olives |
| ▲ fumaric acid | gelatin products, puddings, pie fillings, candy, soft drinks |
| ▲ hydrolyzed vegetable protein | processed meats, gravy, sauces |
| ○ monosodium glutamate (MSG) | oriental foods, soups, foods with animal protein, croutons |
| ○ quinine | tonic water |
| ○ saccharin | some diet soft drinks, diet foods |
| ▲ sodium chloride (table salt) | most processed foods |
| ▲ sugars: corn syrup, dextrose, fructose, glucose, lactose, mannitol, sucrose | soft drinks, candy, baked goods, cereal, nondairy creamers, condiments |

Name ______________________ Sheet 9-6

# TO ADD OR NOT TO ADD

**Directions:** In this activity you will make some decisions as to whether or not certain food additives should be used in three different situations. Write your answers below.

1. What are the four functions of food additives? ______________________

2. Which function is not very important for health or nutrition? ______________________

**Situation A:** Suppose bread is baked and packaged in a bakery. It is then shipped a long distance to supermarkets in many different areas.

3. Do you think preservative food additives like calcium propionate are necessary? Explain your answer.

______________________

4. Perhaps you or someone in your family has baked bread at home. If you ate the bread within a few days after baking, would you need to add preservatives to it? Explain.

______________________

**Situation B:** Refer to Sheet 9-8, "E•N•R•I•C•H." White flour has thiamin, riboflavin, niacin, and iron added to it. It is "enriched" with these nutrients because they are lost when the wheat kernels are refined. Refining is a type of food processing in which the outer covering of the wheat kernel is removed. This is done in order to slow down the spoilage of the grain as well as to change the color and texture of the resulting flour. The flour is enriched in order to replace some of the lost nutrients. Other products that are enriched include rice, spaghetti, buns, rolls, English muffins, macaroni, and cornmeal.

Suppose that you are a food processor who refines flour. Look at Sheet 9-8. Compare the percentage of the U.S. RDAs for enriched bread with those for unenriched white bread.

5. Do you think that enriching your flour with B vitamins and iron is a good idea?

______________________

6. Support your answer by using the figures given in the table. ______________________

Name ______________________________ Sheet 9-7

Instead of refining flour, you have decided to grind the wheat kernels without removing any of their parts. This will give you whole wheat flour.

7. Would you enrich the whole wheat flour? Why? ______________________________

8. Support your answer by using the figures given in the table. ______________________________

**Situation C:** Suppose you made a milkshake at home but didn't like the flavor. You decide to add something to give it more flavor.

9. What flavoring would you add? ______________________________

10. Would the flavoring change the nutritional value of the milkshake? Why? ______

11. Would the flavoring make the milkshake more appealing to others? ______________________________

12. How could you color the milkshake differently? ______________________________

13. Would this color change the nutritional value of the milkshake? Why? ______________________________

14. Would the color make the milkshake more appealing to you? ______________________________

15. Would other students find the color of your milkshake appealing? ______________________________

16. Suppose you decided that you couldn't drink all of the milkshake and put it in the refrigerator. Would the added flavor or color prevent the milkshake from spoiling? ______________________________

17. Which additives could be reduced in the food supply without hurting our health? ______________________________

# E • N • R • I • C • H

| ENERGY | NUTRITIVE ADDITIVES | REFINING | IRON | NUTRITIOUS CHOICES | HEALTH |
|---|---|---|---|---|---|
| Grain and grain products such as flour, rice, bread, and macaroni are enriched with iron and the B vitamins–thiamin, riboflavin, and niacin. These B vitamins help our bodies release energy from the foods we eat. | The B vitamins and iron are nutritive additives used in the enrichment process. As seen in the chart below, enrichment increases the nutritional value of foods. | Refining is the food process that removes the outer layers of grains such as wheat and rice. This is done to change the color and texture of the flour as well as to prevent the spoilage of grains and products made from them. The outer layers contain many of the nutrients. | Iron is the mineral added back to grains and grain products after they have been refined. | White bread, white rice, spaghetti, noodles, and white flour are more nutritious after being enriched. | Enrichment of certain foods is important to health because it provides our bodies with nutrients that are lost during the refining process. |

| | | % U.S. RDA | | | |
|---|---|---|---|---|---|
| **Food** | **Quantity** | **Thiamin** | **Riboflavin** | **Niacin** | **Iron** |
| White bread, enriched | 1 slice | 4 | 3 | 3 | 4 |
| White bread, unenriched | 1 slice | 2 | 2 | 2 | 2 |
| Whole wheat bread | 1 slice | 4 | 2 | 3 | 3 |
| White rice, enriched | 1 cup, cooked | 16 | 8 | 10 | 10 |
| White rice, unenriched | 1 cup, cooked | 2 | 2 | 4 | 2 |
| Brown rice | 1 cup, cooked | 10 | 2 | 12 | 4 |

Name ______________________________ 

# FORTIFIED FOODS

**Directions:** Review the menus for Hardly Fortified Helen and Fortified Frances below. Then calculate the intake in each menu on a separate copy of Chart E. Use Table 9-1, "Mini Food Composition Table," to obtain the figures you will need. Compare the total for each girl to the Recommended Dietary Allowances on Chart A for a female aged 15 to 18 years. Add one additional column to Chart E for Vitamin D.

## HARDLY FORTIFIED HELEN

**Breakfast**
- Oatmeal, cooked, 1 cup
- Milk, skim, 1 cup
- Banana, 1
- Toast, whole wheat, 2 slices
- Margarine, 2 teaspoons

**Lunch**
- Peanut butter, 2 tablespoons
- Jelly, 1 tablespoon
- Whole wheat bread, 2 slices
- Milk, skim, 1 cup
- Chocolate chip cookies, 2

**Snacks**
- Raisins, 1/4 cup
- Peanuts, 1/4 cup

**Dinner**
- Chicken breast, 1/2
- Tossed salad, 1 cup
- Salad dressing, 1 tablespoon
- Potato, baked, 1
- Margarine, 2 teaspoons
- Milk, skim, 1 cup
- Gingerbread cake, 1 piece

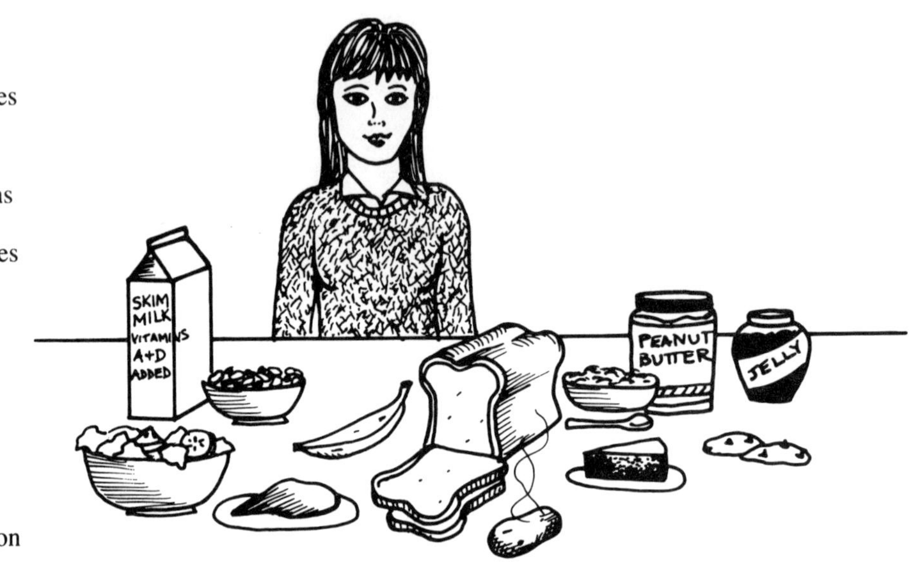


## FORTIFIED FRANCES

**Breakfast**
- Fortified cereal, 1 ounce (about 1 cup)
- Fortified fruit drink, 8 ounce
- Fortified breakfast bar, 1

**Lunch**
- Luncheon meat, 2 slices
- Enriched white bread, 2 slices
- Mayonnaise, 2 tablespoons
- Fortified fruit drink, 8 ounce
- Chocolate chip cookies, 2

**Snack**
- Pop-Tart, frosted, 1

**Dinner**
- Chicken breast, 1/2
- Tossed salad, 1 cup
- Salad dressing, 1 tablespoon
- Potato, baked, 1
- Margarine, 2 teaspoons
- Milk, skim, 1 cup

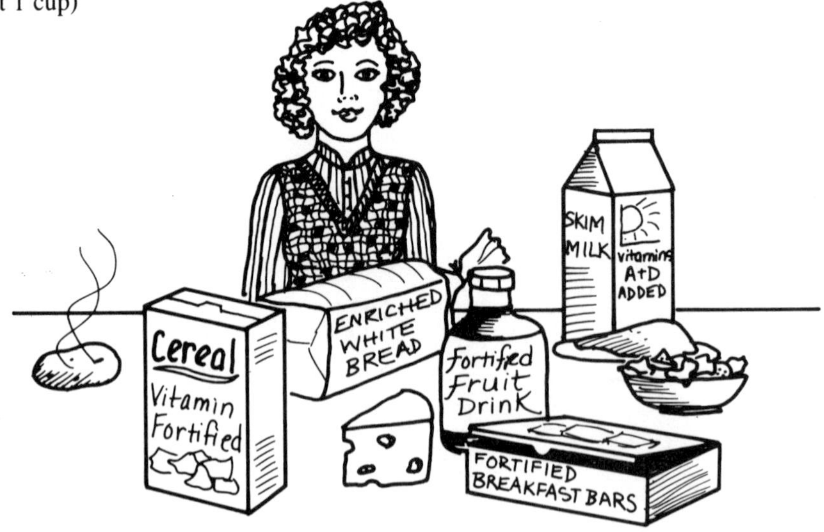

# MINI FOOD COMPOSITION TABLE[1]

| Food | Amount | Energy (cal.) | Protein (g) | Vit A (IU) | Vit C (mg) | Thia. (mg) | Ribo. (mg) | Nia. (mg) | Calcium (mg) | | |
|---|---|---|---|---|---|---|---|---|---|---|---|
| Banana | 1 | 100 | 1 | 226 | 12 | 0.1 | 0.1 | 0.8 | 4 | 0.1 | 0 |
| Bread, enriched white | 2 slices | 140 | 4 | T | T | 0.1 | 0.1 | 1.2 | 42 | 1.2 | T |
| Bread, whole wheat | 2 slices | 110 | 5 | T | T | 0.1 | 0.1 | 1.2 | 44 | 1.0 | T |
| Chicken breast | 1/2 | 245 | 32 | 100 | 0 | 0.1 | 0.2 | 12.4 | 20 | 1.3 | – |
| Chocolate chip cookies | 2 | 120 | 1 | 6 | 0 | T | T | 0.2 | 8 | 0.4 | 6 |
| Fortified breakfast bar | 1 | 190 | 6 | 625 | 8 | 0.2 | 0.2 | 2.5 | 125 | 2.2 | 5 |
| Fortified cereal | 1 oz. | 110 | 2 | 5,000 | 60 | 1.5 | 1.7 | 20.0 | 40 | 18.0 | 400 |
| Fortified fruit drink | 8 oz. | 120 | 0 | 1,974 | 118 | 0.0 | 0.0 | 0.0 | 64 | T | 0 |
| Gingerbread cake | 1 piece | 275 | 3 | 28 | 2 | 0.1 | 0.1 | 1.0 | 134 | 4.1 | 2 |
| Jelly | 1 tbsp. | 55 | 0 | 2 | 1 | T | T | T | 4 | 0.3 | 0 |
| Luncheon meat | 2 slices | 100 | 4 | T | 4 | 0.1 | T | 0.8 | 3 | 0.3 | 17 |
| Margarine | 2 tsp. | 70 | * | 314 | 0 | T | T | 0.0 | 1 | 0.0 | – |
| Mayonnaise | 2 tbsp. | 200 | * | 78 | – | 0.0 | 0.0 | T | 6 | T | – |
| Milk, skim | 1 cup | 85 | 8 | 500 | 2 | 0.1 | 0.3 | 0.2 | 301 | 0.1 | 100 |
| Oatmeat, cooked | 1 cup | 135 | 5 | 0 | 0 | 0.2 | T | 0.1 | 22 | 1.4 | 0 |
| Peanut butter | 2 tbsp. | 175 | 8 | 0 | 0 | T | T | 4.8 | 18 | 0.6 | 0 |
| Peanuts | 1/4 cup | 210 | 9 | T | 0 | 0.1 | 0.1 | 6.2 | 27 | 0.8 | 0 |
| Pop-Tart, frosted | 1 | 220 | 3 | – | 7 | 0.3 | 0.3 | 2.5 | 25 | 2.5 | – |
| Potato, baked | 1 | 145 | 4 | T | 31 | 0.2 | 0.1 | 2.6 | 14 | 1.1 | 0 |
| Raisins | 1/4 cup | 105 | 1 | 7 | T | T | T | 0.2 | 22 | 1.3 | 0 |
| Salad dressing | 1 tbsp. | 70 | * | T | 0 | T | T | T | 1 | 0.1 | – |
| Tossed salad | 1 cup | 30 | 2 | 2,279 | 26 | 0.1 | 0.1 | 0.7 | 48 | 1.1 | 0 |

[1]From *Nutrients in Foods*, Leveille, G. A., Zabik, M. E., and Morgan, K. J. The Nutrition Guild, Cambridge, MA, 1983.
*Less than one gram of protein.
T means food contains only trace amounts of this nutrient.
– means lack of data on this nutrient.

Name ____________________ 

# QUIZ
# INTERPRETING INGREDIENT LABELS: NUTRITIVE FOOD ADDITIVES

____ 1. Food additives are used for:

a. Keeping food safe
b. Making food look good
c. Making food more nutritious
d. All of the above

____ 2. An example of a cosmetic food additive is:

a. Thiamin c. Nitrite
b. Carotene d. Ascorbic acid

____ 3. An example of a nutritive food additive is:

a. Saccharin c. Riboflavin
b. Red dye d. Calcium propionate

____ 4. Calcium propionate is added to bread products to:

a. Preserve the bread
b. Flavor the bread
c. Soften the bread
d. Color the bread

Use the following information from an ingredient label to answer questions 5 and 6.

> "Good Morning Cereal" — Ingredients: Wheat flour, sugar, wheat bran, cellulose, honey, salt, coconut oil, natural flavor, sodium ascorbate, spice, niacinamide, FD&C Yellow #5, artificial color, reduced iron, Vitamin A palmitate, pyridoxine hydrochloride, riboflavin, BHT, thiamin mononitrate, Vitamin $B_2$, and Vitamin $B_{12}$.

____ 5. Which ingredient is a nutritive food additive?

a. Natural flavor c. BHT
b. Niacinamide d. Cellulose

____ 6. Which ingredient is used to enrich this cereal?

a. Reduced iron c. Salt
b. Artificial color d. Sugar

____ 7. The process of adding nutrients to foods is called:

a. Fortification
b. Nutrientization
c. Food processing
d. Enhancement
e. None of the above

____ 8. What nutrients are added when grain products are "enriched"?

a. Calcium, iron niacin, thiamin
b. Riboflavin, iron, protein, niacin
c. Iron, thiamin, riboflavin, niacin
d. Vitamin C, calcium, iron, riboflavin

____ 9. What is food fortification?

a. The same as enrichment.
b. Adding nutrients to food to make it a good source of those nutrients.
c. The combining of two foods to make them more nutritious.
c. A way to preserve foods.

____ 10. Fortified food products are essential for a nutritious diet.

a. True
b. False

____ 11. The Food and Drug Administration:

a. Works on drugs and doesn't care what goes into the food supply.
b. Tests only the safety of drugs.
c. Is a state nutritional program.
d. Tests new additives for safety before they are used.

# Unit 10: Interpreting Ingredient Labels: Cosmetic Food Additives

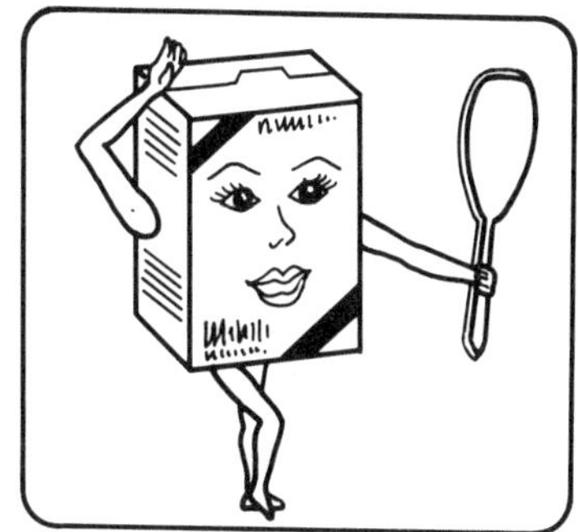

## CONCEPTS

–Cosmetic food additives (colors and flavors) are used in foods for appeal purposes in order to meet consumer expectations.

–In terms of nutrition, cosmetic food additives are generally unnecessary.

–The value and safety of many cosmetic food additives have been questioned.

–A risk/benefit ratio can be examined by consumers in order to help them make decisions about food purchases.

## OBJECTIVES

–Students will be able to describe reasons for using natural and synthetic cosmetic additives in foods.

–Students will be able to assess the benefits and risks of cosmetic food additives.

## TEACHER'S UNIT INTRODUCTION

Cosmetic food additives used to color and flavor foods have often been given special attention recently.

These most widely used additives make food taste and look better. Sugar, salt, and corn syrup are the additives used most extensively, with an average of 130 pounds of added sugar being consumed by each person annually. Together with other substances such as baking soda, vegetable color, citric acid, and pepper, they represent 98 percent of all food additives.

Cosmetic additives have been the focus of great controversy because they are added to food for appeal only. Those against the use of cosmetic additives in food argue that cosmetic additives contribute nothing to the safety or nutritional value of food and that the priority of some food processors may be profit rather than public health. On the other hand, food industries report that consumers want foods that are appetizing and attractive and that sales figures support this.

**Flavor Additives.** Flavor additives are the largest class of food additives and include both natural and synthetic flavors, flavor enhancers, and sweeteners. The terms "natural flavor" and "natural flavoring" mean that the additive was extracted from a spice, fruit or fruit juice, vegetable, edible yeast, herb, bud, bark, root, leaf, meat, seafood, poultry, egg, or dairy product. For example, natural vanilla flavor is extracted from the vanilla bean.

Simply because a chemical occurs naturally in foods, its safety as an additive is not guaranteed. For instance, safrole, a substance extracted from sassafras, is used to flavor root beer. In 1960, the use of safrole as an additive was banned when scientists found that it caused cancer of the liver. Note, however, that food laws have no provision to ban the sale of sassafras even though it contains the banned substance safrole. The law applies only to harmful substances when they are used as additives and not when they occur naturally in foods.

The terms "artificial flavor" and "artificial flavoring" mean any flavoring additive that has not been derived from a plant or animal. After the molecular structure of a natural-flavor compound is identified, food chemists can often synthetically produce an artificial flavor additive that is cheaper, purer, and more consistent in quality than the natural one. The human body cannot always tell if the additive was cultivated in nature or synthesized in the laboratory. The flavor of a cherry, for example, is due to 10 chemical compounds in the fruit. These same chemicals may be manufactured in the laboratory.

Flavors are used in commercially prepared foods for a number of reasons. Here are the primary ones:

- The flavor of the processed food is unacceptable or altered in processing. For example, production of frozen juice concentrate causes a loss of the fresh fruit flavor, so a flavor additive is often used.
- An imitation or an artificial food is created to mimic a real food. For example, flavors are used in fruit drinks to mimic fruit juices, in Baco-Bits to mimic bacon, and in nondairy coffee creamers and whipped toppings to mimic real dairy products.
- A new flavor is desired or added flavoring ingredients are used to complement the basic natural flavor of a food ingredient. For example, the unique flavor of Coca-Cola is laboratory-made, whereas the addition of almond flavor to cherry pie filling enhances the natural flavor of the cherries.

If a product has added flavoring, the law requires that this be stated on the label's ingredient list. Only standardized foods—those foods for which the FDA has established a specific recipe such as ice cream and mayonnaise—are exempt from listing flavors on the label. Natural flavors, such as sugar, salt, pepper, or mustard, are simply listed. In many cases, a manufacturer may choose to use the summary term "natural flavor" in the list of ingredients. For instance, a fruit-punch drink mix may state "natural fruit flavors" in its list of ingredients without listing each extracted fruit juice flavor used. A large number of spices can be listed under the summary term "spices." The summary term "artificial flavors" can also be used instead of listing each chemical compound.

Occasionally, a food's title as it appears on the package will identify the source of the flavor used. For example:

- "Strawberry Yogurt" contains no added flavors other than the flavor from actual fruit pieces.
- "Strawberry-Flavored Yogurt" contains the natural flavor from strawberries although there are no fruit pieces in the yogurt.
- "Artificially-Flavored Yogurt" contains only artificial flavorings or a combination of artificial and natural flavors.

The source of a packaged food's flavor is always found on the label's ingredient list. The following table lists common flavor and sweetener additives. Flavor enhancers are substances that have no flavor of their own but that enhance or bring out a food's natural flavor. There are more than 2,000 flavoring ingredients permitted in foods. [Display the following table on an overhead or opaque projector.]

**Common Flavor, Flavor Enhancer, and Sweetener Additives**

| Flavors | Flavor Enhancers | Sweeteners |
|---|---|---|
| herbs and spices | disodium guanylate | aspartane (NutraSweet) |
| vanilla | disodium inosinate | dextrose |
| salt | disodium inosinate | fructose |
| menthol | hydrolyzed vegetable protein | glucose |
| caprylic acid | MSG (monosodium glutamate) | sucrose |
| ethyl formate | | invert sugar |
| | | corn syrup/solids |
| | | mannitol |
| | | sorbitol |
| | | saccharin |

**Color Additives.** Natural colors are derived from plants in which a pigment occurs, such as orange or red beta-carotene in carrots and caramel in browned sugar. Artificial colors can be defined as synthetic molecules that duplicate the chemical structure of color substances naturally found in foods. For example, beta-carotene can also be made in the laboratory. Artificial colors may also be defined as synthetic molecules that differ from chemicals naturally occurring in foods.

The following table lists some of the colors currently permitted by the FDA for use in foods. Except for Blue #2, Yellow #6, and Green #3, which remain on the provisionally approved list of additives, all color additives used in food have been tested and judged to be safe. [Display the following table on an overhead or opaque projector.]

**Examples of Color Additives**

| Natural | Natural or Synthetic |
|---|---|
| dehydrated beet powder (dark red) | canthaxanthin (orange to red) |
| caramel (dark brown) | beta-carotene (yellow) |
| toasted cottonseed flour (brown) | riboflavin (yellow) |
| grape skin extract (purplish red) | |
| **Synthetic** | **Synthetic—Petroleum-Based** |
| titanium dioxide (white) | FD&C* Red #3 |
| iron oxide (reddish brown) | FD&C* Red #40 |
| ferrous gluconate (black) | FD&C* Blue #2 |
| | FD&C* Yellow #5 |

*FD&C means that the color is acceptable for Foods, Drugs, and Cosmetics.

Artificial colors are used more widely than natural colors because artificial colors are more potent and purer. Consequently, they can be used in smaller quantities at less cost. Recently, the FDA has banned four colors that have either been found to cause cancer or that are suspected of causing cancer in laboratory animals. The colors no longer permitted for use are FD&C Violet #1, used to stamp meats, FD&C Red #2, FD&C Red #4, used in maraschino cherries, and Carbon Black, used in candies. Currently, FD&C Red #40 is under criticism for possibly causing lymph tumors in mice, but a final decision on its continued use has not been reached. FD&C Yellow #5 has been found to cause allergic reactions in some individuals; as a result, the FDA now requires that this color be listed by name on the ingredient label of foods containing it. Except for this color, any other color additives included in foods may be grouped under the general summary term "natural colors" or "artificial colors."

**Consumer Expectations.** Many consumers want convenience products, and many food companies eagerly oblige. Consumers tend to expect each food to have an appropriate taste and color and expect certain standards regarding the appearance of a food to be met before they are willing to even taste the food. This is often understandable. For example, color can mark the difference between fresh and stale food. The fact is, however, that nature does not consistently color foods according to consumer expectations. Experiments have shown that familiar foods are avoided when not colored as expected. For example, most customers will not buy yellow maraschino cherries even though yellow is their natural color. Citrus growers treat oranges with an orange dye to disguise their natural splotchy, mottled green color. Butter may have dye added because it can be an unfamiliar white in winter when dairy cows are not grazing on green grasses containing the yellow carotene pigment.

Color may even outweigh flavor with respect to the impression that a food makes on a consumer. A study of sherbet revealed that color influences a consumer's ability to identify flavors and to estimate their strength and quality. In this study, white sherbet was flavored with lemon, lime, orange, grape, pineapple, or almond flavoring. The taste panel was confused by the color of the sherbet and could not successfully identify the different flavors. When lime-flavored sherbet was deceptively colored purple, only 47 percent of the taste panel could identify the lime flavor. But when the lime sherbet was colored green, 75 percent of the taste panel identified the flavor as lime.

Color and sweetness or tartness are related. The addition of red coloring to a cherry beverage causes an increase in perceived sweetness, and the addition of blue coloring to the same cherry beverage increases perceived tartness.

The federal government has enacted food laws designed to ensure a safe food supply in the United States. It is the job of the Food and Drug Administration to judge an additive harmful or harmless as defined in the Food, Drug, and Cosmetic Act. The FDA also determines the maximum amount, or tolerance limit, of an additive. However, the FDA cannot judge an additive used to make a product look or taste better as necessary and desirable. This controversy has been left to the manufacturer and consumer in the open market system of supply and demand.

When it comes to determining whether consumers or manufacturers are responsible for the use of color additives in the food supply, the question, "What comes first, the chicken or the egg?" applies. Do consumers expect foods to look a certain way, and then industry caters to these expectations? Or does industry use advertising to build expectations that condition and train the consumer to demand a certain food quality?

---

More than 90 percent of the U.S. food supply contains color and flavor additives. What would happen if these were suddenly removed? Would otherwise nutritous foods go uneaten because flavor and color are unacceptable? Questions like these are not easy to answer, but they will be explored by the students in this unit. Although it is very unlikely that color or flavor additives will ever be completely removed from the food supply, it is the right and duty of students to become more informed about the food they are consuming and to express their opinions about additives at least indirectly by casting a food-choice vote in the marketplace.

Although not appropriate for the objectives of this unit, a "Follow-Up Activity" on food preservatives has been included. Because of time constraints, the topic has not been dealt with as a separate unit, but if students demonstrate an interest in preservatives you may want to use this activity as well.

## BASIC ACTIVITY

**Time Needed:** Two class periods
Sheet 10-1: "Is It Natural or Artificial?"
Food package labels
Tables from the "Teacher's Unit Introduction"
Quiz Sheet 10-1

### Class Period 1

1. Prior to this activity, have students bring in labels from food prepared for an evening's dinner or labels from favorite foods at home. Warn students that some "standardized" foods may not list ingredients on the labels because the foods have been processed according to an FDA standard of identity (for example, mayonnaise, margarine, ice cream,

cheese). Also, advise students not to remove a label from a food product without relabeling the container so the family will know what is left in the can or box.

2. Introduce this unit by describing cosmetic food additives as ones added to foods for appeal purposes only. Describe flavorings and colorings by referring to the tables in the "Teacher's Unit Introduction." Encourage students to use this opportunity to study these food additives carefully before forming a definite opinion about them. Ask students to reserve their opinions until the class debate later in this unit.

3. Distribute Sheet 10-1, "Is It Natural or Artificial?" Have students complete the worksheet independently. Provide the tables from the "Teacher's Unit Introduction" as a reference.

4. Conduct a discussion on the students' discoveries. The following questions may be helpful:

- How many food labels listed individual color and flavor additives by name?
- How many labels simply listed "colors added" or "flavors added"?
- Which labels listed only synthetic colors or flavors?
- What foods had no added color? No added flavor? Neither added color nor added flavor?
- Did the front panel of the food specify if the food was natural, artificial, or imitation?

### Class Period 2

1. Students will assess the benefits versus the risks of using cosmetic food additives through a class panel discussion or debate.

2. Divide the class into three groups and assign each group a role to be taken in the viewpoint discussion. The roles are:

**Pro–** Food Industry Representatives. This industry uses flavor and color additives in its food products. This group will emphasize the benefits of cosmetic additives.

**Con–** Objecting Consumers. These consumers object to all color and flavor additives. This group will emphasize the risks of cosmetic additives.

**Neutral–** Undecided Consumers. These undecided consumers want to learn about cosmetic food additives to make a more informed decision about the foods they choose to buy and eat.

One method for organizing the students into three groups according to convictions is to ask "Which do you prefer: foods with or without cosmetic additives?" Assign Pro and Con groups on the basis of the answers, with the undecided students in the Neutral group.

3. Allow each group a brief brainstorming session to organize their viewpoints. The Neutral group should prepare a list of questions to address to each opposing group after the risk and benefit viewpoints have been presented. These questions should be used by the Neutral group to help them come to a concluding opinion.

4. If students are having difficulty coming up with risks and benefits, you may wish to review some risks or benefits with individual groups. Guidelines follow:

**Risks**

- Some additives may be dangerous; in addition, the safety of some others is being challenged.
- Cosmetic additives are unnecessary. They do not improve food safety, storage, or nutritional value.
- Some additives can cause allergic reactions in some people.
- Added colors and flavors can disguise real food color or flavor. Imitation foods that lack the same nutrients as the real foods can be made with colors and flavors to look like these real foods. Consumers may find it hard to know when they are eating "real food."

**Benefits**

- Food products can be made more appealing and are better accepted by consumers. Consumers will not select foods that do not look and taste as they expect.
- Synthetic flavor additives produce more reliable results than do some natural food flavors and are cheaper to use.
- The majority of cosmetic additives are the same ingredients that you use at home in a recipe, such as spices, salt, pepper, and sugar. The commercial food processor saves the consumer time by using these cosmetic additives.

5. Have the Pro group present its case first; then have the Con group make their case presentation.
6. Allow the Neutral group to question the opposing viewpoint groups. Ask the Neutral group to arrive at a concluding opinion.
7. The following questions may be helpful to the Neutral group:

- What do you think would happen if all of the added colors and flavors were removed from food?
- Now that you understand better how to read food ingredient labels, how do you intend to choose your foods in the future?

8. Proceed with the "Advanced Activity" if you wish; otherwise use the quiz mentioned in step 9.
9. **Evaluation:** Distribute Quiz Sheet 10-1 and have students complete it independently. Discuss the answers as a class.

## ADVANCED ACTIVITY

**Time Needed:** One class period

**Materials Needed:** Sheet 10-2: "Creating Synthetic Smells"

- ethanol
- isopentyl alchohol
- glacial acetic acid
- lab apron
- china marker
- glass stirring rods

sulfuric acid
2 beakers
2 test tubes
graduated cylinder
test tube holder
protective gloves
thermometer
2 beakers of warm water
2 beakers, each containing 10 grams of crushed ice
test tube stand

Sheet 10-3: "Creating Natural Colors"

deionized water
acetic acid (vinegar)
sodium bicarbonate (baking soda)
diced beets (16-oz. can)
2 250-milliliter beakers
2 beaker stands
2 Bunsen burners
lab apron
asbestos mitt
china marker
graduated cylinder
lab scale
paper

Quiz Sheet 10-1

1. Introduce the activity by explaining that many colors and flavors can be made in the laboratory that are similar to natural colors and flavors. The experiments on Sheets 10-2 through 10-3 may be done as a teacher demonstration or as a student laboratory experiment. If students participate, try to obtain access to the science laboratory for the experiments if possible, or borrow equipment and supplies from the lab.

2. Distribute Sheet 10-2, "Creating Synthetic Smell." In this experiment esters are formed that produce specific odors. The ester is derived by combining an acid with an alcohol. In the reaction, a hydrogen molecule is released by the alcohol. The remaining parts of the acid and alcohol combine to form an ester, and the hydrogen and hydroxyl group form water.

3. Follow the laboratory methods on the worksheet to complete the experiment.

**Caution: Students must not taste the mixtures—they should only smell them using proper laboratory procedures. While these smells are quite similar to the ones added to foods, they are not the exact smells and can be dangerous if taken internally.** This experiment is *not* intended to produce substances that can be safely added to food. *(See* the "Answer Key" for solutions.)

4. Distribute Sheet 10-3, "Creating Natural Colors." Students should follow the laboratory methods in order to create the two natural colors. *(See* the "Answer Key" for solutions.)

5. **Evaluation:** Distribute Quiz Sheet 10-1 and have students complete it independently. Discuss the answers as a class.

## FOLLOW-UP ACTIVITIES

1. Have students read and report on *The Jungle* by Upton Sinclair. This novel describes the meat-packing industry prior to federal regulation for food quality and safety. Reports can be done in a written or oral format.

2. Visit a natural foods store. Have students check the labels on food products and the prices of five or ten items. They should compare the labels and prices with comparable foods from a regular grocery store. Compare findings through a class discussion.

3. Divide the students into groups. Have each group prepare a meal that uses no color or flavor additives. The group should then write a report about the experience. Included in the report should be the following:

- Ease of finding foods
- Ease of food preparation
- Time involved in food preparation
- Taste of the foods
- Students' feeling about color and flavor additives
- Cost of the meal

4. Distribute Sheets 10-4 and 10-5, "Do You Want to Eat This Food?" Have students complete the sheets and then conduct a poll to determine which food in each pair was chosen by the greater number of students. Ask students to voice their opinions about their choices.

5. Have students keep a three-day food record, reporting all of the foods, beverages, and snacks consumed. Have them count the number of foods with added color (natural or synthetic) and the number of foods with flavors added (natural or synthetic). Discuss the results by asking the students if the colors or flavors were necessary and if there were other similar products that are color- or flavor-free and that could have been substituted.

Name ____________________ **Sheet 10-1**

# IS IT NATURAL OR ARTIFICIAL?

**Directions:** At home, find a food label for a favorite food. Cut out the list of ingredients and attach it to the box below. If the food's name on the front panel of the label includes terms such as *natural, artificial, flavored,* or *imitation,* cut the front panel out also and attach it to the back of this sheet. Complete the questions below based on your food label.

**FOOD INGREDIENT LABEL**

1. Does it contain COLOR additives? ____
2. Name the COLOR additives (if listed): ____________________

   ____________________

   ____________________
3. Can you tell if the additives are natural or synthetic? ____

   If so, which are natural? ____________________

   Which are synthetic? ____________________
4. Does it contain FLAVOR additives? ____
5. Name the FLAVOR additives (if listed): ____________________

   ____________________

   ____________________
6. Can you tell which flavors are natural or synthetic? ____

   If so, which are natural? ____________________

   Which are synthetic? ____________________

Name ____________________________________ Sheet 10-2

# CREATING SYNTHETIC SMELLS

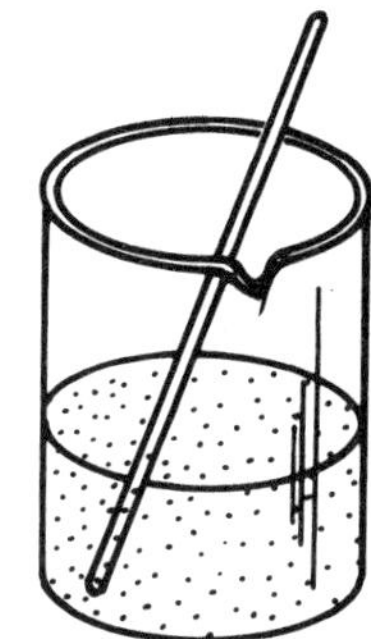

The flavors and fragrances of many fruits are due to the presence of esters. Esters are derivatives of acids in which the acid hydrogen is replaced by an alkyl radical. The general formula for an ester is R-CO-O-R[1]. In this experiment, you will convert two alcohols to their acetate esters by treating them with acetic acid and an acid catalyst (sulfuric acid).

**Materials:**

| | |
|---|---|
| ethanol | lab apron |
| isopentyl alcohol | china marker |
| glacial acetic acid | glass stirring rods |
| sulfuric acid | thermometer |
| 2 beakers | 2 beakers of warm water |
| 2 test tubes | 2 beakers, each containing 10 grams of crushed ice |
| graduated cylinder | test tube stand |
| test tube holder | |
| protective gloves | |



**Procedure:**

1. With a china marker, label the two beakers, one should be marked "ethyl acetate" and the other "3-methyl-1-butarol acetate."
2. Label the two test tubes, #1 "ethanol" and #2 "isopentyl alcohol."
3. Wearing a lab apron, measure 1 milliliter of glacial acetic acid in a graduated cylinder and pour 1 milliliter into each test tube. Rinse the graduate cylinder thoroughly after each use throughout the rest of this experiment.
4. Add 1 milliliter of ethanol to test tube #1 "ethanol."
5. Add 1 milliliter of isopentyl alcohol to test tube #2 "isopentyl alcohol."
6. Wearing protective gloves, gently swirl the contents of each tube in a test tube holder to mix them.
7. While swirling the test tube, cautiously add 1 ml. concentrated sulfuric acid to *each* tube. **(Caution: Handle sulfuric acid with care to avoid burns.)**
8. Place each tube in a beaker of warm (50° C ) water for five minutes.
9. Pour each mixture into a *separate* beaker containing 10 grams crushed ice. Stir each with a separate glass stirring rod.
10. Record the odor you smell from each beaker in the blanks below. Wave the odor toward your nose with your hand—do not smell directly from the beaker. **Caution: Do not taste these mixtures—they are *not* exactly the same as synthetic odor additives used in food and are dangerous if taken internally.**

**Reaction #1**

$$CH_3 - \overset{O}{C} - OH + CH_3 - CH_2 - OH \longrightarrow CH_3 - \overset{O}{C} - OC_2H_5 + H_2O$$

ODOR: _____

glacial acetic acid + ethanol ⟶ ethyl acetate + water

**Reaction #2**

$$CH_3 - \overset{O}{C} - OH + CH_3 - \underset{CH_3}{\overset{H}{C}} - CH_2 - CH_2 - OH \longrightarrow CH_3 - COOCH_2CH_2CH(CH_3)_2 + H_2O$$

glacial acetic acid + isopentyl alcohol ⟶ isopentyl acetate + water

ODOR: ____________________________________

Name ______________________________ Sheet 10-3

# CREATING NATURAL COLORS

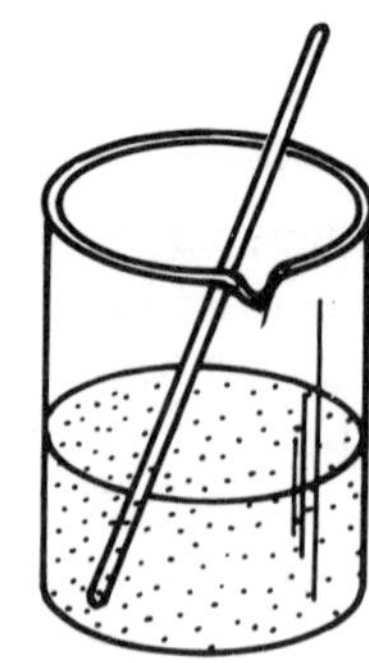

The colors of vegetables are due to naturally occurring pigments that are affected by acidic and basic conditions. Such conditions may occur in food handling and processing. Red anthocyanin, for example, is the main pigment in beets. When an hydroxyl group (-OH) is added to or removed from the pigment's chemical structure, due to acidic or basic conditions, the color changes. In this experiment, you will create two natural colors.

**Materials:** deionized water
acetic acid (vinegar)
sodium bicarbonate (baking soda)
diced beets (16-oz. can)
2 250-milliliter beakers
2 beaker stands
2 Bunsen burners
lab apron
asbestos mitt
china marker
graduated cylinder
lab scale
paper

**Procedure:**

1. With a china marker, label two beakers: #1 acid, #2 base.
2. Wearing a lab apron, measure 45 milliliters of deionized water in a graduated cylinder and add to each of the beakers.
3. Add 10 milliliters acetic acid (vinegar) to beaker #1, the acid. Rinse the graduated cylinder after each use throughout the rest of this experiment.
4. On a piece of paper, weigh 4 grams of sodium bicarbonate (baking soda) and add it to beaker #2, the base.
5. Place 85 grams (or 87 milliliters) of beets in each of the beakers.
6. Place each beaker on a beaker stand and heat with a Bunsen burner.
7. Record the color you observe in each beaker in the blanks below.

**Reaction #1**

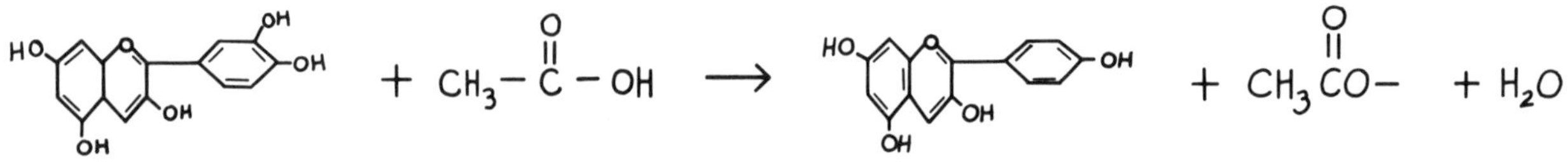

[structure: HO, OH, OH, OH, OH] $+ CH_3-\overset{\overset{O}{||}}{C}-OH \longrightarrow$ [structure: HO, OH, OH, OH] $+ CH_3\overset{\overset{O}{||}}{C}O- + H_2O$

<u>red</u> anthocyanin pigment — acetic acid (vinegar) — COLOR changes to: ____________ anthocyanin pigment

**Reaction #2**

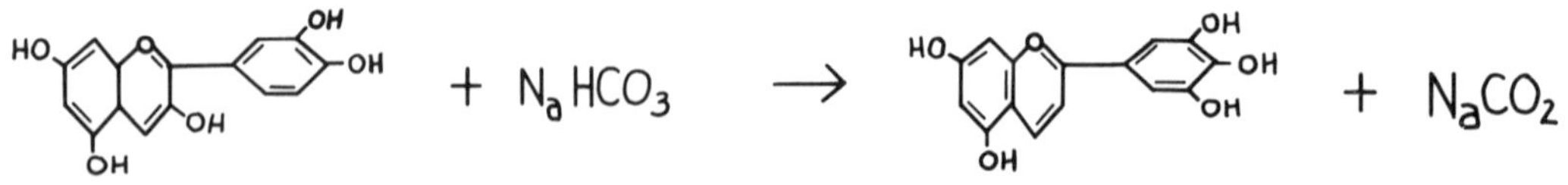

[structure: HO, OH, OH, OH, OH] $+ N_aHCO_3 \longrightarrow$ [structure: HO, OH, OH, OH, OH] $+ N_aCO_2$

<u>red</u> anthocyanin pigment — sodium bicarbonate (baking soda) — COLOR changes to: ______________________________ anthocyanin pigment

Name ______________________ **Sheet 10-4**

# DO YOU WANT TO EAT THIS FOOD?

**Directions:** Given a choice between the foods in each section below, select the one you would rather eat; then defend your choice in writing.

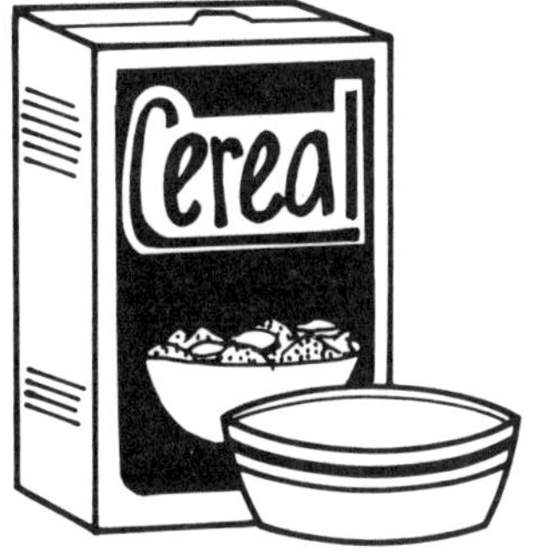


**1. Breakfast Cereals:**

a. ____ Ingredients: Degermed yellow cornmeal, oat flour, sugar, wheat starch, salt, dextrose, calcium carbonate, trisodium phosphate, sodium ascorbate, iron, niacin, Vitamin A palmitate, pyridoxine hydrochloride, riboflavin, thiamin mononitrate, Vitamin $B_{12}$, Vitamin $D_2$.

b. ____ Ingredients: Degermed yellow cornmeal, oat flour, sugar, wheat starch, salt, sodium ascorbate, artificial colors, citric acid, natural and artificial flavors.

Why did you make this selection? ______________________

______________________

______________________

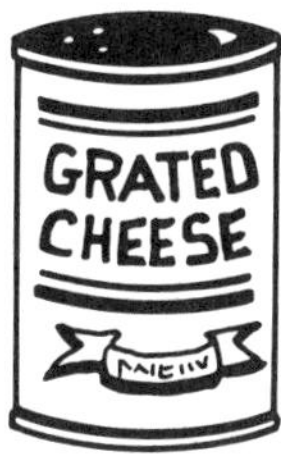


**2. Grated Cheese:**

a. ____ Ingredients: Parmesan cheese, part skim milk, cheese culture, salt, enzymes, calcium chloride.

b. ____ Ingredients: Sharp cheddar cheese, skim milk, whey, salt, sodium phosphate, artificial color, lactic acid.

Why did you make this selection? ______________________

______________________

______________________

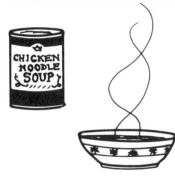

**3. Chicken Noodle Soup:**

a. ____ Ingredients: Water, enriched egg noodles, salt, chicken, chicken broth, natural flavorings, corn syrup, monosodium glutamate, hydrogenated vegetable oil, modified cornstarch, onions, wheat starch, chicken fat, potato starch, parsley, artificial coloring and flavoring.

b. ____ Ingredients: Water, egg noodles, chicken, carrots, salt, dextrose, soy oil, modified food starch, monosodium glutamate, onion powder, natural flavorings, garlic powder, paprika.

Why did you make this selection? ______________________

______________________

______________________

Name ______________________________ Sheet 10-5

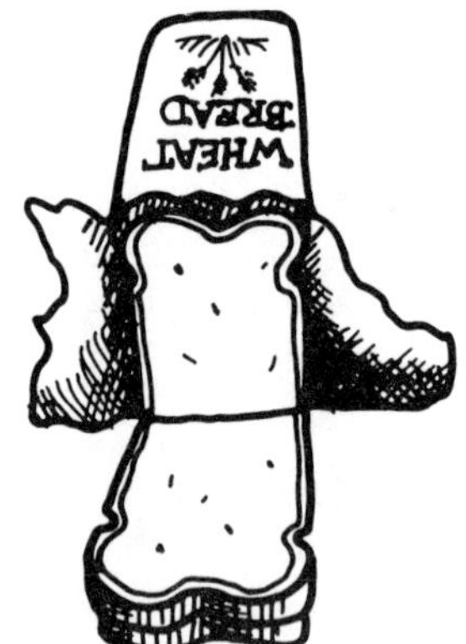


**4. Wheat Bread:**

a. _____ Ingredients: Whole wheat flour, water, whey, molasses, corn syrup, yeast, vegetable shortening, mono- and diglycerides, monocalcium phosphate, calcium propionate, salt, caramel color, barley malt.

b. _____ Ingredients: Wheat flour (bleached flour, malted barley flour), water, whole wheat flour, nonfat milk, brown sugar, yeast, salt, buttermilk, vegetable shortening, wheat gluten, corn syrup, honey, whey, yeast nutrients (calcium sulfate, ammonium chloride, potassium bromate), mono- and diglycerides, dough conditioner, corn flour, soy flour, calcium propionate, calcium peroxide (a bleaching agent).

Why did you make this selection? ______________________________

______________________________

______________________________

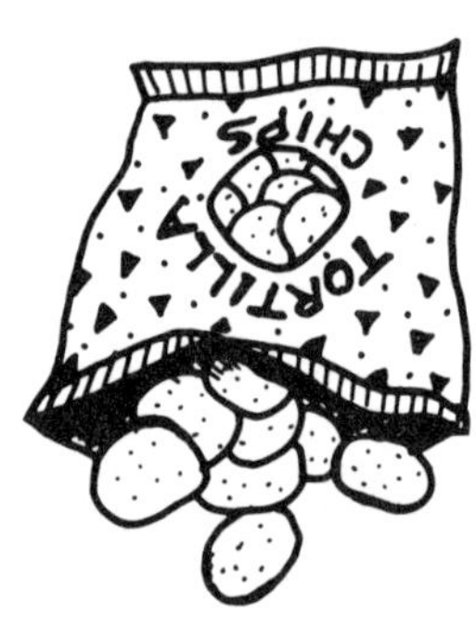


**5. Tortilla Chips:**

a. _____ Ingredients: Corn, soybean oil, salt, yeast, onion, spices, corn flour, carob powder, garlic, monosodium glutamate, caramel color, citric acid, paprika extract.

b. _____ Ingredients: Corn, vegetable oil, whey solids, salt, Romano cheese, wheat flour, onion, tomato, monosodium glutamate, Parmesan cheese, dextrose, cheddar cheese, sugar, citric acid, extract of tumeric, garlic, hydrolyzed cereal solids, artificial color, spice, bleu cheese, disodium inosinate, and guanylate.

Why did you make this selection? ______________________________

______________________________

______________________________

# QUIZ
# INTERPRETING INGREDIENT LABELS: COSMETIC FOOD ADDITIVES

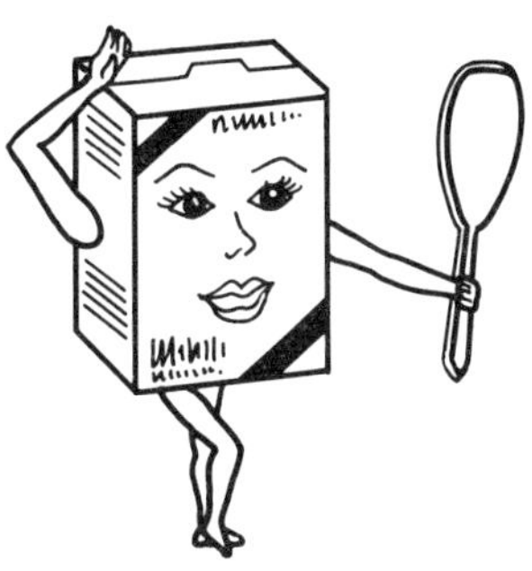

____ 1. Which group of food additives is not important to good health?

a. Preservatives
b. Colorings
c. Nutrients
d. All of the above

____ 2. Which of the following is a food additive?

a. FD&C Yellow #5
b. Caramel flavoring
c. Salt
d. All of the above

____ 3. Which of the following is a cosmetic food additive?

a. Natural flavor
b. Reduced iron
c. FD&C Red #3
d. Both (a) and (c)

____ 4. Which of the following would be most likely to appear on a cereal box?

a. D&C Yellow #5
b. FD&C Red #3
c. Ext D&C Orange B
d. FD&A Brown #2

____ 5. Which of the following is one benefit of using cosmetic additives in foods?

a. Makes the food look and taste better
b. Increases its nutritional quality
c. Makes it safer to eat
d. Helps keep the food fresh longer

____ 6. When is it illegal to use color and flavor additives?

a. When they allow the food to be processed more cheaply
b. When they increase the food's appeal to the customer
c. When they cover or disguise spoiled or impure food
d. When the additive is not natural

# Unit 11: Getting the Most for Your Food Dollar

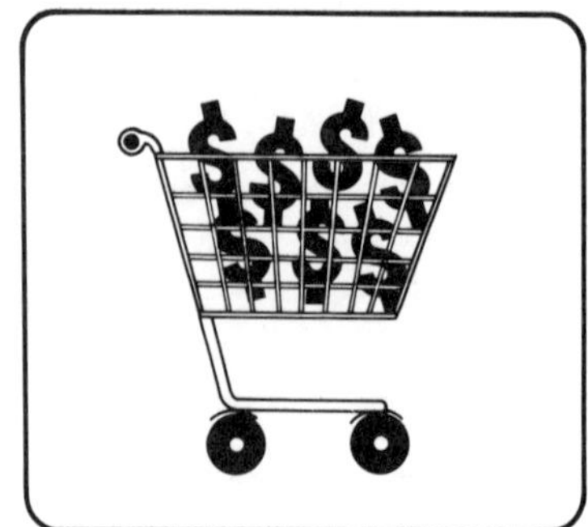

## CONCEPTS

–Comparative food shopping means comparing the cost of food to its nutritive value in order to get more nutrition at lower prices.

–Foods of limited nutritional value ("empty-calorie" foods) are usually poor buys because they offer few nutrients at high prices.

–The food purchaser must analyze the availability and price of foods at different markets.

## OJBECTIVES

–Students will compare different types of food stores.

–Students will calculate the cost of a nutrient from different food markets and the cost of a nutrient from various types of food.

–Students will be able to discriminate between good shopping habits and poor ones.

–Students will be able to categorize foods on a shopping list as either nutritious or empty-calorie foods.

## TEACHER'S UNIT INTRODUCTION

Shopping for groceries when a person is unprepared or impulsive can lead to disastrous results in terms of both nutrition and costs. This style of grocery shopping can sometimes lead to dissatisfied feelings and a sense of being "ripped off." You can avoid these unpleasant feelings by learning to shop wisely.

Planning menus and preparing a shopping list will help prepare you for an efficient shopping trip. Once the meals are planned and a shopping list is made, the consumer can enter the grocery store with some degree of confidence. However, there are many things to be aware of once you begin your actual shopping. To make the most of your food dollar, there is one important guideline to follow: *compare nutrients to cost.* Being a comparative food shopper allows you to buy the most nutritious foods for the least amount of money.

Customers can comparison shop by comparing the cost of foods per serving and the cost of certain nutrients per serving of food. It is important to remember that a food might be nutrient-dense in more than one nutrient, so the higher price might still be worth the money. Formulas for comparison shopping include:

$$\text{Cost per serving} = \text{Total price of food} \div \text{Number of servings}$$

$$\text{Cost of nutrient per serving} = \frac{\text{Total price of food} \div \text{Amount of nutrient in food}}{\text{Number of servings}}$$

The cost per serving, or the price of nutrients in a serving, are not the only ways to measure cost. As we all know, convenience foods have become an important part of many persons' daily food intake; hence, the cost of convenience should also be measured. Convenience foods reduce the amount of time and work needed to prepare a meal. Food preparers spend less time shopping, less time preparing meals, and less time cleaning up afterwards when using convenience foods. Saving time is appealing to many people. The working mother who has a limited amount of time or the person who dislikes cooking are perfect examples. There are many reasons why people choose to use convenience foods. Nevertheless, a wise consumer has to decide if the convenience is worth the price.

Today's supermarkets, with their enormous variety and selection, can confuse even the most conscientious comparative shopper. Similar foods come in different-sized packaging, different forms (frozen, canned, dried, fresh), different combinations, and from different manufacturers. Comparing nutrients to cost is not always an easy task. In addition to comparing nutrients to cost, it is important to compare nutrients to calories for the most nutritious bargain. To do this, remember our definition of empty-calorie foods. Empty-calorie foods are ones that offer little nutritionally, except for calories. Empty-calorie foods include the following:

alcoholic beverages
cake icings (depending on ingredients)
some cakes, pies, and other sweetened baked goods (depending on ingredients)
candy (especially hard candies, licorice, gumdrops, taffy, caramels)
chewing gum
corn syrup
frozen ices, unfortified
fruit drinks, unfortified
honey
jam
jelly
ketchup
maple syrup
soft drinks
sugar, brown sugar, or raw sugar

When shopping for nutrition, it is important to remember to limit the amount of empty-calorie foods purchased. Nutritious foods are usually a better bargain, in the long run, than empty-calorie foods. They are economical and significant contributors to nutritious meals.

There are a variety of stores where a person can shop for food. Knowledge of the differences among the stores can be very beneficial to you as a consumer. One type, the convenience store, is usually located in neighborhoods and is open long hours. Even though a convenience store has many advantages, its major disadvantage is that its prices are higher than those in supermarkets. Cost is also higher in specialty stores such as bakeries and delicatessens. A supermarket is a retail store that is less expensive than the convenience or specialty store. This is where the majority of consumers shop for food each week. A discount supermarket, as the name implies, is even less expensive than the regular supermarket. The lower prices found there are possible only because consumers are provided fewer conveniences. For example, at discount supermarkets shoppers have to bag groceries themselves (sometimes providing their own bags or purchasing them). In addition, the discount store is usually open fewer hours, and it provides less variety in the sizes, styles, and selection of products. Discount stores are only a bargain if the cost of getting to the store is not great and if the store offers you the food you want to buy in the quantities you want to buy it in.

Selecting the store is not the only problem in food shopping. You may also encounter some problems once inside the store. These problems may prevent you from getting the most nutrients for the lowest price. Some include:

**1. Problems in the Marketplace**

a. *Placement of foods:* Marketers strategically place high-profit food items on the shelf so that the consumers are tempted to buy the foods they do not really need. For example, highly sugared cereals are generally placed at eye level (or at children's eye level), whereas less-sugary cereals are placed on very low or very high shelves. Often, the more nutritious choices, which are often lower-profit items as well, are placed on lower shelves in the store.

b. *Specials:* Items are often displayed with "Special" tags at the ends of aisles or amidst the aisles. Some of these really are specials and are reduced in price; others are selling at the regular price. Consumers are enticed into buying the items because they think they are getting a bargain. The foods that are placed on "special" may not always be the most nutritious or even the most economical.

c. *Cost:* Today it seems that nutritious foods are the "in" thing. Marketers are jumping on the bandwagon by advertising foods as "nutritious," "all-natural," or "wholesome." While many of these products may be more nutritious choices, their advertisements and popularity have pushed the prices up. Many of these foods are not nutritious bargains at the current prices. In addition, the nutrient densities of these foods may be relatively low. For example, the natural-style granolas have so much honey, brown sugar, or other sweeteners that they are high in calories compared to their other nutrient contributions.

**2. Weaknesses in the Consumer:**

a. *Impulse buying:* One of the biggest problems facing the wise shopper is his or her own tendency to buy impulsively. To avoid impulse buying, remember these hints:

- Avoid shopping when hungry.
- Use a shopping list.
- Buy only necessary items; select only one or two luxury items.
- Shop alone or with a conscientious partner.
- Allow enough time for careful decision making.
- Read labels.
- Be aware of the effects of advertisements.

b. *Habits:* Consumers often buy out of habit. They buy what their mother or father bought, or what they have been buying for years. Food items change, and so can eating habits. It is important to be flexible enough to change brands or types of foods in order to get the most nutritious bargains.

---

The problems listed above are only a sampling of those consumers encounter in the supermarket. Teenagers may be especially susceptible to impulsive buying and subtle advertising. Unit 11 is designed to teach students some of the ways to make shopping a "nutritious" and satisfying experience.

The following activities attempt to show how important it is to be a wise consumer in today's high-priced world. It should be kept in mind, however, that the lower price is not always the best bargain. Some foods may cost more but they could also be more nutrient-dense. If the "cook" lacks culinary skills to prepare a meal, using a convenience food to improve the palatability of the meal might be worth the extra money. It is also important to remember that there are still some convenience foods that are cheaper than their homemade or fresh counterparts. For instance, some vegetables are cheaper when they are canned or frozen compared to similar fresh produce, especially when the fresh produce is out of season. Besides saving time in preparation, there are other reasons why canned or frozen vegetables are useful. The extended shelf life of these products can be a convenience to the consumer.

While completing this unit, it should become clear to students that consumerism is a skill that has to be learned and practiced before it is mastered. For increasing numbers of people, this skill is becoming a way to ease the impact of higher prices.

## BASIC ACTIVITY

**Time Needed:** One class period

**Materials Needed:** Food composition table (*see* References/Resources")
Sheet 11-1: "Grocery Price List" (five copies for entire class)

Sheets 11-2 through 11-6: "Shopping for Bargains" (one copy of each for the entire class)
Calculators *(optional)*
Sheet 11-7: "Grocery Shopping Hints"
Quiz Sheet 11-1

1. Divide the class into five groups.

2. Distribute one copy of Sheet 11-1, "Grocery Price List," to each group and Sheets 11-2 through 11-6, "Shopping for Bargains," by giving Sheet 11-2 to group one, Sheet 11-3 to group two, and so on so that each group is assigned to a different nutrient.

3. Explain to students that they are going to compare the prices of nutrients from various food sources.

4. Student groups should complete Sheets 11-2 through 11-6 as follows:

- Complete column 1 by using Sheet 11-1, "Grocery Price List."
- Complete column 2 by filling in the amount of nutrient per food-consumption unit using a food composition table.
- Complete column 3 by calculating the amount of nutrient in the purchased unit. For example, if there are 6 grams of protein in one egg, how much protein is contained in a dozen eggs?

$$\frac{6 \text{ grams of protein}}{1 \text{ egg}} = \frac{\times \text{ grams of protein}}{12 \text{ eggs in a dozen}}$$

$$\times = \frac{12 \text{ eggs} \times 6 \text{ grams of protein}}{1 \text{ egg}}$$

$$\times = 72 \text{ grams of protein}$$

- For column 4 calculate what portion of the purchased food would have to be consumed in order to receive one-half of the U.S. RDA for that nutrient (see table on Sheet 11-1). [We do not calculate for 100 percent of the U.S. RDA because most individuals do not require the entire U.S. RDA (refer to Unit 7 of *Nutrition Curriculum Activities Kit, Level 1,* for a description of the U.S. RDA). One-half of the U.S. RDA is adequate for most students because the U.S. RDAs represent the highest RDAs for any age or sex group (usually 18-year-old males.] The students should round their answer to the nearest hundredth. For example, what portion of the dozen eggs would be required to supply one-half of the daily requirement for high-quality protein? (Divide 22.5 by the answer in column 3.)

$$\times = \frac{22.5 \text{ grams of protein}}{72 \text{ grams of protein}}$$

$$\times = .31 \text{ dozen eggs would provide 22.5 grams of protein}$$

- For column 5 calculate what it costs to consume the specified amount of nutrient in column 4. For example, what does it cost to consume .31 dozen eggs? (Multiply column 4 by the cost found in column 1.)

| .31 × 99¢ = 31¢ |
|---|

5. Have students rank each food from 1 to 8 according to the best buy, with 1 being the best buy. Have them look at the amount that must be consumed to meet ½ of the RDA as well as the price for that amount.

6. Discuss the results. Do the students find this to be useful information? Why? Are there any products that are rich sources of more than one nutrient? What other foods would students like to compare?

7. Distribute Sheet 11-7, "Grocery Shopping Hints."

8. Discuss each grocery shopping hint and have students explain why each hint would help them save food dollars.

9. Have students add to the list other hints for saving food dollars.

10. Proceed with the "Advanced Activity" if you wish; otherwise use the quiz mentioned in step 11.

11. **Evaluation:** Distribute Quiz Sheet 11-1 and have students complete it independently. Discuss the answers as a class.

## ADVANCED ACTIVITY

**Time Needed:** One class period

**Materials Needed:** Sheets 11-8 through 11-9: "Tips for Cutting Food Costs"
Sheets 11-10 through 11-11: "Comparison Food Shopping"
Food containers from:
(1) eggs–different sizes and/or grades
(2) canned foods–different brands and/or sizes of the same food
(3) milk–different forms (fresh, dry, evaporated)
(4) snack foods–different sizes or brands of similar types
(5) juice or juice drinks–frozen, canned, fresh, powdered
Quiz Sheet 11-1

1. Conduct an "either/or" forced choice activity in the following manner:

- Have all of the students stand in the middle of the room.
- Read the choices below (*a* through *h*), one at a time.

- Have students move to one side of the room if they identify with the first word and to the other side of the room if they identify with the second word.
- Have them pair off with someone on the same side of the room and discuss why they made that choice.
- Before the next pair of choices is read, students should return to the middle of the room.
- Here are some pairs of choices to use:

"When you go to the grocery store, do you usually buy... (Or, "...would you buy..."):

a. soft drinks or fruit juices?
b. packaged cookies or whole-grain crackers?
c. piece of fruit or candy bar?
d. presweetened cereal or oatmeal?
e. peanuts or hard candy?
f. caramels or raisins?
g. oatmeal-raisin cookies or vanilla wafers?
h. [create other pairs]

2. Review with students the concept of empty calories. Ask: What are empty-calorie foods? How do they compare in cost to other foods? Are they a good choice for people on a low budget?

3. Have students read Sheets 11-8 through 11-9, "Tips for Cutting Food Costs," independently. Then discuss each item as a class.

4. Set up a "mock grocery store." In order to save time, you may want to set up the store before class or while students are reading Sheets 11-8 and 11-9. Collect food containers of the five types of food items that students might want to purchase (see "Materials"). Try to provide containers that represent different forms of the same food (for example, frozen, dried, fresh, canned), or different brands of the same food.

5. Have students comparison shop in the mock grocery store using Sheets 11-10 through 11-11, "Comparison Food Shopping."

6. Students should determine the food that would be the best selection for them from among similar foods in the mock grocery store. To arrive at each food-purchase selection, have students consider factors, in addition to economy, such as convenience of preparation and storage, and attractiveness.

7. In a large-group discussion, ask them questions like these: Which food item in each group was the most economical buy? Which food items did you decide to buy? Why? Would your answers be different if you had a limited (or unlimited) food budget? Would they be different if you had little time (or a lot of time) to prepare meals? Which would you select if you had no refrigerator or had limited freezer or storage space?

8. Review shopping behaviors that may or may not lead to nutritious bargains.

9. **Evaluation:** Distribute Quiz Sheet 11-1 and have students complete it independently. Discuss the answers as a class.

## FOLLOW-UP ACTIVITIES

1. Have students, independently, make a shopping list for a family (or group) of four for a week. Alternatively, have them make a shopping list for one meal, or for one day, for their own family. Have them record food items and amounts. Then conduct a large-group discussion to decide which foods are of limited nutritional value and which foods are nutritious. Then have them find the costs of several brands or forms (for example, canned, frozen, fresh) of each item by visiting a local grocery store. This type of real-life experience is important for many reasons. The most important reason is the fact that an experimental activity better prepares the students for real-life experiences. However, if a field trip or individual excursions to the grocery store are not possible, collect food containers of the food items students might want to "purchase" prior to the activity. Be sure the prices are marked on the containers. Then have students calculate the total cost of their menus. Have students calculate the cost of their menus per person. Once students have gathered this information, have them return to a large-group discussion. Ask them questions like these: What was the cost of your menu? Compare that cost to other students' menu costs. Was your menu cost higher or lower? Why? Also, discuss shopping behaviors that may or may not lead to nutritious bargains.

2. Have each student make a list of ten food products that are sold in different-sized packages in a supermarket. As an outside assignment, have them go to the market and locate these products. They should record:

- The product–type and brand name
- The size and cost per unit (ounce, gram, etc.) of the large package
- The size and cost per unit of the small package

In class, have students calculate how much it costs per unit to buy the amount in the larger packages and the per-unit cost of the smaller packages. They should then calculate the differences between the per-unit costs. An example is given below:

A pound of processed cheese spread costs $1.87, or 11.7¢ per ounce for the pound container. An 8-oz. box costs $1.08, or 13.5¢/ounce for the half-pound container. How much more does it cost to buy 1 pound of cheese spread in 8-oz. boxes than in a 1-pound box?

| | | | |
|---|---|---|---|
| half-pound box | = | 13.5¢/oz. or | $2.16 per pound |
| pound box | = | 11.7¢/oz. or | 1.87 per pound |
| | | | $ .29 more per pound |

Discuss the results of the comparisons. Is there a savings in all cases? Did the smaller package ever turn out to be less expensive per unit than the larger package? Do students find this to be useful information?

3. Invite a manager of a food corporation to discuss alternative marketing systems.

4. Conduct an open discussion of "What is a nutritious bargain?" Is it more important to compare nutrients to cost? Or to compare nutrients to calories? Or both?

5. Have different groups of students visit different food markets. Have them draw floor plans of the store layouts, including where the various foods are shelved. Also have them note end-of-aisle displays, music, announcements, or other promotional techniques. Have them return to class for a large-group discussion of their findings. Are stores designed the way they are for a reason? Why?

6. Invite a grocer to class to discuss the marketing and retail business. Perhaps the grocer would also lead the students on a guided tour of the market.

Name ____________________ Sheet 11-1

# GROCERY PRICE LIST

| Product | Purchase Unit | Price |
|---|---|---|
| Bacon (20 slices/pound) | 1 pound | $1.79 |
| Beef, regular ground | 1 pound | 1.69 |
| Eggs, Grade A, large | 1 dozen | .99 |
| Liver, beef | 1 pound | .99 |
| Tuna, light, oil-packed | 6½ ounces | 1.15 |
| Cottage cheese, small curd | 12 ounces | .79 |
| Ice cream, chocolate | ½ gallon | 2.69 |
| Milk, whole | 1 gallon | 2.07 |
| Milk, 2% butterfat | 1 gallon | 2.05 |
| Milk, nonfat dry | 4 pounds (20 qts. fluid) | 5.63 |
| Milk, evaporated | 13 ounces | .49 |
| Pasteurized processed cheese spread | 1 pound | 1.89 |
| Swiss cheese | 1 pound | 2.89 |
| Corn flakes | 12 ounces | .83 |
| Graham crackers | 1 pound | 1.19 |
| Oatmeal, quick oats | 1 pound 2 ounces | .65 |
| White bread, enriched (22 slices/loaf) | 1 loaf (23 ounces) | .79 |
| Margarine (32 tbsp./pound) | 1 pound | .57 |
| Applesauce (9 oz./cup) | 25 ounces | .83 |
| Orange | 8 | .99 |
| Orange juice, frozen, store brand | 16 ounces (64 oz. diluted) | 1.29 |
| Orange juice, frozen, name brand | 16 ounces (64 oz. diluted) | 1.67 |
| Prune juice | 40 fluid ounces | 1.15 |
| Raisins, seedless | 15 ounces | 1.69 |
| Broccoli, frozen, chopped (6.6 oz./cup) | 10 ounces | .53 |
| Carrots, canned, sliced (5.6 oz./cup) | 1 pound | .40 |
| Green beans, frozen (5.7 oz./cup) | 9 ounces | .55 |
| Peas, canned (6.6 oz./cup) | 1 pound | .44 |
| Pumpkin, canned (8.6 oz./cup) | 16 ounces | .49 |
| Sauerkraut, canned (6.6 oz./cup) | 16 ounces | .39 |
| Spinach, frozen, leaf (6.7 oz./cup) | 20 ounces | .89 |

**U.S. RDAs**

| | |
|---|---|
| Protein–high-quality only | 45 g. |
| –low-quality only | 65 g. |
| Vitamin A | 5,000 IUs |
| Vitamin C | 60 mg. |
| Thiamin | 1.5 mg. |
| Riboflavin | 1.7 mg. |
| Niacin | 20 mg. |
| Calcium | 1.0 g. |
| Iron | 18 mg. |

# SHOPPING FOR BARGAINS
## PROTEIN

| Food Source | 1 Cost / Purchase Unit | 2 Amount Protein / Food Composition Unit | 3 Amount Protein / Purchase Unit | 4 Portion of Purchased Unit Consumed to Receive 1/2 U.S. RDA of Protein | 5 Cost of 1/2 U.S. RDA Protein | 6 Rank |
|---|---|---|---|---|---|---|
| Bacon, fried crisp (low-quality) | | | | | | |
| Beef, regular ground, broiled (high-quality) | | | | | | |
| Swiss cheese (high-quality) | | | | | | |
| Milk, whole (high-quality) | | | | | | |
| Tuna, light, oil-packed (high-quality) | | | | | | |
| Liver, beef, fried (high-quality) | | | | | | |
| Oatmeal, quick oats (low-quality) | | | | | | |
| Eggs, Grade A, large (high-quality) | | | | | | |

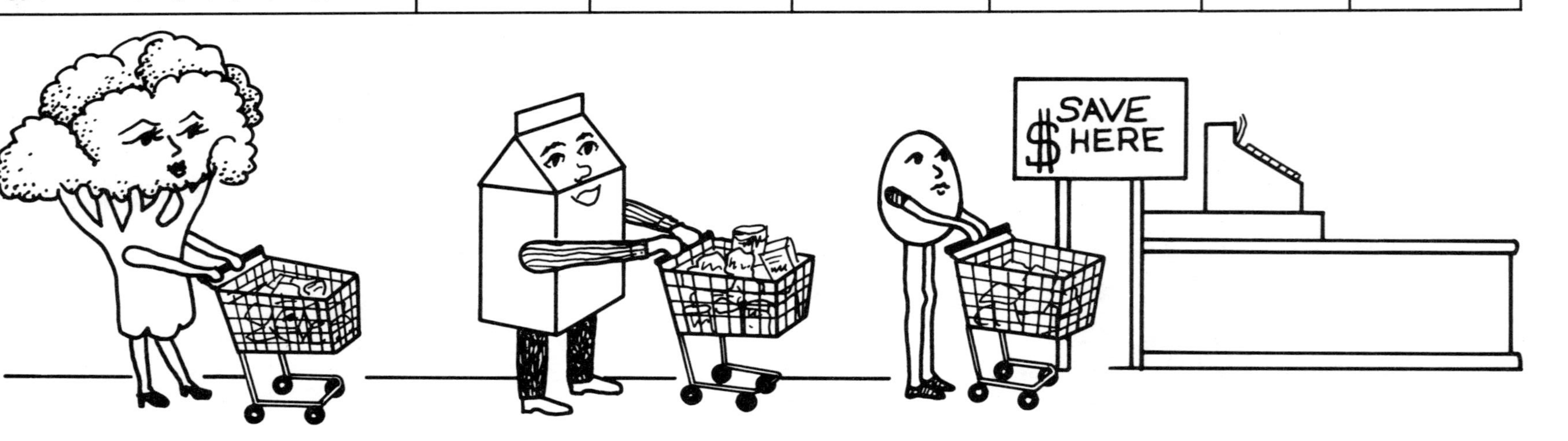

# SHOPPING FOR BARGAINS
# IRON

| Food Source | 1 Cost / Purchase Unit | 2 Amount Iron / Food Composition Unit | 3 Amount Iron / Purchase Unit | 4 Portion of Purchased Unit Consumed to Receive 1/2 U.S. RDA of Iron | 5 Cost of 1/2 U.S. RDA Iron | 6 Rank |
|---|---|---|---|---|---|---|
| Liver, beef, fried | | | | | | |
| Beef, regular ground, broiled | | | | | | |
| Peas, canned | | | | | | |
| White bread, enriched | | | | | | |
| Corn flakes | | | | | | |
| Graham crackers, 2½″ squares | | | | | | |
| Prune juice | | | | | | |
| Raisins | | | | | | |

# SHOPPING FOR BARGAINS
# CALCIUM

| Food Source | 1 Cost / Purchase Unit | 2 Amount Calcium / Food Composition Unit | 3 Amount Calcium / Purchase Unit | 4 Portion of Purchased Unit Consumed to Receive 1/2 U.S. RDA of Calcium | 5 Cost of 1/2 U.S. RDA Calcium | 6 Rank |
|---|---|---|---|---|---|---|
| Milk, whole | | | | | | |
| Milk, 2% butterfat | | | | | | |
| Milk, evaporated | | | | | | |
| Milk, nonfat, dry | | | | | | |
| Cottage cheese, small curd | | | | | | |
| Swiss cheese | | | | | | |
| Processed cheese spread | | | | | | |
| Ice cream, chocolate | | | | | | |

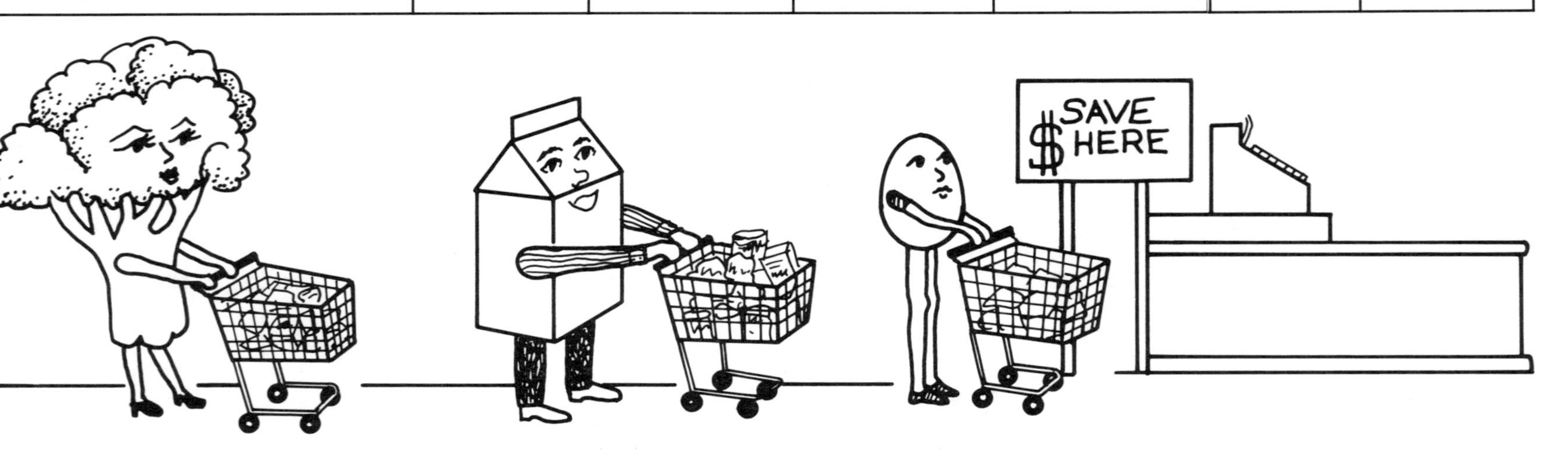

# SHOPPING FOR BARGAINS
# VITAMIN C

| Food Source | Cost / Purchase Unit [1] | Amount Vitamin C / Food Composition Unit [2] | Amount Vitamin C / Purchase Unit [3] | Portion of Purchased Unit Consumed to Receive 1/2 U.S. RDA of Vitamin C [4] | Cost of 1/2 U.S. RDA Vitamin C [5] | Rank [6] |
|---|---|---|---|---|---|---|
| Orange | | | | | | |
| Orange juice, frozen, diluted, store brand | | | | | | |
| Orange juice, frozen, diluted, name brand | | | | | | |
| Broccoli, frozen | | | | | | |
| Sauerkraut, canned, solids, and liquids | | | | | | |
| Applesauce | | | | | | |
| Prune juice | | | | | | |
| | | | | | | |

# SHOPPING FOR BARGAINS VITAMIN A

| Food Source | Cost / Purchase Unit (1) | Amount Vitamin A / Food Composition Unit (2) | Amount Vitamin A / Purchase Unit (3) | Portion of Purchased Unit Consumed to Receive 1/2 U.S. RDA of Vitamin A (4) | Cost of 1/2 U.S. RDA Vitamin A (5) | Rank (6) |
|---|---|---|---|---|---|---|
| Milk, whole | | | | | | |
| Margarine, Vitamin A fortified | | | | | | |
| Green beans, frozen | | | | | | |
| Spinach, frozen, leaf | | | | | | |
| Carrots, canned, sliced | | | | | | |
| Liver, beef, fried | | | | | | |
| Eggs, Grade A, large | | | | | | |
| Pumpkin, canned | | | | | | |

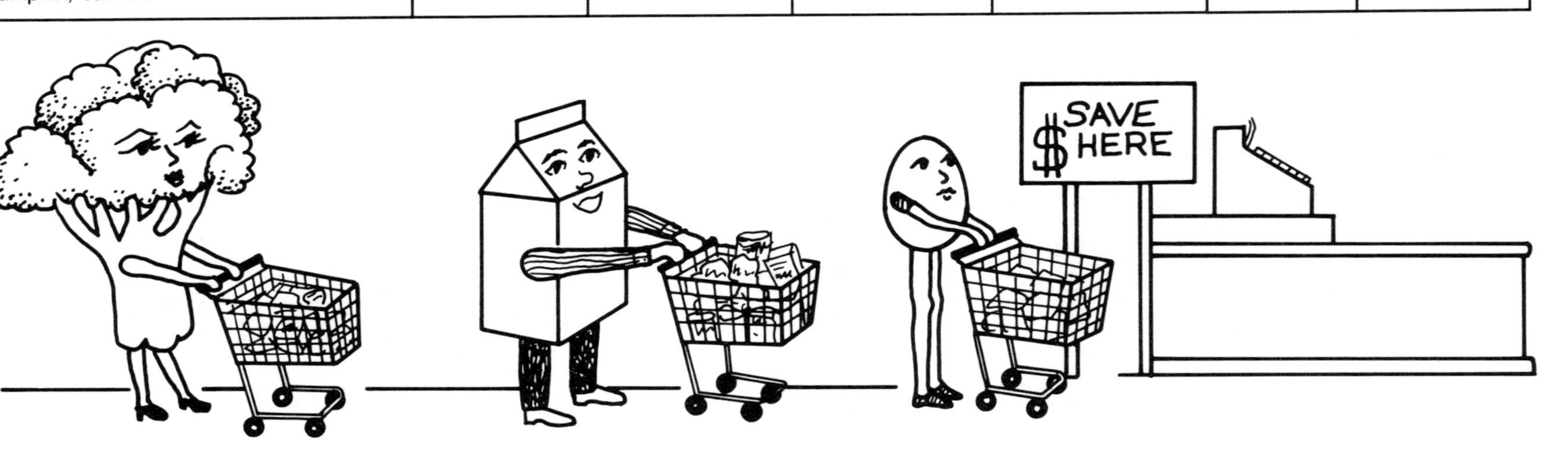

# GROCERY SHOPPING HINTS

1. Look for coupons in the local paper. These are useful *only* if the item will be used in the household. Beware that sometimes, even with coupons, name brands are still more expensive than generic brands.
2. Shop on sale days.
3. Shop as infrequently as possible.
4. Try not to stop in convenience stores. Take advantage of discount grocery stores.
5. Make a grocery list before going to the store. However, it's wise to be flexible with the list in order to take advantage of special sales.
6. Avoid shopping on an empty stomach.
7. Avoid impulse purchasing or "luxury" items.
8. Try to shop alone in order to decrease outside influences.
9. Minimize the use of convenience foods as much as possible (for example, frozen dinners) to save money. However, if saving time is important, convenience foods may be a solution.
10. Buy larger packages if you can properly store these items and if they are less expensive than multiple smaller units.
11. Decrease the amount of prime cuts of meat purchased.
12. Decrease the purchase of out-of-season fruits and vegetables.

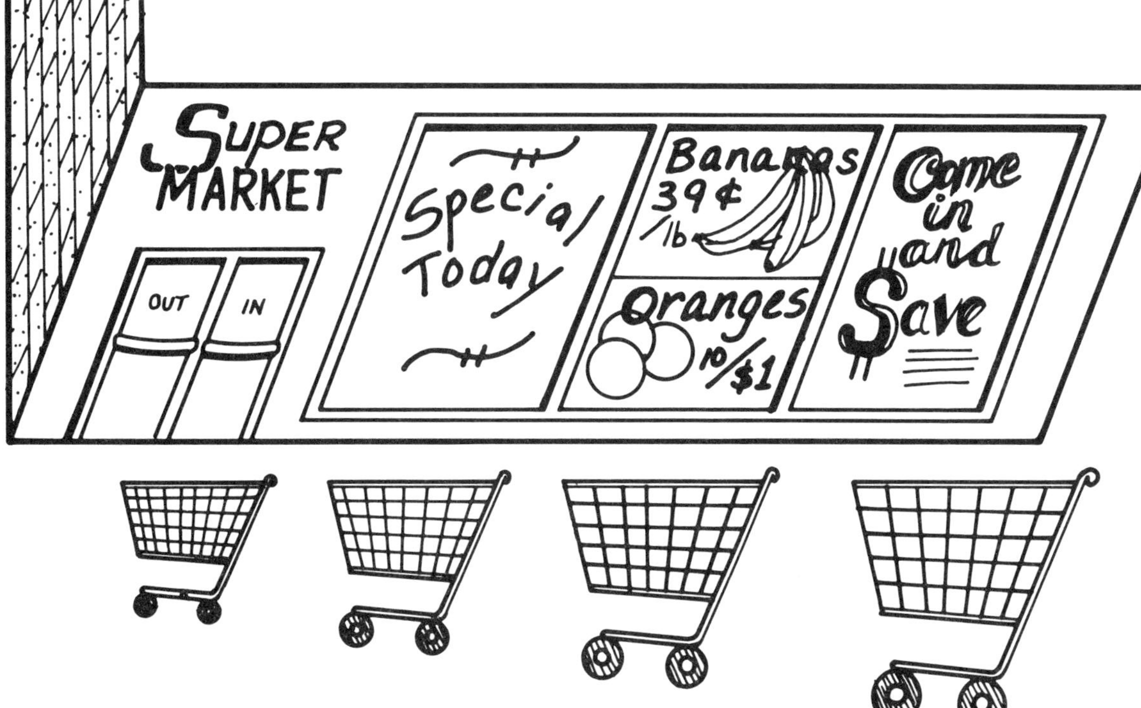

# TIPS FOR CUTTING FOOD COSTS

★ Select from cuts and types of meat, poultry, and fish that provide the most cooked meat for the money spent.

★ The "USDA Good" grade of beef is more lean and usually costs less per serving than "USDA Choice" or "USDA Prime" grades. The "USDA Good" grade is not quite as juicy or flavorful, however.

★ Use small servings of meat, poultry, and fish, and rely on more economical foods—potatoes, rice, macaroni, breads—to fill in meals.

★ Buy fresh fluid milk at a grocery or dairy store. Home-delivered milk and milk at convenience stores usually cost more.

★ Buy fresh milk in 1/2-gallon or 1-gallon sizes if you can use the milk before it spoils. The larger sizes of milk are usually a little cheaper than the quart size.

★ Use nonfat dried milk in cooking and as a beverage.

★ Check different forms of a food (fresh, canned, dehydrated, frozen) to see which is the best buy.

★ Buy only as much fresh food as you can use before it spoils.

★ Buy fruits and vegetables in season.

★ If you have room to store them, stock up on good buys of frozen or canned foods.

★ Try lower-priced brands of canned or frozen foods. Chain stores and less-advertised brands may be similar in quality to widely known products, yet cost less.

★ When shape, color, and uniformity of size are not important, try to select grade B ("Choice") or grade C ("Standard") canned products. Not all graded vegetables have the grade on the label.

★ Season and prepare sauces for frozen vegetables yourself, if you have the time. Frozen vegetables that come with sauce or butter are usually more expensive than plain, frozen vegetables.

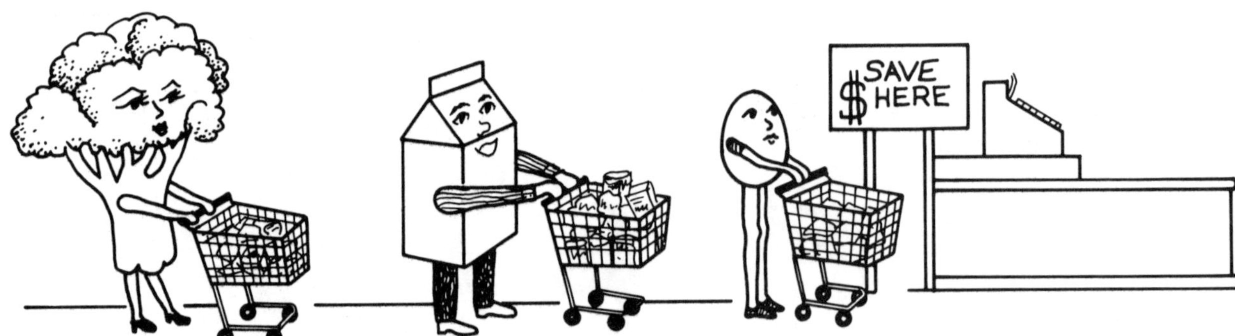

★ Buy regular rice instead of instant rice for the best buy.

★ Specialty breads often cost more than wheat bread with similar nutritional value.

★ Cereals you cook yourself are usually less expensive than the ready-to-serve ones.

★ Day-old breads and baked goods are often available at a great savings.

★ Buy ingredients and make homemade goods at less cost than ready-baked products.

★ Ground beef blended with textured soy protein is less expensive, is juicier, shrinks less, and has comparable flavor and nutrition as plain ground beef.

★ Buy whole chickens and cut them up yourself for savings over precut ones.

★ Buy large eggs when their price is no more than 7 cents higher than the medium size.

★ Buy cheese in large pieces or slice it yourself.

★ Buy juice instead of juice drinks or soft drinks for better nutritional value.

★ Avoid foods with sugar as the first or second ingredient.

★ Processed meats, such as bologna and frankfurters, have more fat and less protein than fresh meats, which makes processed meats a poor nutritional buy.

★ Avoid "gimmicky" or "novelty" foods. You are paying for the advertising and for the idea rather than for food value.

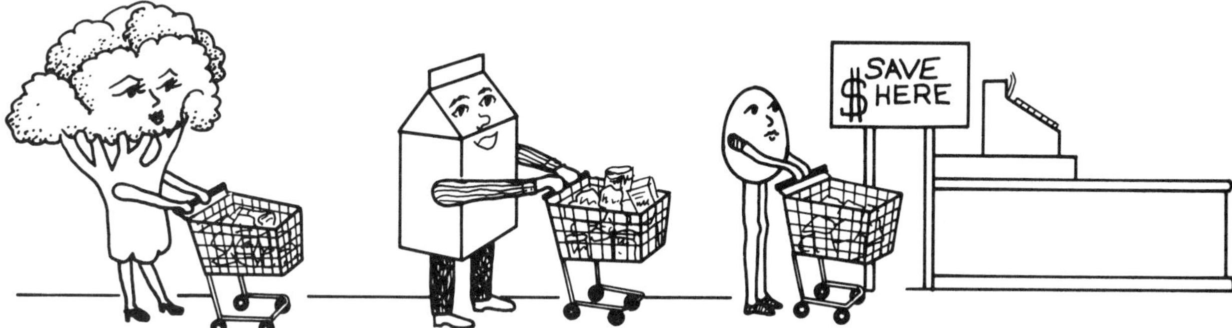

Name ______________________________ 

# COMPARISON FOOD SHOPPING

**Directions:** For each group of similar foods, determine the item that is the best selection for you. In addition to dollars and cents, also consider the convenience of food preparation and storage, taste, and attractiveness.

| Food Item | No. of Servings | Total Cost | Price per Serving |
|---|---|---|---|
| **Example** | | | |
| Orange Juice (food item) | | | |
| Choice 1 frozen | 6 | $ .48 | $ .08 |
| Choice 2 fresh | 16 | $1.44 | $ .09 |
| Choice 3 canned | 8 | $ .96 | $ .12 |
| 1. ________ | | | |
| Choice 1 ________ | ___ | ___ | ___ |
| Choice 2 ________ | ___ | ___ | ___ |
| Choice 3 ________ | ___ | ___ | ___ |
| 2. ________ | | | |
| Choice 1 ________ | ___ | ___ | ___ |
| Choice 2 ________ | ___ | ___ | ___ |
| Choice 3 ________ | ___ | ___ | ___ |
| 3. ________ | | | |
| Choice 1 ________ | ___ | ___ | ___ |
| Choice 2 ________ | ___ | ___ | ___ |
| Choice 3 ________ | ___ | ___ | ___ |
| 4. ________ | | | |
| Choice 1 ________ | ___ | ___ | ___ |
| Choice 2 ________ | ___ | ___ | ___ |
| Choice 3 ________ | ___ | ___ | ___ |
| 5. ________ | | | |
| Choice 1 ________ | ___ | ___ | ___ |
| Choice 2 ________ | ___ | ___ | ___ |
| Choice 3 ________ | ___ | ___ | ___ |

Name ______________________________



Remember: Price per serving = $\frac{\text{Total Cost}}{\text{Total number of servings}}$

Sample calculation: If one 32-oz. can of orange juice costs $.96, what is the price per serving?

32-oz. can = eight 4-oz. servings

price per serving = $\frac{\$.96 \text{ total cost}}{8 \text{ servings}}$

price per serving = $.12

For Food Item Example: Orange Juice
Which choice is the most economically priced? __1__
Which choice would you select? __2__
Why? Choice 2 is not much more expensive than Choice 1, and I have very little freezer space. Choice 2 would be the best selection for me.

For Food Item 1:
Which choice is the most economically priced? ____
Which choice would you select? ____
Why?

For Food Item 2:
Which choice is the most economically priced? ____
Which choice would you select? ____
Why?

For Food Item 3:
Which choice is the most economically priced? ____
Which choice would you select? ____
Why?

For Food Item 4:
Which choice is the most economically priced? ____
Which choice would you select? ____
Why?

For Food Item 5:
Which choice is the most economically priced? ____
Which choice would you select? ____
Why?

Name ______________________________ Quiz Sheet 11-1

# QUIZ
# GETTING THE MOST FOR YOUR FOOD DOLLAR

1. Select the shopping behaviors that you think are good ones by placing a check mark beside each item:

____ Eating before you shop
____ Buying soft drinks
____ Buying fruit drinks instead of fruit juices (for the same price)
____ Buying the same foods every week
____ Buying foods that are heavily advertised
____ Taking young children or friends shopping with you
____ Buying items that are ready-made
____ Using a shopping list
____ Buying whatever your mother or father buys
____ Shopping alone
____ Selecting products that catch your eye
____ Shopping when you are hungry
____ Reading labels

2. Here is Bill's shopping list for the week. He has less money than he expected, so he needs to eliminate some of the items on his list. He knows that foods of limited nutritional value are usually not nutritious bargains. To help Bill, place an EC next to each food that is an empty-calorie food.

____ Blackberry jelly
____ Bananas
____ Spinach
____ Carrots
____ Tomatoes
____ Potatoes
____ Canned corn
____ Eggs
____ Milk, skimmed
____ Granulated sugar
____ Nondairy creamer

____ Swiss cheese
____ Oatmeal
____ Maple syrup
____ Flour
____ Red Hots (cinnamon candies)
____ Canned buttercream frosting
____ Chocolate cake mix
____ Maraschino cherries
____ Ketchup
____ Dried navy beans
____ Rice
____ Lifesavers

3. On the back of this sheet, describe the distinct characteristics of convenience stores and of discount supermarkets that make them different from regular supermarkets. Discuss how the price of food is affected by the type of store in which it is purchased.

4. Name another cost that can be measured besides the cost per serving of a food:

______________________________________________

5. When comparing the cost of a nutrient in different foods, what has to be considered before they are ranked in a special order?

______________________________________________

______________________________________________

# Unit 12: Storing Foods to Preserve Nutrients

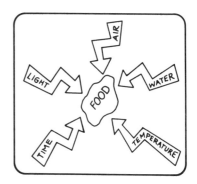


## CONCEPTS

–Improper storage of food can cause changes of food, including loss of nutrients and quality.

–These food losses may be affected by several factors such as light, temperature, water, air, and time.

–Properly wrapped and stored foods will retain their nutrients and quality.

–Some nutrients are lost more easily than others.

## OBJECTIVES

–By participating in a food-wrapping activity and completing the worksheets in this unit, students will

(1) practice a variety of methods for wrapping and storing foods
(2) identify which nutrients are most affected by improper storage
(3) name the factors that could lead to loss of these nutrients (light, temperature, water, air, time)

## TEACHER'S UNIT INTRODUCTION

How a food is stored determines how long it will keep its nutrients and quality. Improper or extended storage may lead to the loss of several nutrients or may cause the food to spoil and become unfit to eat.

Proper storage protects both the nutrients and the quality of a food. Quality can be judged by four important characteristics of food: flavor, odor, color, and texture. If a food maintains its quality, it usually maintains its nutrients.

Some nutrients in food are more likely to be lost than others. Of the Iron CaPAC nutrients, the ones that are the most likely to be lost are Vitamin C, Vitamin A, and the minerals calcium, and iron. Protein is not generally destroyed by normal, routine kitchen procedures. There are other nutrients in foods that may also be lost by improper storage, but we will focus only on the Iron CaPAC nutrients.

A variety of factors may cause the loss of each of these nutrients. These factors include light, heat, air, and water. Additionally, "time" could be considered a factor that encourages nutrient losses. All nutrient losses increase with time. The longer a food is stored, especially if it is stored improperly, the greater the nutrient losses will be.

Vitamin C is the most easily lost nutrient. It tends to be lost with exposure to air, heat, or water. The type of food, the maturity of the plant at harvest, the storage temperature, and other similar factors will determine exactly how much Vitamin C will be lost. If surfaces of foods containing Vitamin C are exposed to air, such as when a food is cut, some of the vitamin will be lost. More Vitamin C will be lost, for example, in the shredding of cabbage than when cabbage is cut in large wedges. Storage at high temperatures destroys Vitamin C and also causes more rapid losses into the air. Storage of Vitamin C-rich foods in the freezer causes very little loss of this vitamin. Vitamin C is a water-soluble vitamin, and if foods are stored or cooked in water or other liquid, the Vitamin C will dissolve and be lost if the liquid is discarded.

Vitamin A is not lost as easily as Vitamin C. Vitamin A may be lost if foods are exposed to air at room temperature for too long. Foods that are cut, bruised, or physically damaged in other ways may also lose some Vitamin A. Exposure to high temperatures or to water does not affect this vitamin.

Minerals such as iron or calcium may be lost by soaking foods in water. The minerals will leach out of food and into the water. If the water is discarded, these nutrients will be lost. Few other factors will destroy these minerals.

To prevent nutrient losses, foods should be stored in proper areas and in appropriate packaging or containers. Proper storage should keep foods at the proper temperature, protected from heat, light, and moisture, and clean and free from insects and other pests.

Three types of storage are appropriate for preserving the nutrients, quality, and safety of foods. Foods can be stored in dry storage, in a refrigerator, or in a freezer.

Dry storage is recommended for foods that are not perishable. Foods should be kept in a cool, dry area. Nonperishable items and unopened packaged foods, such as canned foods, cereals, sweeteners, oil, or spices can be kept in dry storage. Most items stored in dry storage should be kept in their original containers. If the containers have been opened, they should be tightly reclosed, transferred to clean, airtight containers, or refrigerated, if necessary.

The second type of storage is refrigeration. Perishable foods, such as dairy products, meat, poultry products, ripe fruits, and most vegetables (except potatoes, onions, and beets), are stored in the refrigerator. Potatoes, onions, and beets are best stored in a cool, *dry* place. Unripe fruits should be allowed to ripen before refrigerating them. The proper temperature for the maintenance of nutrients and freshness is 32°F to 45°F. Most foods stored in the refrigerator should not be kept for more than one week. Foods stored in the refrigerator should be tightly wrapped or placed in airtight containers. Improperly wrapped foods are likely to dry out and lose nutrients and flavor.

Freezing is the third method used for storage. Freezers are for long-term storage. The proper temperature is below 32°F (0°C). Many foods may be frozen from six months to one year without any great nutrient or quality losses. When packaging foods for freezer storage, it is important to do it properly because otherwise they have a tendency to dry out. Foods that are purchased already frozen may be stored in their original unopened containers. Other foods should be tightly packaged in plastic-coated freezer wrapping paper, heavy-duty aluminum foil, heavy plastic wrap or freezer bags, plastic-coated freezer cartons, or plastic containers with tight-fitting lids. To avoid exposing the nutrients to air, force as much air as possible out of the package and secure it tightly with freezer tape. When plastic containers are used, leave about one inch of space at the top between the food and the lid. This practice allows space for the food to expand during freezing without forcing the lid off and exposing the food to air. Label all frozen foods with the food name and the date of freezing. Use those foods with the oldest date first and regularly check them for length of storage time.

Remember that the importance of storing foods is to maintain three vital aspects of food: the nutrients in the food, the quality of the food in terms of color, odor, texture, and flavor, and the safety of the food.

---

Unit 12 illustrates changes in the quality of foods that may occur during storage. In this unit, a variety of different foods are stored properly and improperly to illustrate the changes that can take place. Foods are also wrapped differently to show how wrapping may affect a food.

The purpose of this unit is to show

- the changes that occur in foods that are improperly stored
- proper methods of storing and wrapping foods to preserve their nutrients as well as their quality and safety
- how some nutrients may be lost by improper storage

Before conducting discussions in the classrooom, take a look at the "Answer Key" to Quiz Sheets 12-1 and 12-2. Make sure to emphasize the words appearing in the word search puzzle during discussions.

Although this unit focuses mainly on storing foods to preserve nutrients and quality, it is important to point out to students that the most important reason for proper storage is to protect food from contamination and spoilage and to keep it safe to eat.

## BASIC ACTIVITY

**Time Needed:** Two class periods, one week apart

**Materials Needed:** Sheet 12-1: "The Case of the Lost Nutrients"
Sheets 12-2 through 12-4: "Wrapping It Up" (one copy of each for the class)

11 slices bread
3/4 pound cheddar cheese
6 carrots
3–4 bananas
6 ounces ground meat
6 ounces ice cream
lemon juice
plastic wrap
heavy plastic wrap (or freezer wrap)
aluminum foil
heavy-duty aluminum foil
waxed paper
3 plastic freezer or storage containers with lids
2 plastic sandwich bags
1 small bowl of water
1 small paper bag
5 paring knives
storage space in refrigerator, freezer, and dry storage area
10 china markers

Sheet 12-5: "Wrapping It Up Evaluation" (10 copies for class)
Quiz Sheets 12-1 through 12-2

**Class Period 1**

1. Discuss the importance of proper storage for the retention of nutrients. Include a discussion of how Iron CaPAC nutrients might be lost during storage.

2. Distribute Sheet 12-1, "The Case of the Lost Nutrients." Have students complete the worksheet independently; then discuss the answers as a class. Include in your discussion the ways to store or handle each food differently to minimize nutrient losses.

3. Divide the class into 10 groups. Cut apart and distribute one of the ten food-wrapping exercises on Sheets 12-2 through 12-4, "Wrapping It Up," and one copy of Sheet 12-5, "Wrapping It Up Evaluation," to each group. Also distribute to each group the appropriate food item and wrapping materials that go with each exercise.

4. Instruct the students to observe their fresh food item and record their initial observations on Sheet 12-5. They should use the food descriptors for accuracy.

5. Then each group should prepare and wrap the food item according to the exercise directions. Remind students to wrap foods intended for the freezer tightly in order to preserve their nutrients. (Or, you may add an additional variable to the exercise involving freezing by having one item wrapped tightly and one wrapped loosely.)

**Class Period 2** (1 week after Class Period 1)

1. Return the stored food items to the groups.

2. Have each group record its observations on Sheet 12-5, "Wrapping It Up Evaluation" and complete the questions at the end of the sheet. Students should use the food descriptors provided on the sheet for accurate descriptions.

3. Have the groups share their observations informally with students moving from one group station to another to examine the food item and read the "Wrapping It Up Evaluation" sheet results. Conduct a class discussion with the entire group and point out that although we cannot see nutrient losses, deterioration of the quality of a food and its nutrient losses usually occur together. In addition, the longer a food is stored, especially unsealed, the greater are the nutrient losses.

4. **Evaluation:** Distribute Quiz Sheets 12-1 and 12-2 and have students complete them independently. Present the answer key for the word search on an opaque or overhead projector or on the chalkboard. Discuss the answers as a class.

## FOLLOW-UP ACTIVITIES

**Materials Needed:** Sheet 12-6: "Storage Life of Food" (for activities #1 and #4)

1. Have students bring in empty food containers or use food models (*see* "References/ Resources" for this unit at the end of this kit). Be sure the food containers are clean and intact if you use them. Arrange the containers on a counter. Have students label three sheets of paper with the name of each major storage area: dry, refrigerator, freezer. Have students pretend to store each container by listing it on the appropriate sheet. Then discuss why each food is stored in that area and the proper length of time for storage (refer to Sheet 12-6, "Storage Life of Food").
2. Bring in samples of different types of packaging materials or storage containers for food. Discuss the types of storage that the packaging or containers are appropriate for and the advantages and disadvantages of each.
3. Take a field trip to a food-processing plant or a supermarket. Ask for a description of the food-wrapping and packaging procedures, if available. View the procedures; then discuss them in class.
4. Have students guess how long foods may be stored in each of the three different ways (dry, refrigerator, freezer). Confirm their answers with Sheet 12-6.

Name ______________________________ 

# THE CASE OF THE LOST NUTRIENTS

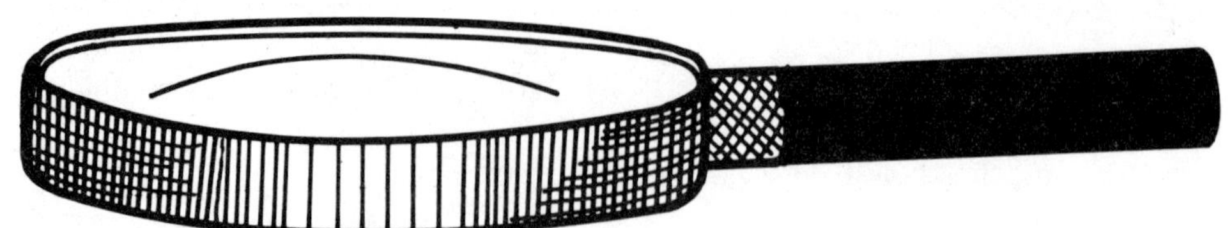

**Directions:** Below are six cases where a food was improperly handled or stored. Indicate in the chart at the bottom of the page which nutrients may have been lost and how they were lost. One case has been done for you as an example.

**Example:** Forgetful Fred forgot to put the orange juice in the refrigerator after breakfast. It sat out all day while he was at school.

1. Jean likes to munch on crisp, raw broccoli. She stores cut up broccoli in a bowl of water in the refrigerator to keep it crisp.
2. Henry is learning to juggle by practicing with apricots from the fruit basket. Unfortunately, he frequently drops them and then puts them back in the fruit basket.
3. Martha lost the lid to the orange juice jar, but doesn't have time to look for it. She puts the juice back in the refrigerator uncovered.
4. George found a "quick and easy" way to clean spinach. He soaks it overnight in a tightly closed bowl in the refrigerator and then discards the dirty water.
5. Margie buys stick margarine and then stores it in the cupboard to keep it soft enough to spread.
6. Jennifer was having a party. She wanted to make the fruit punch early, so she mixed it up and left it out on the kitchen counter while she continued to prepare some other snacks.

| Case | Food | Nutrient | How Lost? |
|---|---|---|---|
| Example | Orange juice | Vitamin C | Destroyed by warm temperature |
| | | | |
| | | | |
| | | | |
| | | | |
| | | | |
| | | | |

# WRAPPING IT UP

Buttery Bread

GROUP 1

FOOD ITEM: Bread

**Directions:** For each example, wrap and store one slice of bread as indicated. Number each example:

(1) freeze, unwrapped
(2) freeze, wrapped in heavy plastic wrap
(3) refrigerate, unwrapped
(4) refrigerate, wrapped in plastic wrap
(5) store in dry storage area, unwrapped

Buttery Bread

GROUP 2

FOOD ITEM: Bread

**Directions:** For each example, wrap one slice of bread as indicated and store in a *dry* storage area. Number each example.

(1) wrap in plastic wrap
(2) wrap in aluminum foil
(3) wrap in waxed paper
(4) store in plastic sandwich bag, closed
(5) store in paper bag, closed
(6) store in plastic container with lid

GROUP 3

FOOD ITEM: Cheddar Cheese

**Directions:** For each example, cut, wrap, and store 1 or 2 slices of cheese as indicated. Number each example.

(1) freeze, wrapped in heavy plastic wrap
(2) refrigerate, unwrapped
(3) store in dry storage area, wrapped in plastic wrap
(4) store in dry storage area, unwrapped

GROUP 4

FOOD ITEM: Cheddar Cheese

**Directions:** For each example, cut and wrap 1 or 2 slices of cheese as indicated and store in the refrigerator. Number each example.

(1) wrap in waxed paper
(2) wrap in aluminum foil
(3) store in plastic sandwich bag, closed
(4) wrap in plastic bag
(5) store in plastic container with lid
(6) leave remaining cheese in original wrapper and fold it over

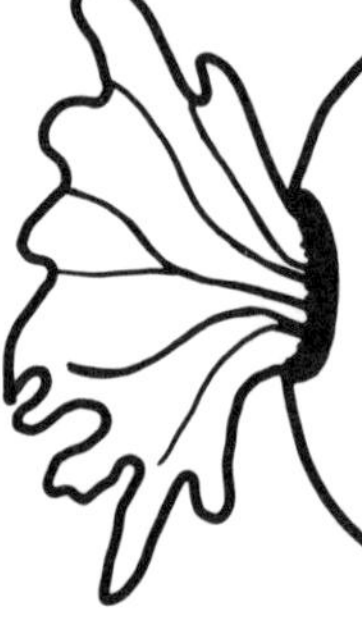

GROUP 5
FOOD ITEM: Carrot
**Directions:** For each example, wrap and store one carrot as indicated. Number each example.

(1) freeze, wrapped in heavy plastic wrap
(2) refrigerate, wrapped in plastic wrap
(3) refrigerate, unwrapped
(4) refrigerate in bowl of water (cut up if necessary)
(5) store in dry storage, wrapped in plastic wrap
(6) store in dry storage, unwrapped

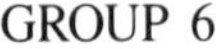

GROUP 6
FOOD ITEM: Banana
**Directions:** For each example, wrap and store banana prepared as indicated. Number each example.

(1) freeze slices, wrapped in heavy plastic wrap
(2) freeze half a banana, unwrapped, with peel
(3) coat slices with lemon juice and freeze, wrapped in heavy plastic wrap
(4) refrigerate half a banana, unwrapped, with peel

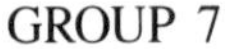

GROUP 7
FOOD ITEM: Banana
**Directions:** For each example, wrap a few slices of banana as indicated and store in the refrigerator. Number each example.

(1) unwrapped
(2) dip in lemon juice to coat, store unwrapped
(3) wrap in plastic wrap
(4) dip in lemon juice to coat, wrap in plastic wrap

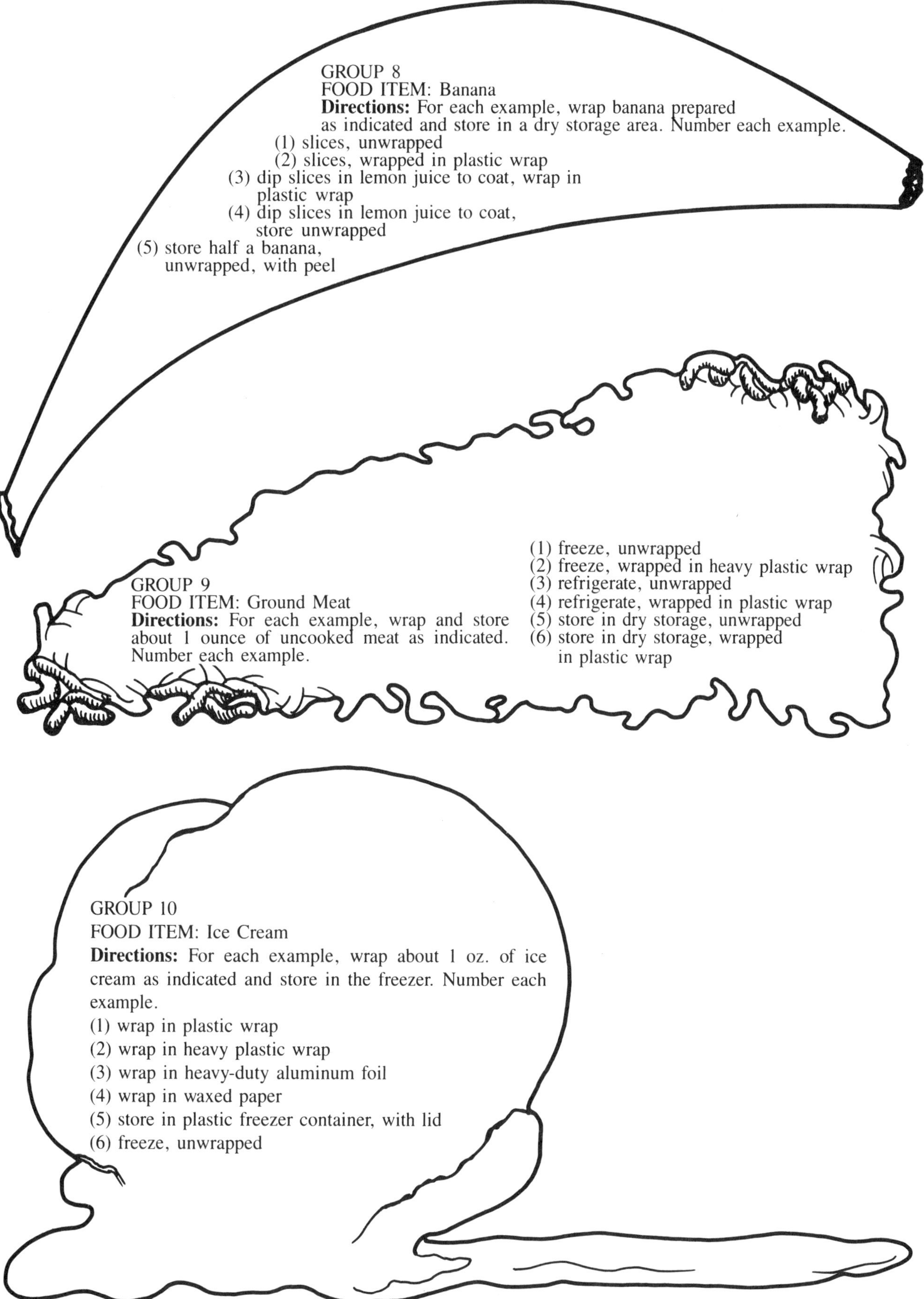

GROUP 8
FOOD ITEM: Banana
**Directions:** For each example, wrap banana prepared as indicated and store in a dry storage area. Number each example.

(1) slices, unwrapped
(2) slices, wrapped in plastic wrap
(3) dip slices in lemon juice to coat, wrap in plastic wrap
(4) dip slices in lemon juice to coat, store unwrapped
(5) store half a banana, unwrapped, with peel

GROUP 9
FOOD ITEM: Ground Meat
**Directions:** For each example, wrap and store about 1 ounce of uncooked meat as indicated. Number each example.

(1) freeze, unwrapped
(2) freeze, wrapped in heavy plastic wrap
(3) refrigerate, unwrapped
(4) refrigerate, wrapped in plastic wrap
(5) store in dry storage, unwrapped
(6) store in dry storage, wrapped in plastic wrap

GROUP 10
FOOD ITEM: Ice Cream
**Directions:** For each example, wrap about 1 oz. of ice cream as indicated and store in the freezer. Number each example.

(1) wrap in plastic wrap
(2) wrap in heavy plastic wrap
(3) wrap in heavy-duty aluminum foil
(4) wrap in waxed paper
(5) store in plastic freezer container, with lid
(6) freeze, unwrapped

Name ______________________________ 

# WRAPPING IT UP EVALUATION

**Directions:** Record the characteristics of your food item when fresh. After one week of storage, record the characteristics of the food for each wrapping or storage method. Use the descriptive words in the box or use additional ones.

FOOD ITEM: ______________________ GROUP NUMBER: __________

| | Food Appearance/Color | Food Odor | Food Texture |
|---|---|---|---|
| Fresh | | | |
| One Week Later: | | | |
| (1) | | | |
| (2) | | | |
| (3) | | | |
| (4) | | | |
| (5) | | | |
| (6) | | | |

On the back of this sheet write:
- –Which treatment(s) preserved the quality of the food?
- –Would this preserve the nutrients?
- –How long could the food be stored this way and still maintain its quality and nutrients?
- –What are your suggestions for storing this food?

| | |
|---|---|
| Appearance/Color | bleached<br>blotchy<br>bright<br>clear<br>color, any<br>colorless<br>dark<br>deep-colored<br>discolored<br>dull<br>faded<br>fresh<br>intense<br>light<br>moldy<br>muddy<br>pale<br>shrunken<br>vivid<br>wilted |
| Odor | faint<br>fragrant<br>fruity<br>grassy<br>moldy<br>musty<br>offensive<br>perfumed<br>pleasing<br>pungent<br>rancid<br>rotten<br>scentless<br>sour<br>stench<br>strong<br>sweet<br>yeasty |
| Texture | coarse<br>crumbly<br>crusty<br>curdled<br>crystalline<br>dense<br>dry<br>fluffy<br>hard<br>liquefied<br>mushy<br>rubbery<br>runny<br>slick<br>slimy<br>smooth<br>soft<br>solid<br>spongy<br>thick |

# STORAGE LIFE OF FOOD

| NR: not recommended | Dry (55°–70°F) | Refrigerator (38°–40°F) | Freezer (0°F or below) |
|---|---|---|---|
| Bacon | NR | 5–7 days | NR |
| Beef, lamb, veal | NR | 4–6 days | 8–12 months |
| Breads, quick, baked | 5–7 days | 1–2 weeks | 2 months |
| Breads, yeast, unbaked | NR | 2–3 months | 1/2 month |
| Butter | NR | 2 weeks | 5–6 months |
| Cakes | 5–7 days | 1–2 weeks | 6 months |
| Cereal, ready-to-eat | 6–8 months | NR | NR |
| Cheese, cottage | NR | 3–5 days | 1 month |
| Cheese, hard or semi-hard | NR | 3–6 months | 6–12 months |
| Cheese, soft | NR | 2 weeks | 4 months |
| Cookies, baked | 5–7 days | 2 weeks | 6 months |
| Cookies, unbaked | NR | 1–2 weeks | 4 months |
| Eggs | NR | 1 week | 12 months |
| Fish | NR | 1–3 days | 2–3 months |
| Fruits, apples | 1 month (cool) | 1 month | 12 months |
| Fruits, canned | 24–36 months | 3–5 days | NR |
| Fruits, citrus | 2 weeks (cool) | 2 weeks | 3–4 months |
| Fruits, except apples & citrus | 3–5 days | 3–7 days | 12 months |
| Ground meat | NR | 1–2 days | 3–4 months |
| Ice cream | NR | NR | 1–3 months |
| Luncheon meats | NR | 1 week | NR |
| Margarine | NR | 2 weeks | 5–6 months |
| Milk, fluid | NR | 1 week | 1 month |
| Pasta, dry | 6–12 months | 6–12 months | NR |
| Pies, baked | NR | 5–7 days | 1 month |
| Pies, unbaked | NR | NR | 3 months |
| Pork, cured | NR | 1 week | 1–2 months |
| Pork, fresh | NR | 4–6 days | 6–8 months |
| Poultry | NR | 2 days | 12 months |
| Prepared main dishes | NR | 2–3 days | 3–8 months |
| Soups | NR | 2–3 days | 4–6 months |
| Vegetables, canned | 24–36 months | 3–4 days | NR |
| Vegetables, cooked | NR | 3–4 days | 1 months |
| Vegetables, raw (except potatotes, onions, beets) | 1–2 days | 5–10 days | 12 months |
| Vegetables, raw–potatoes, onions, beets | 3–4 weeks (cool) | NR | NR |
| Vegetable oil, liquid | 3–4 months | 6 months | NR |

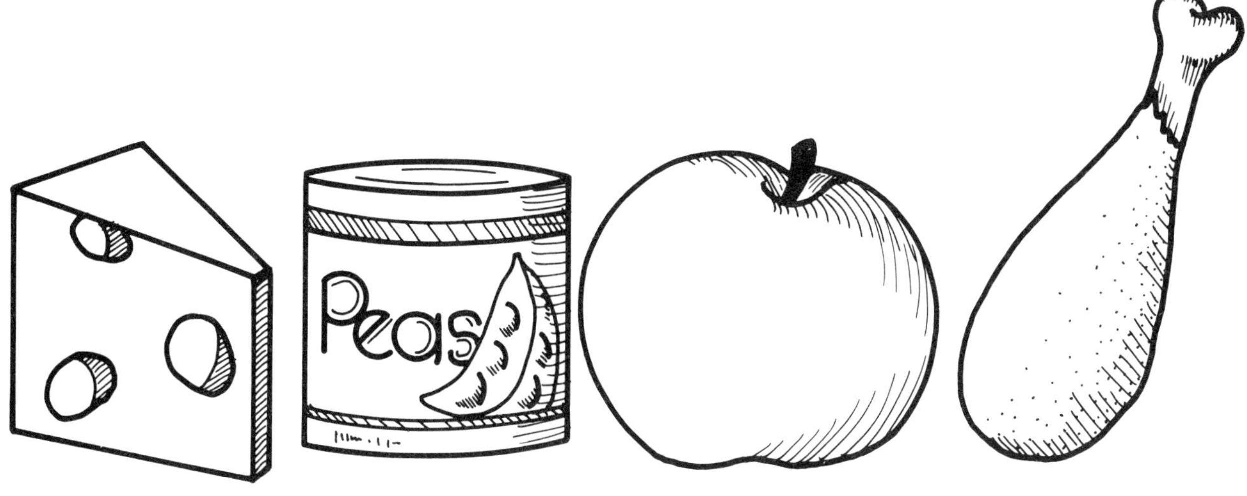

Name ______________________ Quiz Sheet 12-1

# QUIZ
# STORING FOODS TO PRESERVE NUTRIENTS

**Directions:** In the word search puzzle below find and circle the words related to proper food storage and the preservation of nutrients. Words appear across the box, up and down, and diagonally. Words are spelled forwards and backwards. Clues are given in the fill-in-the-blank questions below the puzzle. If you know the answer but cannot find it in the puzzle, write the correct answer in the blanks provided.

| | | | | | | | | | | | | | | |
|---|---|---|---|---|---|---|---|---|---|---|---|---|---|---|
| A | O | T | N | K | E | Y | W | C | A | L | C | I | U | M |
| E | D | H | U | O | T | M | A | S | Q | I | J | V | T | V |
| N | O | K | S | E | B | A | T | C | B | G | D | M | R | I |
| B | R | W | F | M | R | F | E | N | G | H | N | R | H | T |
| U | J | A | V | L | N | O | R | I | E | T | U | G | Y | A |
| C | S | Y | M | D | Z | G | K | M | U | S | T | W | P | M |
| R | E | F | R | I | G | E | R | A | T | O | R | F | Q | I |
| Y | X | T | L | H | U | E | Z | T | W | J | I | E | T | N |
| T | K | O | W | A | Z | H | L | I | R | O | E | R | I | A |
| I | X | N | G | E | V | J | D | V | O | C | N | U | G | B |
| L | Q | A | E | R | T | O | M | S | L | N | T | T | H | S |
| A | W | R | S | L | I | X | R | K | O | Z | S | X | T | G |
| U | F | X | A | R | M | L | S | E | C | U | R | E | L | Y |
| Q | T | E | M | P | E | R | A | T | U | R | E | T | Y | A |

1. If a food has a fresh, wholesome, and pleasant appearance, it is said to be of highest (1) Q _ _ _ _ T Y.
2. Storing foods properly prevents spoilage and protects the (2) S _ _ _ T Y of the food.
3. The (3) N _ _ _ _ _ _ T S in food are preserved through proper storage.

Name three main types of storage areas:

4. ______________________
5. ______________________
6. ______________________

**Name** ________________________________ **Quiz Sheet 12-2**

Which Iron CaPAC nutrients are most likely to be lost during improper storage?

7. ________________________________
8. ________________________________
9. ________________________________
10. ________________________________

Name five factors that lead to loss of nutrients:

11. ________________________________
12. ________________________________
13. ________________________________
14. ________________________________
15. ________________________________

It is important to wrap foods (16) T __ __ __ __ L Y in order to maintain freshness and quality.

An important step in sealing foods is to make sure lids fit (17) S __ __ __ __ __ L Y.

Name four indicators of the quality of food:

18. ________________________________
19. ________________________________
20. ________________________________
21. ________________________________

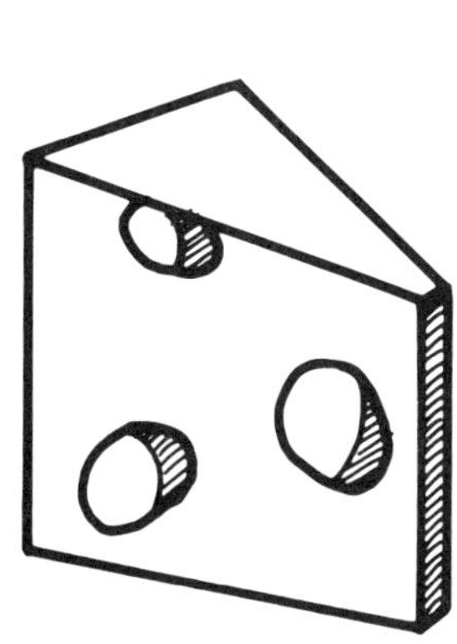

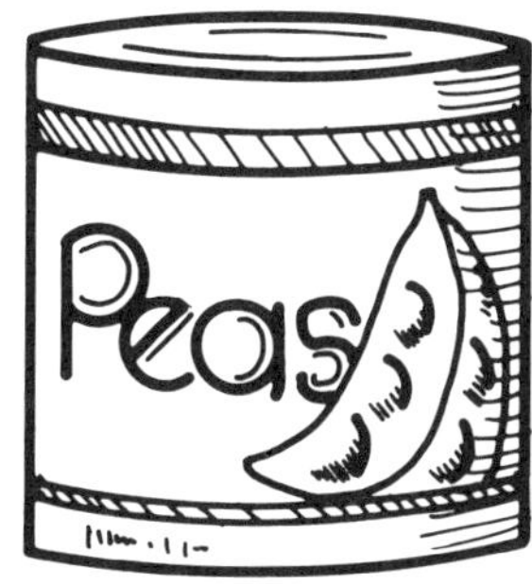



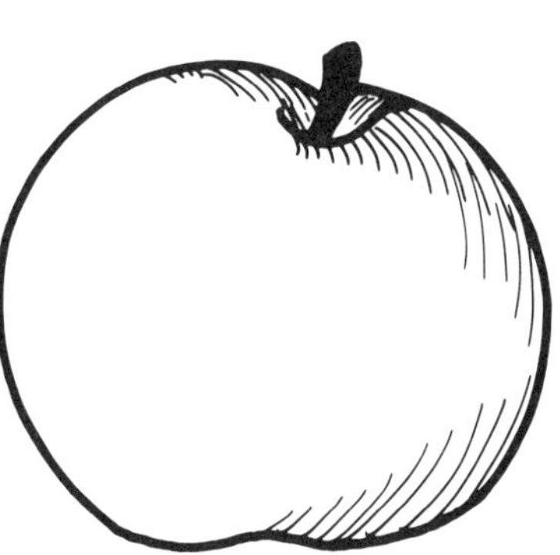

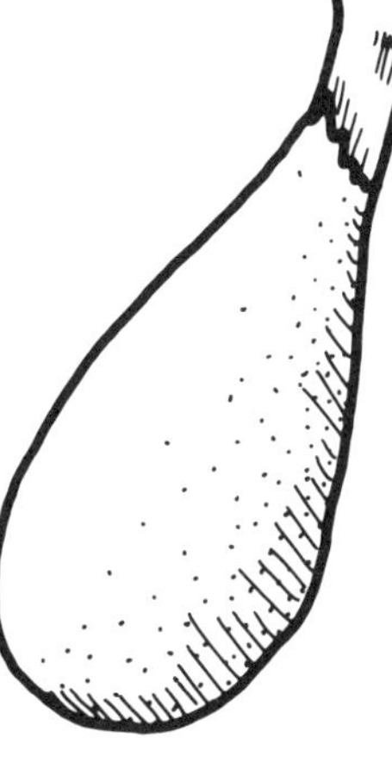

# Unit 13: Budgeting Resources in Meal Planning

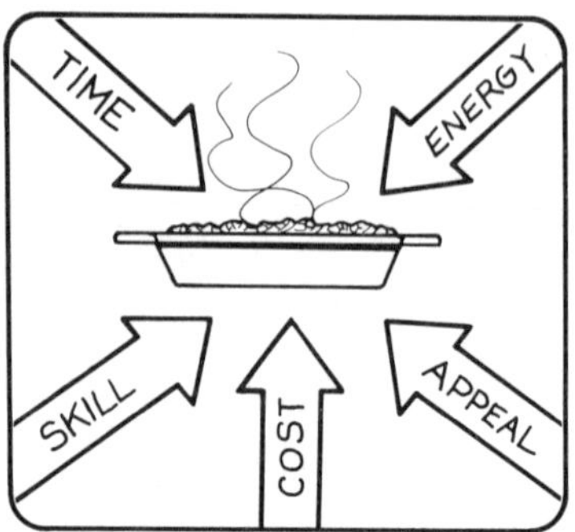


## CONCEPTS

–There are five factors to be considered when planning and preparing meals: energy, time, cost, skill, and appeal.

## OBJECTIVES

–Students will plan and evaluate a meal according to nutrition guidelines, as well as in terms of energy, time, cost, skill, and appeal.

–Students will plan and prepare a nutritious meal that demonstrates budgeted resources.

## TEACHER'S UNIT INTRODUCTION

Up to this point, you have been looking at meals and snacks based on a nutritional point of view. In this and in the following two units you will be looking at five other factors involved in meal planning—energy, time, cost, skill, and appeal. Here's a brief description of each one:

**Energy.** In today's energy-conscious society, this resource is of utmost importance in planning meals. The meals chosen by the population can influence not only their health but also the conservation (or consumption) of precious and nonrenewable resources. Energy can be conserved at various stages of food production, including growing, processing, transporting, storing, and preparing. For example, buying local produce rather than produce that has been transported many miles conserves diesel fuel used in transportation, as well as electrical energy for the refrigeration of perishables during transportation. In the marketplace, buying food with little or no packaging conserves energy by eliminating the need to produce, and ultimately waste, packaging materials such as plastic, aluminum, tin, paper, or glass. At home, consumers can conserve energy by reducing their use of electrical and gas appliances (in length of time and total number used), by limiting shopping to fewer visits to the grocery store (saving personal time), by growing as much food as possible, or by using reusable items such as cloth napkins and dish towels. There are many other examples of energy conservation, as you can imagine.

In addition to conserving energy through the food system from farm to table, different types of diets use different amounts of energy. The concept of a food chain or web demonstrates the idea of energy-efficient diets. Simply described, energy passes from sunlight to green plants, to microbes and small animals, to larger animals, and finally to people. In order to move from one level to another, energy is expended. For example, in order for people to eat beef, plant food must be eaten by the cattle and converted to their flesh. The cattle are then slaughtered, butchered, and the beef finally prepared and consumed by people. If the cattle were mainly range-fed (grazing on grass) rather than grain-fed, they would then be a more energy-efficient food source. Refrigeration is also needed from the time the cattle are slaughtered until the beef is cooked. Each process requires energy in one form or another. However, when people consume plant foods directly, they eliminate many stages of energy consumption. Thus, eating foods lower on the food chain conserves energy. [See *Diet for a Small Planet,* in the "References/Resources" section for this unit.]

**Time.** Individuals have varying interests in food and nutrition. The amount of time they are willing to spend in planning, shopping for, preparing, and consuming nutritious meals will vary greatly. These personal interests must be taken into account in meal planning. Nutritious meals may be achieved in minutes or they may take hours of preparation. Many individuals want to be able to do both, depending on their schedule or their mood. Whatever the case, the amount of time involved in getting a meal on the table and consuming it must be considered.

**Cost.** The cost of food today is a major factor affecting meal planning. However, cost need not limit the nutritional value of a meal. In fact, people who can afford to spend a lot of money on food are not always healthier than people on a limited budget. Affluence that leads to an excess of food can be nearly as bad as not having enough money for food. Meal planning on limited expenses requires thought and deliberate planning. Many of the lower-cost food items are nutritious bargains.

**Skill.** Every individual has different abilities when it comes to food preparation, depending upon his or her background, interest, and the availability of equipment. Skills depend on (1) whether or not you have had training in food preparation techniques; (2) frequent or recent experience in using the techniques; (3) interest in learning new skills and techniques; and (4) exposure to the variety of kitchen equipment available. Accommodation must be made for varying skill levels. For example, consider a young person who has recently left home for the first time and is living in a roominghouse with only a few pieces of kitchen equipment. This young person would need to plan and prepare meals that are quite different from those prepared by an older person with a complete kitchen who has been cooking in a gourmet restaurant for many years. Nevertheless, meals prepared by either person can be nutritious and appealing.

**Appeal.** The appeal of meals depends completely on individual taste. In some countries, a plate of rice and fried ants might look appealing. To most people in this country, it would not! However, meals can be planned and served with the tastes of the family or guests in mind. A variety of colors, textures, temperatures, tastes, and shapes will add to the appeal of most meals.

In addition to these five areas of concern—energy, time, cost, skill, and appeal—it is important to remember the nutritional guidelines when planning and preparing meals. You need to budget your resources, but you also need to plan nutritious meals.

---

Meal planning is a task that appears with regularity in many lessons. It is a task which is also addressed in popular food magazines and cookbooks. Many of these sources, however, focus on the appeal of the food rather than on giving attention to other issues. During Unit 13 it is important to emphasize these other issues, particularly the idea of conserving energy and maintaining high nutritional quality. In this fast-paced, pleasure-seeking society, issues other than time and appeal must be brought to the forefront.

## BASIC ACTIVITY

**Time Needed:** Two class periods

**Materials Needed:** Sheet 13-1: "Practice Menu"
Chart B: "Daily Food Guide"
Sheets 13-2 through 13-3: "Meal Planning Budget Checklist"
Sheet 13-4: "Energy-Savers in the Kitchen"
Ingredients for meals to be prepared
Quiz Sheet 13-1

### Class Period 1

1. Introduce this activity by briefly describing the factors that can be taken into consideration during the planning and preparation of meals in the "Teacher's Unit Introduction." These factors include energy, time, cost, skill, appeal, and of course, nutrition.

2. Distribute Sheet 13-1, "Practice Menu," and have students plan one meal for the day, keeping the factors above in mind. The students should be familiar with the "Daily Food Guide" from the exercises in previous lessons. If not, distribute Chart B, the "Daily Food Guide," and briefly discuss the principles of a well-balanced diet. When planning a single

well-balanced meal based on the "Daily Food Guide," it is recommended to include approximately ⅓ of the total recommended number of servings. Thus, one meal should contain:

1–2 servings from the Fruit-Vegetable group
1–2 servings from the Bread-Cereal group
1–2 servings from the Milk-Cheese group
0–1 serving from the Meat-Poultry-Fish-Beans group

Remind students that there is no recommendation for servings from the Fats-Sweets-Alcohol group. The practice menus for this activity should follow these nutrition guidelines. Have students work on the menus individually or in pairs.

3. Following the menu planning and nutritional evaluation, distribute Sheets 13-2 and 13-3, "Meal Planning Budget Checklist," and Sheet 13-4, "Energy-Savers in the Kitchen." These forms are designed to help students evaluate their use of resources, including energy, time, cost, and skill. Students should complete the "Meal Planning Budget Checklist" for their "Practice Menu," keeping their own habits and skills in mind. The "Checklist" is meant to be an approximation, of course, and does not provide exact calculations. For example, under the section describing "time," it is not possible to know exactly how much time is spent shopping for the meal. Students should take an average shopping trip as the model for "time."

4. During the final part of this class, students should be given situations that involve certain limits on their resources. The following are examples of situations. Create other situations that may be more relevant to the students in your classroom, if necessary. Read one or more of these situations to the students and have them create a practice menu in accordance with the limited resources. The students may work in pairs for this activity. You may want to give different groups of students different situations for variety.

a. Jim plays soccer for the high school team. He practices in the early morning and again in the afternoon following school. He rushes home from practice. He has only half an hour to prepare and eat dinner every evening and must prepare it alone since his parents both work late. He has a part-time job at the shopping mall and is expected to report to work by 6:30. Plan Jim's daily diet.

b. Annie works after school to help her mother support the family. She has two sisters who are too young to work. They have just enough money to make ends meet. Annie is helping her mother plan the menus and food budget this week. They have only $38.00 to spend on food this week. That means they have about $2.75 to spend on each night's supper for the four of them. Plan the family's evening meal.

c. Sarah is moving to a roominghouse this week. She has never cooked a meal before in her life. She has a hot plate, a small refrigerator, one pot, a table knife, fork, spoon, one plate, and a drinking cup. Give Sarah suggestions for meals and snacks she could prepare.

5. In a large-group discussion, have students describe how they managed to cut back on resources in each of the examples in step 4 and also how effective they believe these cutbacks will be. Ask them if they would be willing to follow their own recommendations.

### Class Period 2

1. Have small groups of students prepare one of the meals they planned in step 2 of Class Period 1, selecting one based on limited resources. Either all groups can prepare the same meal, or each can prepare a different one. Have each group evaluate the meal in terms of appeal.

2. **Evaluation:** Distribute Quiz Sheet 13-1. Have students answer the questions independently. Then conduct a discussion of question #1.

## FOLLOW-UP ACTIVITIES

1. Have students plan a grocery list for a family of any size using a specific maximum amount of money they may spend to provide a nutritionally adequate diet. Reproduce and distribute the following "Cost of Food at Home" chart for suggested dollar limits.

**Cost of Food at Home***

| Sex-age group | Cost for 1 week | | | |
|---|---|---|---|---|
| | Thrifty plan | Low-cost plan | Moderate-cost plan | Liberal plan |
| FAMILIES | | | | |
| Family of 2: | | | | |
| 20–50 years | $36.50 | $45.90 | $56.50 | $ 69.50 |
| 51 years and over | 34.50 | 43.80 | 53.90 | 64.10 |
| Family of 4: | | | | |
| Couple, 20–50 years and children— | | | | |
| 1–2 and 3–5 years | 53.20 | 65.90 | 80.50 | 98.10 |
| 6–8 and 9–11 years | 61.00 | 77.60 | 96.90 | 116.10 |
| INDIVIDUALS | | | | |
| Child: | | | | |
| 1–2 years | 9.60 | 11.50 | 13.40 | 16.10 |
| 3–5 years | 10.40 | 12.70 | 15.70 | 18.80 |
| 6–8 years | 12.70 | 16.80 | 21.00 | 24.50 |
| 9–11 years | 15.10 | 19.10 | 24.50 | 28.40 |
| Male: | | | | |
| 12–14 years | 15.80 | 21.70 | 27.00 | 31.70 |
| 15–19 years | 16.50 | 22.60 | 27.80 | 32.20 |
| 20–50 years | 17.50 | 22.20 | 27.80 | 33.30 |
| 51 years and over | 15.90 | 21.00 | 25.80 | 30.80 |
| Female: | | | | |
| 12–19 years | 15.70 | 18.80 | 22.70 | 27.30 |
| 20–50 years | 15.70 | 19.50 | 23.60 | 29.90 |
| 51 years and over | 15.50 | 18.80 | 23.20 | 27.50 |

*From *Family Economics Review,* No. 1. USDA, Science and Education Administration, Beltsville, MD 20705, 1985

2. Conduct a discussion of a meat-based versus a vegetarian diet in terms of nutrition, energy, time, cost, skill, and appeal. Which factors are more demanding in a meat-based diet? Which ones are more demanding in a vegetarian diet?

3. Have students role-play situations in which one person is trying to convince another to limit his or her food preparation energy consumption, to cut back on the amount of money spent on food, to devote more time to food preparation, to improve food-related skills, or to prepare food more efficiently to save time.

Name ______________________ Sheet 13-1

# PRACTICE MENU

ENERGY TIME CO$T SKILL APPEAL

| Food | Amount | Fruit-Vegetable Group | Bread-Cereal Group | Milk-Cheese Group | Meat-Poultry-Fish-Beans Group | Fats-Sweets-Alcohol Group |
|---|---|---|---|---|---|---|
| | | | | | | |
| TOTAL NUMBER OF SERVINGS: | | | | | | |
| RECOMMENDED NUMBER OF SERVINGS PER MEAL: | | | | | | |

Name ______________________________ Sheet 13-2

# MEAL PLANNING BUDGET CHECKLIST

**Time**

I spent ____ minutes planning this meal.
I will spend approximately ____ minutes shopping for this meal.
I will spend approximately ____ minutes preparing for this meal.
I will spend approximately ____ minutes cleaning up after this meal.

TOTAL TIME SPENT: ____ minutes

The approximate time I will spend planning, shopping, preparing, and cleaning up after this meal is:
too much too little just about right.

***********************************************************************************

**Cost**

| FOOD ITEM | PURCHASE UNIT COST | SERVING SIZE | COST/SERVING |
|---|---|---|---|
| | | | |
| | | TOTAL COST FOR ONE PERSON: | |

The money I spent purchasing food for this meal was: too much too little just about right.

Name ________________________  Sheet 13-3

## Skills

Place a check mark in front of each food preparation skill you possess:

_____ baking
_____ barbecuing
_____ basting
_____ beating
_____ blanching
_____ blending
_____ boiling
_____ braising
_____ breading
_____ broiling
_____ candying
_____ canning
_____ carmelizing
_____ chopping
_____ creaming
_____ crisping
_____ cutting in
_____ dicing
_____ dredging
_____ egging and crumbing
_____ folding
_____ freezing
_____ fricasseeing
_____ frizzling
_____ frying
_____ glacéing
_____ grilling
_____ grinding
_____ kneading
_____ larding
_____ marinating
_____ melting
_____ microwaving
_____ mincing
_____ mixing
_____ pan-broiling
_____ pan-frying
_____ parboiling
_____ parching
_____ paring
_____ peeling
_____ planking
_____ poaching
_____ pot-roasting
_____ pressure cooking
_____ reconstituting
_____ rehydrating
_____ rendering
_____ roasting
_____ sautéing
_____ scalding
_____ scalloping
_____ scoring
_____ searing
_____ simmering
_____ steaming
_____ steeping
_____ stewing
_____ stirring
_____ toasting
_____ whipping

Place a check mark in front of each piece of kitchen equipment to which you have access. On the back of this sheet describe the pieces noted.

_____ electric/gas range
_____ electric/gas oven
_____ microwave oven
_____ convection oven
_____ broiler
_____ toaster oven
_____ toaster
_____ dishwasher
_____ garbage disposal
_____ refrigerator
_____ freezer
_____ food processor
_____ electric mixer
_____ hand mixer
_____ blender
_____ pressure cooker
_____ saucepans (describe)
_____ skillets/frying pans (describe)
_____ baking pans (describe)
_____ cutting board
_____ knives
_____ knife sharpener
_____ measuring cups
_____ measuring spoons
_____ flour sifter
_____ vegetable steamer
_____ strainers
_____ can opener
_____ bowls
_____ spatula
_____ whisk/whip
_____ garlic press
_____ candy/meat thermometers
_____ baster
_____ pastry brush
_____ rolling pin
_____ coffee percolator
_____ teapot
_____ others (describe)

The skills I have to prepare this meal are: completely adequate almost adequate not adequate

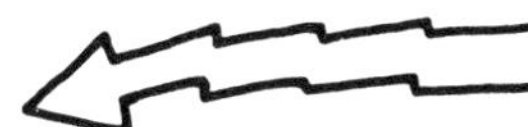
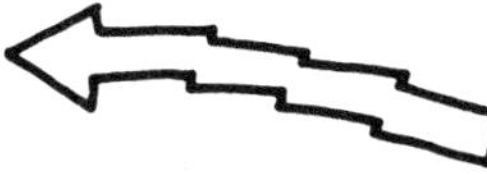
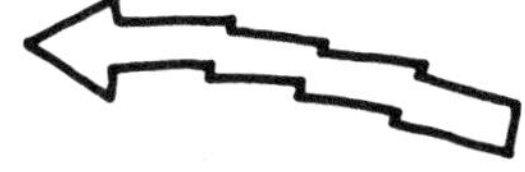

# ENERGY–SAVERS IN THE KITCHEN

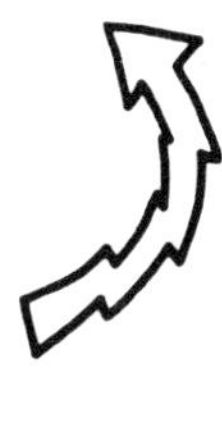
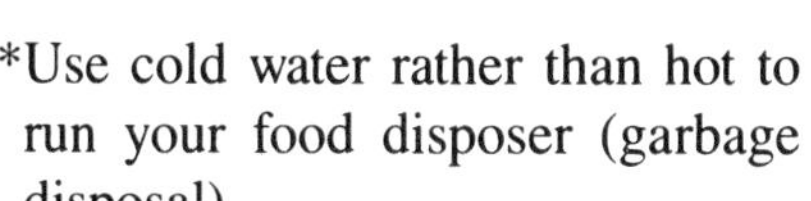
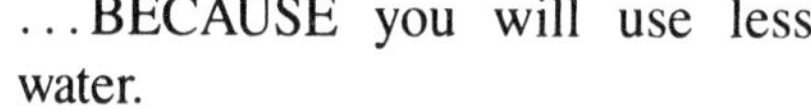

*Use cold water rather than hot to run your food disposer (garbage disposal)... ...BECAUSE hot water requires additional electricity for gas.

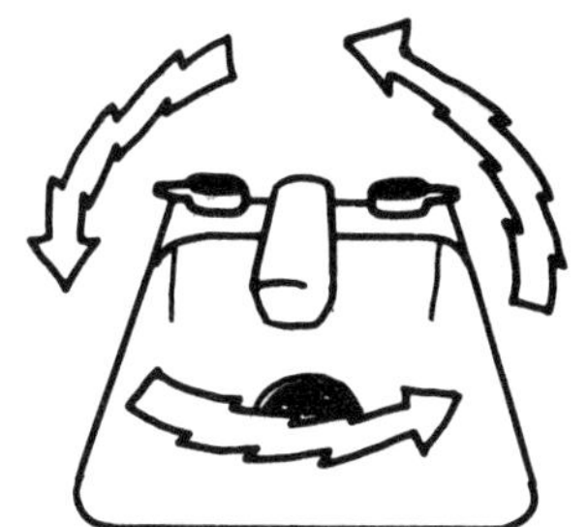

*Install an aerator in your kitchen sink faucet... ...BECAUSE you will use less water.

*Use gas ovens or ranges with an automatic (electronic) ignition system instead of a pilot light... ...BECAUSE you will save up to 30 percent on gas that normally burns away in a constant gas pilot light.

*If you have a gas stove, make sure the pilot light is burning efficiently (a blue flame instead of yellow)... ...BECAUSE less gas is used when the pilot light burns with the proper ratio of oxygen to gas.

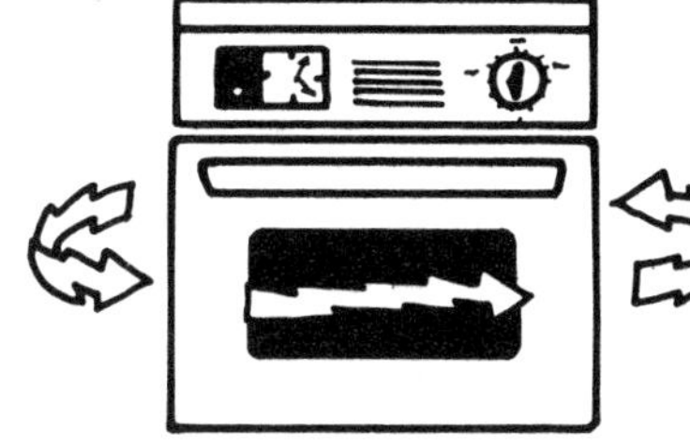

*Boil water in a lid-covered pan... ...BECAUSE the lid conserves heat to boil the water faster.

*Keep range top burners and reflectors clean... ...BECAUSE more heat will be distributed to the pots and pans.

*Match the size of the pan to the size of the heating element... ...BECAUSE less heat will escape unused around the sides of the pan.

*If you cook with electricity, turn off burners several minutes before the end of the allotted cooking time... ...BECAUSE you will continue to cook with burners that remain hot long after being turned off.

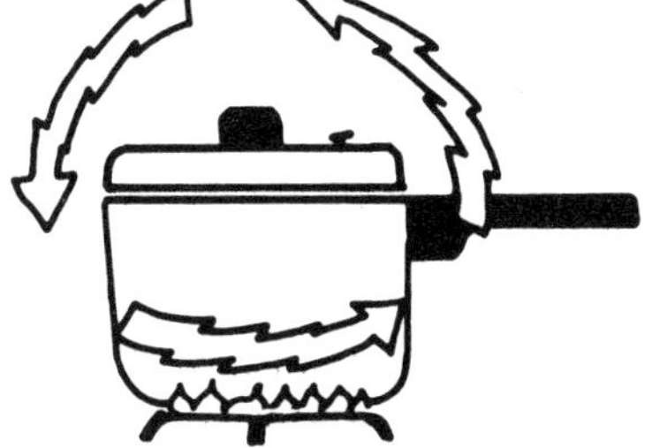

*When using the oven, make the most of the heat from that single source by cooking several foods at once... ...BECAUSE you will make the most efficient use of the oven.

*Watch the clock or use a timer. Do not open the oven door continually to check for doneness... ...BECAUSE cooking heat will escape and your oven will waste fuel maintaining an even temperature.

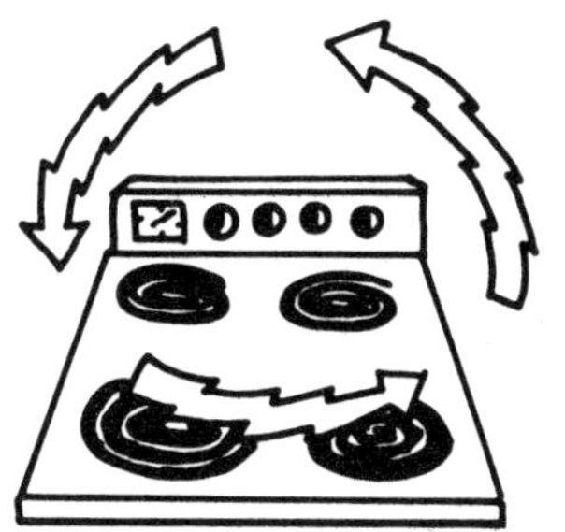

*Use small electric pans or ovens for small meals... ...BECAUSE you will not be heating an unused cooking area.

*Use a pressure cooker or a microwave oven if you have one... ...BECAUSE these appliances require shorter cooking time and less energy.

Name ________________________________________ 

# QUIZ
# BUDGETING RESOURCES IN MEAL PLANNING

1. When planning a meal, you must consider five factors: Energy (E), Time (T), Cost (C), Skill (S), and Appeal (A). For each of the following descriptions, place the appropriate letters to show which factor(s) is (are) being considered.

    _____ a. Use fresh peas in June instead of frozen.

    _____ b. Use canned peaches in December instead of fresh.

    _____ c. Make buttered noodles instead of macaroni and cheese.

    _____ d. Plan a meal with three colors instead of two.

    _____ e. Make twice as much casserole as you need and save leftovers.

    _____ f. Make instant soup instead of homemade soup.

    _____ g. Make homemade soup instead of instant soup.

    _____ h. Make biscuits instead of croissants.

    _____ i. Serve cool mint jelly with roast lamb instead of serving gravy.

    _____ j. Use cold water instead of hot water whenever possible.

_____ 2. All of the following methods help to cut food costs *except:*

a. Using protein-extended dishes
b. Using nonfat dry milk
c. Using pasta
d. Using prime-grade meat

_____ 3. Which of the following hints would help to save food dollars?

a. Purchase only canned fruits and vegetables
b. Make a grocery list before going to the grocery store
c. Shop with a friend
d. Buy only advertised brands of foods

_____ 4. If you bought apples from a wholesaler, you would expect the apples to:

a. Be very expensive
b. Be of poor quality
c. Cost the same as apples in the grocery store
d. Cost less than apples in the grocery store

_____ 5. To decrease the number of times a food is handled between its origin and me, I could:

a. Use fresh foods
b. Use frozen foods
c. Buy packaged food
d. Eat in restaurants

# Unit 14: Menu Planning Using the "Daily Food Guide"

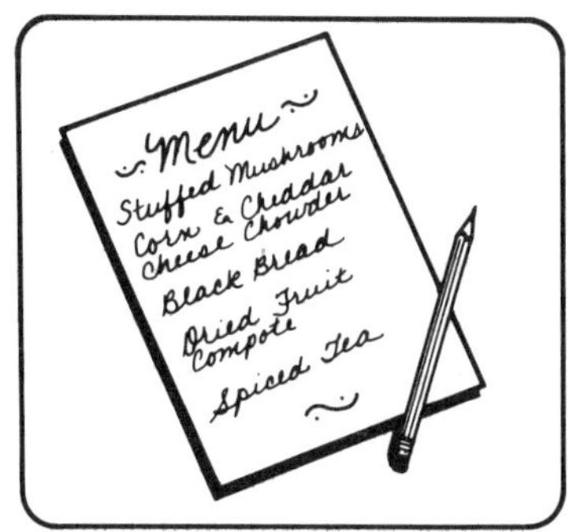
Menu
Stuffed Mushrooms
Corn & Cheddar Cheese Chowder
Black Bread
Dried Fruit Compote
Spiced Tea

## CONCEPTS

–A nutritious meal generally includes at least one serving of food from each food group in the "Daily Food Guide."

–Planning and preparing nutritious meals and snacks can be a creative challenge.

## OBJECTIVE

–Students will demonstrate creativity by planning, preparing, and evaluating a unique and nutritious meal.

## TEACHER'S UNIT INTRODUCTION

Prior to the 1960s, most meals were eaten in the home. Usually, families ate meals that the mother had prepared. Meals eaten away from home were usually prepared at home, and bagged or boxed for traveling. With the advent of the fast-food restaurant, eating-on-the-run became popular, and people began eating more and more meals prepared and consumed away from home. Today, nearly one-third of the dollars spent on food are spent on food prepared away from the home. This change in eating habits has caused the food preparer of the family to have less influence on the quality and quantity of food consumed by family members and has given the food industry more influence.

Previously, if the family's major food preparer knew the basics of planning nutritionally balanced meals, the family members could be fairly well assured of having a nutritious diet to eat. The major food preparer could plan the family's diet not only meal by meal, but also week by week, in order to assure adequate intake of a variety of nutritious foods. Now, however, each family member may be planning at least one meal, if not more, independently.

Each family member must be responsible for his or her own nutritional needs. The emphasis in planning must switch from a week-by-week family orientation to a day-to-day individual orientation in order to accommodate this shift in meal-planning responsibilities.

The big concern is: What does a nutritionally balanced meal look like? How does a family member know when he or she has planned a nutritious meal? Using the "Daily Food Guide" or the Nutrient Analysis Method, a person can plan the types and amounts of foods needed for a full day's nutritious diet. But a single nutritionally balanced meal is more difficult to plan because it needs to fit into (or complement) the rest of the foods consumed during the day. Thus, if one meal contains four servings of the Milk-Cheese group, another meal contains four servings of the Bread-Cereal group, and a third meal contains the required servings from the other two food groups, the day's total diet would be nutritious. Each meal individually would not be nutritious, however. Most nutritionists agree that it is better to spread out the types of foods consumed throughout the day rather than lumping them together in one meal. Absorption of nutrients can take place only at a certain pace; if the body receives too much of one nutrient at one time, it may be "overloaded" and will be unable to efficiently absorb the nutrient. But if foods are spread out throughout the day, the absorption of nutrients can be maximized.

So, to plan a nutritionally balanced meal, we can use the same guidelines as we do when planning a nutritious diet. Depending upon how many meals you eat in a day, divide that number into the number of servings of a food group (or the amount of nutrients) that you need for the day. Roughly, this translates into one serving from each of the food groups in the "Daily Food Guide" for each meal. A serving from the Meat-Poultry-Fish-Beans group may be eliminated at one meal since only two servings per day are required for adequate protein and other nutrients. Keep in mind that the Milk-Cheese group and the Bread-Cereal group also contribute protein; in fact, the protein quality of the latter is improved when consumed with foods from the Meat-Poultry-Fish-Beans group or the Milk-Cheese group.

---

In order for students to accept nutrition as important, good-tasting food must be fully appreciated. No matter how much people know about nutrition, it will not do any good until they use their nutrition knowledge to select a nutritious diet. Unit 14 is designed to create in the students a desire to prepare and eat good-tasting and nutritious foods.

Some students will feel that good-tasting foods are different from nutritious foods. Many people equate nutritious foods with bland soybean loaves, dry whole wheat bread, or bitter salad greens. In reality, nutritious foods can be delightfully appealing if they are planned, prepared, and served creatively.

How do you teach creativity and still teach acceptable menu planning? Many teachers believe that students should be given standard recipes and definite guidelines to follow when planning and preparing meals. They feel that the evening meal is not complete without an appetizer, an entree, two vegetables, some form of bread, beverage, and dessert. Appropriate and traditional place setting and service styles are often encouraged. This form of standardization may stifle creativity and imagination. Traditional meals have their place but should be supplemented by a variety of self-designed and imaginative ones.

Imagine an easy and festive meal such as this one:

Raw Vegetable Chunks
Swiss Cheese Fondue
Cubed French Bread
Tossed Green Salad
Pastries or Fruit
Coffee or tea

For a wintertime favorite, imagine a hearty soup dinner such as this one:

Hot Stuffed Mushrooms
Corn and Cheddar Cheese Chowder
Black Bread
Dried Fruit Compote
Spiced Tea

Or, why not have sandwiches play a major role in the evening meal? Try French-style sandwiches or hot open-faced sandwiches with a variety of fillings such as salmon spread, soybean spread, hummus (Middle Eastern chickpea spread), sliced meats and cheeses, marinated vegetables, anchovies or herring, bean sprouts, grated carrots or beets, sliced hard-cooked eggs, or sliced mushrooms. Add to the sandwiches a salad or soup plus fresh fruit for dessert and your meal is complete.

The assortment of foods and combinations of foods used for a meal is limited only by individual preferences and nutritional considerations. After these details have been attended to, the sky is the limit! Creativity in the students can be sparked by the creativity displayed by their teacher, as well as by books and magazines pertaining to food. *Bon Appetite, Cuisine, Gourmet,* and other magazines offer many recipes and menus to create enthusiasm among the students. Cookbooks with color and flair will be of use, too. However, the most trusted tool in stirring up creativity in the students is the students themselves. A bit of encouragement, support, and open-mindedness go a long way in allowing the students to expand their horizons regarding meal planning.

## BASIC ACTIVITY

**Time Needed:** Two class periods

**Materials Needed:** Sheet 14-1: "Creative Kitchen Cupboard"
Sheet 14-2: "Creative Menu"

Cookbooks, gourmet magazines, recipe files, pictures of food
Chart B: "Daily Food Guide"
Sheet 14-3: "Creative Practice Menu"
Quiz Sheet 14-1

**Class Period 1**

1. This activity is designed to encourage students to be resourceful and creative in planning menus. Begin the activity with a brief description of creative meal planning.

2. Distribute Sheet 14-1, "Creative Kitchen Cupboard." Have the students "fill" the cupboard by naming seasonings, foods, and equipment that they wish to use in planning a creative menu. Write students' suggestions on a copy of Sheet 14-1 and display it on an overhead transparency or on the chalkboard. (A sample completed "Kitchen Cupboard" is found in the "Answer Key" at the end of this kit.)

3. Delete or add items to the list of seasonings, foods, and equipment on Sheet 14-1 according to either the exigencies of the situations in which the students are living or according to what is available in the classroom. All students should then record the final list on individual copies of Sheet 14-1.

4. Distribute Sheet 14-2, "Creative Menu." Using additional resources such as cookbooks, gourmet magazines, recipe files, or pictures of foods, have students individually create a menu using only the food items found on Sheet 14-1, "Creative Kitchen Cupboard." Make sure students know that their menus must meet the guidelines for a nutritious diet. Distribute Chart B, "Daily Food Guide," if students do not already have a copy from previous units.

**Class Period 2**

1. Distribute Sheet 14-3, "Creative Practice Menu," for students to record their menus.

2. Have them evalute their menus according to Chart B, "Daily Food Guide."

3. If time permits, have students calculate the cost of each of their meals. Have students obtain prices from a local grocery store as homework, or have available a price list for a variety of food items.

4. After students have completed their menu evaluation with Chart B, bring them back to a large-group discussion. Have students share the menu plans with one another. Discuss problems, shortcomings, and imaginative ideas that present themselves during the activity. Rate the creativity of the menus both by observing the variety of colors, tastes, textures, shapes, and temperatures in the meals as well as by determining if the food combinations have been planned or prepared previously in the class. This type of rating is extremely subjective; it is important to be open-minded during this evaluation.

5. If possible, have students vote on the menus and decide on one or more meals to prepare in class. Prepare and evaluate the chosen meal(s) during a later class period.

6. Proceed with the "Advanced Activity" if you wish; otherwise use the quiz mentioned in step 7.

7. **Evaluation:** Distribute Quiz Sheet 14-1 and have students complete it independently. Discuss the answers as a class.

## ADVANCED ACTIVITY

**Time Needed:** One class period

**Materials Needed:** Sheet 14-3: "Creative Practice Menu" (completed)
Chart E: "Dietary Calculation Chart"
Sheet 14-4: "I Would Rather . . . "
Calculators (*optional*)
Food Composition tables (*optional*) (*see* "References/Resources" at the end of this kit)
Chart B: "Daily Food Guide"
Quiz Sheet 14-1

1. Begin this activity with a values-ranking activity by having students complete independently Sheet 14-4, "I Would Rather. . . ." In a large-group discussion, help students explore the relative importance that they give to taking the time to plan nutritious meals. There are no correct answers for the sheet, but individuals should come to a better understanding of their personal food intake styles from it.

2. Have students perform a nutrient analysis of the menus written in the "Basic Activity." They should use Chart E, "Dietary Calculation Chart," for this analysis. Have on hand food composition tables and, possibly, calculators to complete this evaluation.

3. Have students compare their evaluations based on the "Daily Food Guide" versus the Nutrient Analysis method. Ask: How do the two methods compare? Is one method or the other more favorable? Which one took longer to calculate? Are the results worth the additional time?

4. **Evaluation:** Distribute Quiz Sheet 14-1 and have students complete it independently. Discuss the answers as a class.

## FOLLOW-UP ACTIVITIES

1. Select one or more of the creative menus from the "Basic Activity" to prepare in class. Have students rate the meal in terms of nutrition and creativity. You may also want to have the students evaluate the meal in terms of resources used (energy, cost, time, skill).

2. Have students plan a creative food experience for a group of students in a local preschool or elementary school. If they carry it out, have them evaluate the children's response to the food.

3. Invite a chef or head cook from a restaurant or cooking school to speak to the students about creative expression with food.

4. Have students write a short paragraph describing their favorite meal. Have them answer questions like these: Why do you like that meal above all others? How much creativity does that meal exhibit? Is it important to be creative in meal planning and preparation? Why?

5. Discuss some unusual foods that might be considered in creative meal planning. One group of foods often overlooked is edible flowers and herbs. Flower cookery was popular in

ages past, but it may be experiencing a revival. The added colors and textures of flowers lend appeal to otherwise drab meals. Try borage flowers, nasturtiums, dandelions, or violets in green salads. Or, how about fried squash blossoms or lily buds? Several books on the topic of flower cookery are available, including one by Mary MacNicol entitled *Flower Cookery: The Art of Cooking with Flowers*. **Caution** should be exercised in this activity because some flowers are poisonous.

Another group of foods often ignored is edible insects. Although insect-eating is not popular in this country, it is a common practice in some other areas of the world such as Latin American, South America, and Africa. And, as our world food resources become more scarce, we may need to turn to insects, ourselves, as an alternative source of nutrients. Books with titles such as *Insects in Human Nutrition* and *Entertaining with Insects* and many others may be found in the public library and will be extremely useful and entertaining.

6. Conduct a "What's Wrong with This Meal?" activity. Display one menu at a time. The menus should lack variety in either color, shape, texture, temperature, or flavor. Displays should consist of menus written on the chalkboard or on an overhead projector transparency, photos of foods, or food models. Have students select which factor is causing the meal to be unappealing. Have students alter each menu so that it becomes more appealing. You might also have students create additional sample menus that challenge the class to evaluate "What's Wrong with This Meal?"

Name ______________________ Sheet 14-1

# CREATIVE KITCHEN CUPBOARD

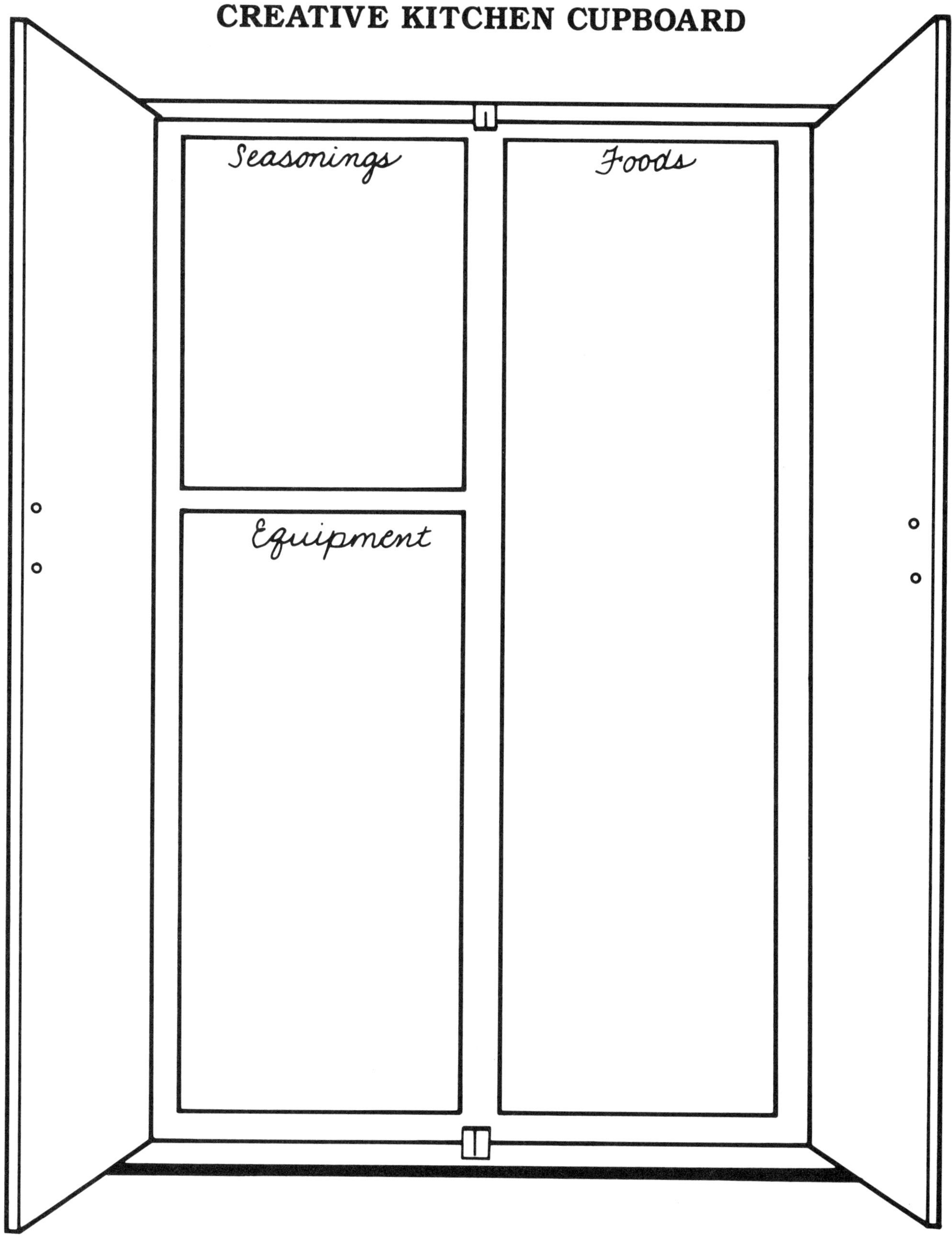

Name ______________________________ 

# CREATIVE MENU

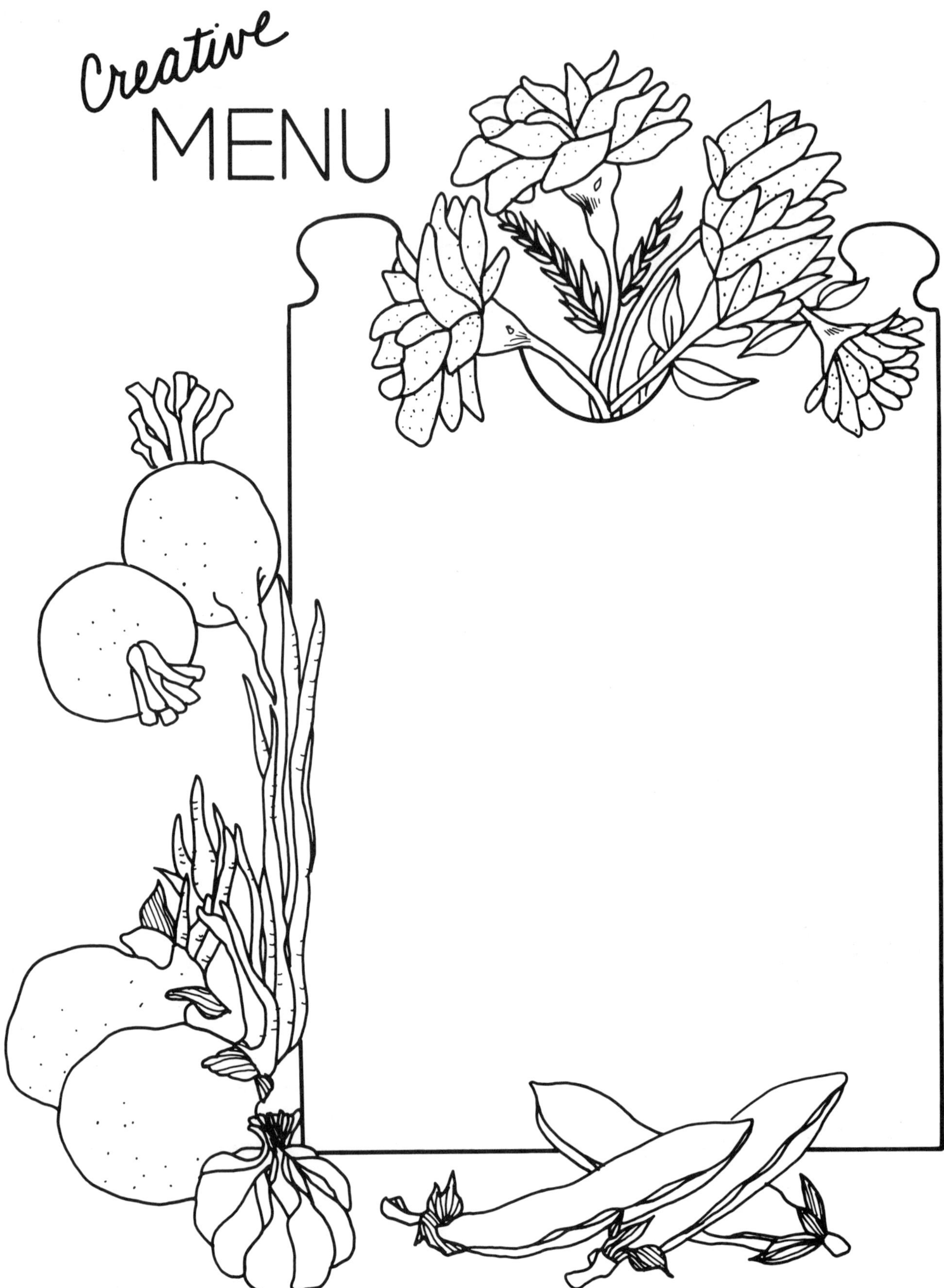

Name ______________________





# CREATIVE PRACTICE MENU

| Food | Amount | Fruit-Vegetable Group | Bread-Cereal Group | Milk-Cheese Group | Meat-Poultry-Fish-Beans Group | Fats-Sweets-Alcohol Group |
|---|---|---|---|---|---|---|
| | | | | | | |
| TOTAL NUMBER OF SERVINGS: | | | | | | |
| RECOMMENDED NUMBER OF SERVINGS PER DAY: | | | | | | |

Name ______________________________ **Sheet 14-4**

# I WOULD RATHER...

**Directions:** This exercise will help you to better understand your personal food intake style. In each group below, place a "1" beside your first choice, a "2" beside your second choice, and a "3" beside your last choice. Answer: "I would rather...

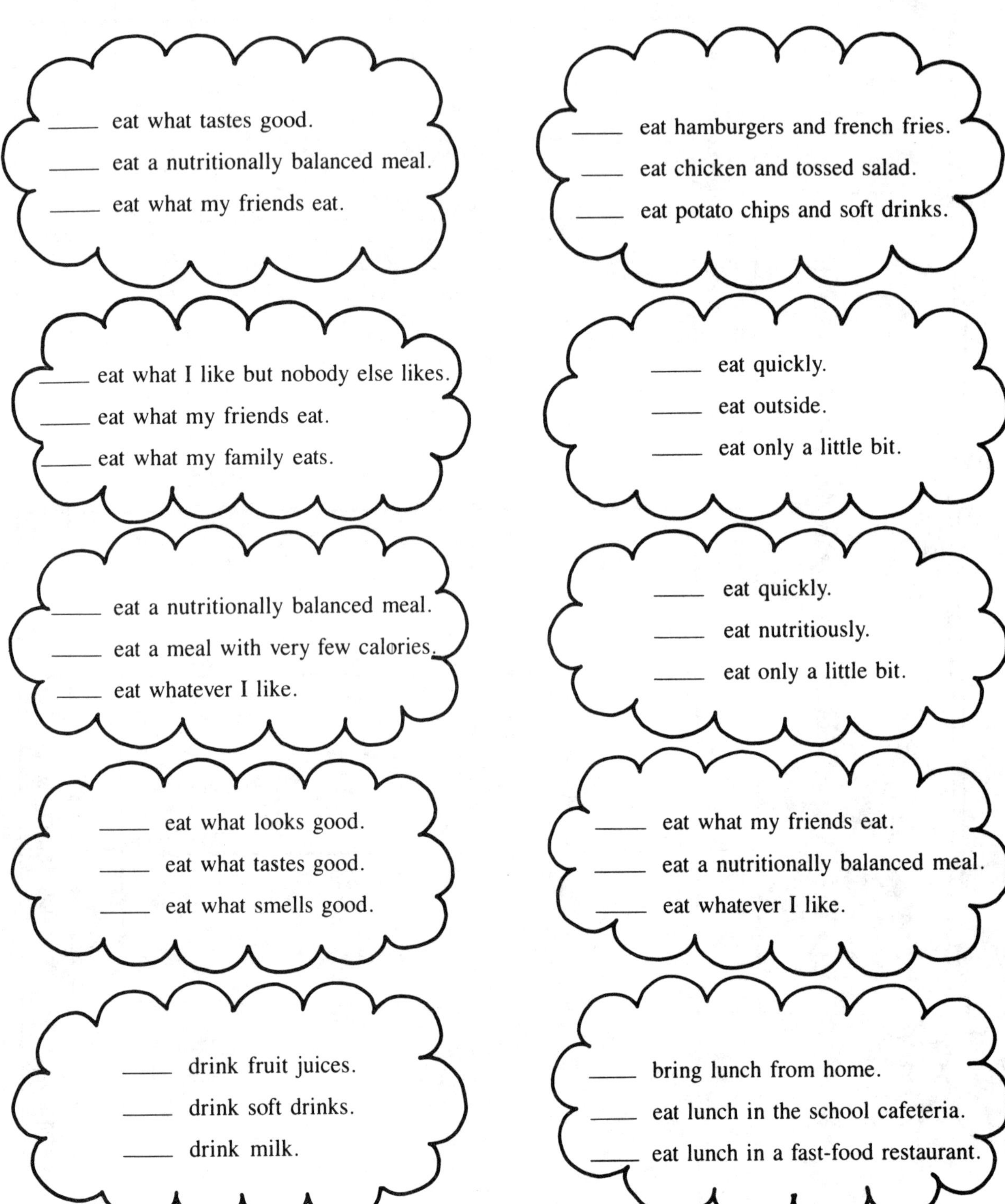

____ eat what tastes good.
____ eat a nutritionally balanced meal.
____ eat what my friends eat.
____ eat hamburgers and french fries.
____ eat chicken and tossed salad.
____ eat potato chips and soft drinks.
____ eat what I like but nobody else likes.
____ eat what my friends eat.
____ eat what my family eats.
____ eat quickly.
____ eat outside.
____ eat only a little bit.
____ eat a nutritionally balanced meal.
____ eat a meal with very few calories.
____ eat whatever I like.
____ eat quickly.
____ eat nutritiously.
____ eat only a little bit.
____ eat what looks good.
____ eat what tastes good.
____ eat what smells good.
____ eat what my friends eat.
____ eat a nutritionally balanced meal.
____ eat whatever I like.
____ drink fruit juices.
____ drink soft drinks.
____ drink milk.
____ bring lunch from home.
____ eat lunch in the school cafeteria.
____ eat lunch in a fast-food restaurant.

Name ____________________ Quiz Sheet 14-1

# QUIZ
# MENU PLANNING USING THE "DAILY FOOD GUIDE"

_____ 1. Which of the following menus provides one-third of the recommended servings from the "Daily Food Guide?"

a. 1 slice of toast with jelly, bowl of cereal, milk
b. 1 slice of bread, lettuce and tomato salad, salad dressing, juice
c. 1 egg, orange juice, muffin, milk
d. Hamburger with bun, mustard, ketchup, chocolate milk

_____ 2. Suppose you had this breakfast:

small glass of orange juice
3 slices of bacon
2 eggs
1 slice of rye bread

How could you change this menu to make it more nutritious?

a. Add a cup of tea
b. Remove the bacon and add sausage
c. Remove the bacon and add a glass of milk
d. Add a vegetable

Use this menu for questions 3 and 4:

hamburger on a bun
french fries
soft drink

_____ 3. Which food group is not represented in this meal?

a. Milk-Cheese group
b. Bread-Cereal group
c. Fruit-Vegetable group
d. Meat-Poultry-Fish-Beans group

_____ 4. What changes could you make in this menu the next time so that each food group is represented?

a. Order cole slaw instead of fries
b. Order milk instead of a soft drink
c. Order lettuce, tomato, and pickle on the hamburger
d. Order a fish sandwich instead of a hamburger

_____ 5. You should eat the suggested number of servings from the "Daily Food Guide" to:

a. Lose weight
b. Gain weight
c. Get needed minerals and vitamins
d. Meet the daily needs for the four major nutrients

_____ 6. A nutritious meal is one that:

a. Includes several types of food
b. Contains few carbohydrates
c. Includes no fat
d. Includes mostly protein

# Unit 15: Menu Planning for the Family

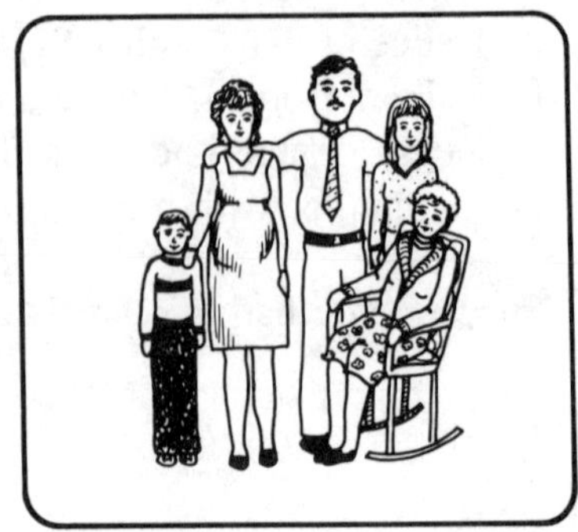

## CONCEPTS

–Each member of a family or household may have different nutritional needs.

–Planning a diet for individual family members requires an investigation of each person's nutritional needs, food preferences, budget, skill in food preparation techniques, and the amount of time each can spend preparing food.

## OBJECTIVES

–Students will plan and conduct a short interview of individual family members regarding each one's nutritional needs and food preferences, budget, skill in food preparation techniques, and the amount of time each can spend preparing food.

–Students will plan a day's or a week's menu for the family using the data collected during the interviews.

–Students will share this plan with the family and will report the family's reaction to the recommended menus.

## TEACHER'S UNIT INTRODUCTION

As you grow older, you want to and are expected to become more self-reliant in your food selection. Often teenagers are responsible not only for selecting their own food, but also for helping to plan and prepare foods for other family members. Anyone who is planning meals for groups of people should be aware of several aspects of meal planning. These are:

- **Nutritional Needs.** Every individual has special nutritional needs that must be taken into consideration when planning menus. Serving sizes are especially important to keep in mind, especially with young children. Most people need the same variety of foods, that is, several servings from each group in the "Daily Food Guide." [Refer to

Sheet 7-8, "Special Nutritional Needs at Different Life Stages," in Unit 7 for more information.]

- **Food Preferences.** Food likes and dislikes vary from person to person, with age, and with the passage of time. When planning meals for groups of people, it is difficult to please everyone all of the time. Occasionally compromises must be made by everyone.
- **Budget.** This aspect of meal planning probably demands the most time and thought. Although some families have unlimited food budgets, most families do not. As food prices rise, families need to learn how to shop economically and how to find nutritious bargains for their food dollars. Here is a list of ideas to help in budgeting. [Also refer to Sheet 11-7, "Grocery Shopping Hints," and Sheet 11-8, "Tips for Cutting Food Costs."]

–Establish limits on what certain foods should cost.

–Buy seasonal foods whenever possible. Some "staple" foods are good buys all year around (oats, wheat flour, nonfat dried milk, canned tomatoes, etc.).

–Compile an on-going shopping list of foods as they are used at home.

–Plan shopping trips ahead of time. Avoid frequent and unnecessary trips to the grocery store.

–Avoid impulse buying. Buy only necessary items.

–To avoid impulse buying, eat before you shop.

–Watch out for displayed products. They often encourage impulse buying and may not be on special sale.

–Avoid convenience foods, which are more expensive than the made-from-scratch variety.

–Buy store brands or generic brands.

–Compare prices of fresh, frozen, and canned versions of the same item.

–Shop alone or with a conscientious partner.

–Buy larger sizes, which are usually less expensive. Check unit pricing.

–Check ads and use coupons for bargains.

–Compare various stores' prices. Choose the store without gimmicks and heavy advertising. The costs of these extras are passed on to the consumer.

–Buy direct from local producers whenever possible to eliminate transportation costs.

- **Skill in Preparation Techniques.** Some people can whip up a spinach souffle without batting an eye; others struggle over a fried egg. The degree of skill possessed by family members influences the types of menus that can be planned and prepared.
- **Amount of Time to Spend.** Different families allot different amounts of time to the planning, preparation, and consumption of food. Some people enjoy devoting a large part of their day to food. Other people plan, prepare, and eat their meals as quickly as possible.

Meal planning in Unit 15 depends upon the use of Chart B, "Daily Food Guide." This method is not problem-free. One of the major problems occurs when students try to fit combination dishes into the meal pattern. For example, beef-barley soup contains some meat, some grain, and some vegetables, but not full servings of each. To accommodate these types of combinations, students must learn to break the foods apart and then to approximate the percentage of a serving size which the dish contributes. Using the same example, in one cup of soup there might be one ounce of beef (1/2 to 1/3 serving Meat-Poultry-Fish-Beans group), 1/2 cup of cooked barley (1 serving Bread-Cereal group), and 1/8 cup of vegetables (approximately 1/4 to 1/5 serving Fruit-Vegetable group). Thus, when planning meals with combination dishes, percentages of servings must be taken into account.

## BASIC ACTIVITY

**Time Needed:** Two class periods

**Materials Needed:** Sheet 7-8: "Special Nutritional Needs at Different Life Stages"
Chart A: "Recommended Dietary Allowances"
Sheet 15-1: "Planning a Diet for Everyone"
Sheet 15-2: "Family Practice Menu"
Quiz Sheet 15-1

### Class Period 1

1. This activity revolves around students talking with family members about their dietary habits. A family, for this purpose, is defined as any small group of individuals who share the planning, preparation, and consumption of some or all of their meals together. It is important for the students to actually interview the individuals in order to find out about other people's habits, preferences, and restrictions.

2. Have students engage in small-group planning sessions. Each group should decide the kinds of questions they would like to ask.

3. Bring students back to a large group. Try to get the large group to agree on most of the questions to be included in the interviews. Some questions may be added to individual interviews if there is not a consensus, as long as the questions are reasonable.

4. Students should practice interviews by questioning each other in dyads. Interviews should be limited to 15 to 20 minutes in length. Examples of the kinds of questions to be asked follow:

a. Do you have any special nutritional needs or restrictions?

b. What are some of your favorite foods?

c. What are some of your least favorite foods?

d. Does the rest of the family like or dislike these foods?

e. How much money does your family usually spend on groceries each week?

f. How much could you afford to spend on groceries?

g. How much would you like to spend on groceries?

h. How long have you been cooking?

i. Does your kitchen have: an oven? stove-top burners? a broiler? a microwave? a toaster? pots? pans? a spatula? a whisk/whip? a freezer? a mixer? a blender?

j. How much time do you usually spend preparing each meal?

k. Do you enjoy preparing meals?

These questions are only suggestions. Be aware that some of these questions are personal, especially those regarding money. Consider your own students and their families before encouraging them to ask personal questions during the interviews.

5. Distribute copies of Sheet 7-8, "Special Nutritional Needs at Different Life Stages," or Chart A, "Recommended Dietary Allowances," in order to investigate individual family members' nutritional needs.

6. Students should conduct the interviews at home, keep notes, and complete Sheet 15-1, "Planning a Diet for Everyone," and Sheet 15-2, "Family Practice Menu."

**Class Period 2**

1. Students should report informally to the class the results of their interviews. If there is some information that they do not wish to report, allow for abstention.

2. Divide the students into small groups. Have each group pick their favorite practice menu and, if possible, prepare that meal. Alternatively, use the small groups of students as hypothetical families and have them plan, prepare, and evaluate a meal accordingly.

3. Proceed with the "Advanced Activity" if you wish; otherwise use the quiz mentioned in step 4.

4. **Evaluation:** Distribute Quiz Sheet 15-1 and have students complete it independently, either in class or as homework. Discuss the answers as a class.

## ADVANCED ACTIVITY

**Time Needed:** One class period

**Materials Needed:** Sheet 15-2: "Family Practice Menu" (completed)
Chart A: "Recommended Dietary Allowances"
Chart E: "Dietary Calculation Chart"
Food composition tables (*See* "References/Resources" at the end of this kit)
Calculators *(optional)*
Quiz Sheet 15-1

1. Distribute Chart A, "Recommended Dietary Allowances," and Chart E, "Dietary Calculation Chart."

2. Have students record their foods from Sheet 15-2 onto Chart E.

3. Have students calculate the nutrient content of their menu and compare it to the RDAs for at least one family member. Remind students that each meal should provide one-third of the RDAs for the day.

4. Have students compare the two methods of evaluating the menus: the one that uses the "Daily Food Guide" and the one that uses the Nutrient Analysis Method.

## FOLLOW-UP ACTIVITIES

1. Look at the Recommended Dietary Allowances (RDAs) for several nutrients to compare levels for males and females and also for several different age levels. Why is there a difference? What does the difference mean in terms of food? Have students compare their own food intake to that of others of the opposite sex and of different ages. Do their comparisons look like the differences in the RDA tables?

2. Have students plan an evening meal that will satisfy food preferences for a vegetarian and for a nonvegetarian at the same meal.

3. Have students plan a menu for a family of four (two teenagers and two parents) using a low-cost food plan. Have them adapt the menu to a holiday menu, an outdoor menu, a low-calorie menu, and a time-saving menu.

Name ______________________________ Sheet 15-1

# PLANNING A DIET FOR EVERYONE

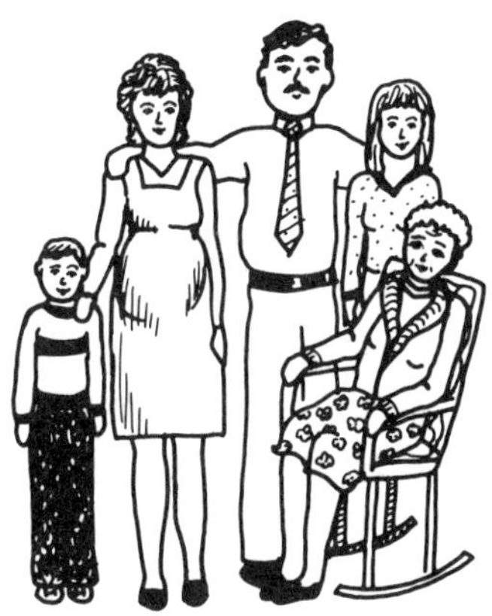

### A. Family Profile

Take into account the nutritional needs of each family member when planning a family diet. (1) Fill in the number of people in your family in the appropriate categories on the chart. (2) Use Sheet 7-8, "Special Nutritional Needs at Different Life Stages," and figure out how many servings of each food is needed. Total the number of servings in the right-hand column.

| FOOD GROUPS | Pregnant Women #_____ | Infants #_____ | Children #_____ | Teenagers #_____ | Adults #_____ | Elderly #_____ | TOTAL #_____ |
|---|---|---|---|---|---|---|---|
| MILK-CHEESE GROUP | | | | | | | |
| MEAT-POULTRY-FISH-BEANS GROUP | | | | | | | |
| FRUIT-VEGETABLE GROUP | | | | | | | |
| BREAD-CEREAL GROUP | | | | | | | |

(3) Interview each family member and record your notes on the back of this sheet.

### B. Practice Menu

Now that you know how many servings of each type of food your family needs, you can plan a menu. Keep in mind the information you gathered about which foods family members prefer, your family budget, individual skills in the kitchen, and the amount of time your family spends on food preparation. Complete Sheet 15-2.

### C. Evaluation

Take the menu on Sheet 15-2 to your family and ask them to tell you what they think of it. Ask them these questions:

1. Do you like the foods on this menu?
2. Do you think it provides a nutritious selection of foods?
3. Would the cost of the foods be within your budget?
4. Do you know how to prepare, or could you learn how to prepare, all of the foods on this menu?
5. Do you have the time to prepare this menu?
6. Will you use this menu some day next week or next month? Why or why not?

Name ______________________ Sheet 15-2

# FAMILY PRACTICE MENU

**Directions:** Write a practice menu for one day on the sheet below and count the number of servings from each food group. Write in the "Total Number of Servings for the Family" using your "Family Profile." Now compare your menu to your family's needs. Do you have the right number of servings per day from each food group? Are the foods ones your family likes? Will the menu fit their budget? Are the preparation time and skill right for the family? If there are problems with the menu, alter it until it seems just right. Then continue to plan daily menus for the rest of a full week.

| Food (M) MEAL OR (S) SNACK | Amount | Fruit-Vegetable Group | Bread-Cereal Group | Milk-Cheese Group | Meat-Poultry-Fish-Beans Group | Fats-Sweets-Alcohol Group |
|---|---|---|---|---|---|---|
| | | | | | | |
| TOTAL NUMBER OF SERVINGS FOR THE FAMILY: | | | | | | |
| RECOMMENDED NUMBER OF SERVINGS PER DAY: | | | | | | |

# QUIZ
# MENU PLANNING FOR THE FAMILY

____ 1. What would be the most important thing to know when planning a meal for your family?

a. The type of bread, vegetable, meat, dessert, and drink they like
b. How much calcium, Vitamin C, protein, iron, and calories they need
c. How much money and time the family has available for food preparation
d. All of the above

2. Write a short paragraph describing the results of your family interviews. Remember to include descriptions of food preferences, nutritional needs of family members, budget, preparation time, and the skills and interests of the food preparers.

______________________________________________________________________

______________________________________________________________________

______________________________________________________________________

______________________________________________________________________

______________________________________________________________________

______________________________________________________________________

______________________________________________________________________

______________________________________________________________________

______________________________________________________________________

______________________________________________________________________



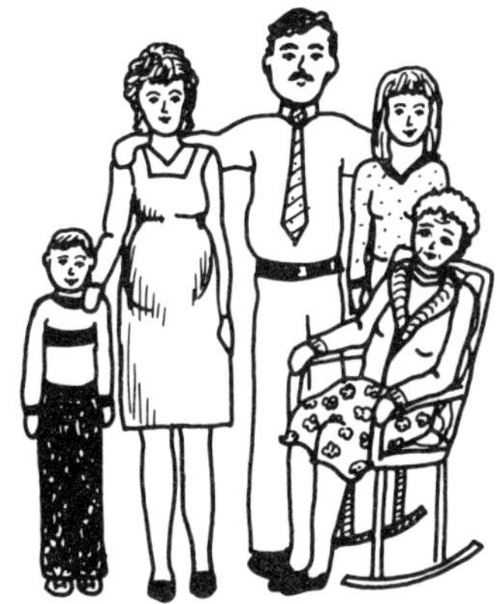

# SECTION V

# NUTRITION ISSUES

# Unit 16: Evaluating Nutrition Information

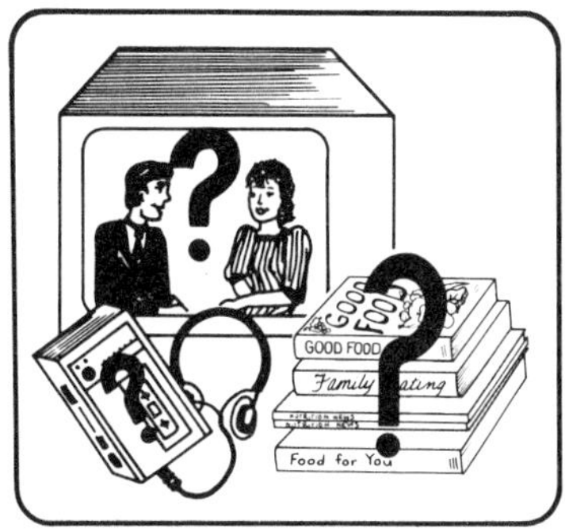


## CONCEPTS

–Many diet and health claims promote the acceptance of a particular mode or method of attaining optimal nutritional health.

–Awareness of unreliable and reliable sources of nutrition information is the basis for making well-planned decisions concerning nutritional intake.

–Reliable sources of nutrition information can be obtained from many public and private organizations.

–Reliable sources of nutrition information are ones that are trustworthy, dependable, and consistent and that promote only up-to-date, scientifically based information.

## OBJECTIVES

–Students will be able to assess the reliability of specific nutritional claims and to explain why each is either reliable or unreliable.

–Students will be able to identify reliable sources of nutrition information.

## TEACHER'S UNIT INTRODUCTION

With all of the nutrition information available today from books, magazines, TV personalities, radio talk shows, and other sources, it is important for you to be able to tell which information is reliable and which is unreliable. You must be especially wary of many of the food fads that are being marketed. The topics that are currently very popular among many segments of the population are the various questionable methods of weight control that offer quick cures for obesity.

The Food and Drug Administration has set standards for truth in labeling, product purity, and the testing and use of food additives. The Federal Trade Commission takes action against advertisements that are misleading or untruthful, but often the process is drawn out in the courts. However, these two organizations cannot make decisions for you as to which food products you will choose to use on a daily basis. You must be able to make those choices yourself. This unit will give you the tools to make informed food product selections on your own.

---

The student is faced with many problems in trying to make a proper assessment of nutritional claims. Since nutrition is a relatively young science, new trends and information are beginning to appear daily, and the need for research continues to grow. Many consumers of all ages lack basic nutrition knowledge. Today's school-aged children are fortunate to be in school during a time when there is more emphasis being placed on nutrition education in the classroom. However, many who are beyond school age find themselves having to search out nutrition information, not knowing how to selectively choose their sources nor which sources to believe. Therefore, it is wise for a person to be aware of guidelines to follow in determining the reliability of a source. In Unit 16, a reproducible sheet of questions to screen nutrition information has been provided for this purpose. Review Sheet 16-3, "The Reliability Detector," before reading further.

An example of an unreliable nutrition claim and how it can be detected follows:

> VITAMINS FOR HAIR CARE! Is your hair dry, brittle, or falling out? Then you need some of our special formula vitamins at $5.95 for a jar of 30. You'll see improvements in your hair condition in no time!

To evaluate this claim, apply the following screening questions from Sheet 16-3:

#1 Is fear a tactic? Are you urged to buy something you would not have otherwise bought? (Yes)

#3 Does the promoter attribute most diseases to a faulty diet and state that his or her special product(s) or diet will cure your ills dramatically? (Yes)

#8 Are magical or secret properties about certain food products or nutrients suggested? (Yes)

In addition to using these questions, you can also consult reliable nutrition books, journals, and booklets listed in the "References/Resources" section for this unit at the end of this kit, as well as long-established, reputable agencies concerned with the dissemination of reliable nutrition information. Examples are voluntary health agencies, such as the American Diabetes Association, the American Heart Association, and the National Foundation-March of Dimes. Some of the material produced by these agencies is aimed at specific target groups such as expectant mothers (American Heart Association and March of Dimes), persons with high blood pressure, cardiovascular disease, and obesity (American Heart Association), and diabetics (American Diabetes Association). Other reliable professional organizations that provide nutrition information include: the American Dietetic Association, the Society for Nutrition Education, the American Medical Association, and the American Dental Association. These associations publish professional journals for members and other health professionals as well as provide service projects such as National Nutrition Week and messages to the public on radio and television.

Many trade associations, such as the National Potato Board, the Cereal Institute, and the National Livestock and Meat Board, also provide a variety of nutrition information. One should be aware, however, that some of the material promoting their food products may be biased, although nutritionally accurate.

## BASIC ACTIVITY

**Time Needed:** One class period

**Materials Needed:** Sheets 16-1 through 16-2: "Which Nutrition Claims Are Reliable?"
Sheet 16-3: "The Reliability Detector"
Quiz Sheet 16-1

1. Distribute Sheets 16-1 through 16-2, "Which Nutrition Claims Are Reliable?" Using their previous nutrition knowledge, students should be given about ten minutes to independently determine and identify:

   a. Which claims are reliable (marked OK).

   b. Which claims are unreliable (marked UR).

2. As a class, discuss which claims are reliable and why. (*See* the "Answer Key" for Unit 16 at the end of this kit.) Have students suggest reasons to explain why these claims seem unreliable. Lead students to the idea that a set of questions can be used to screen nutrition claims and to determine their reliability.

3. Distribute Sheet 16-3, "The Reliability Detector." For each claim marked "UR" on Sheets 16-1 through 16-2, students should identify the specific questions from Sheet 16-3 that would be used to detect unreliability.

4. Conduct a brief discussion regarding the questions that indicate the unreliability of each claim. Suggest that one way to further check the reliability of each claim is to consult a reliable nutrition textbook, journal, or the informational literature of a voluntary agency concerned with the dissemination of reliable nutrition information. Cite several of these agencies, relating some of them to specific claims on the worksheet. Samples are:

   a. claim 7: American Heart Association

   b. claim 9: March of Dimes, American Heart Association

   c. claim 10: American Medical Association

   d. claim 4: American Diabetes Association, American Dietetic Association

5. Proceed with the "Advanced Activity" if you wish; otherwise use the quiz mentioned in step 6.

6. **Evaluation:** Distribute Quiz Sheet 16-1 and have students complete it independently. Discuss the answers as a class.

## ADVANCED ACTIVITY

**Time Needed:** One class period

**Materials Needed:** Samples of nutrition information, both reliable and unreliable, from magazines, newspapers, and books
Sheet 16-3: "The Reliability Detector"
Quiz Sheet 16-1

1. Give small groups of students samples of nutrition information in printed form, including one or two paragraphs of both reliable and unreliable information taken from popular magazines, local newspapers, and books.
2. Have each group evaluate its nutrition information according to the criteria on Sheet 16-3, "The Reliability Detector."
3. Have each group present its findings to the class. Then conduct a large-group discussion about which sources students should use to obtain nutrition information.
4. Present the following cases to the whole class and have students discuss where they would go to find reliable and unbiased nutrition information to solve each one:
    a. Your best friend is going on a crazy-sounding diet called "The Flab Fighter's Food Feast." You want to try to convince your friend not to try it. Where would you go for more information about the diet? (*Sample answers:* local health department, hospital dietitian, family doctor)
    b. Your mother told you about an article she read that said teenagers need extra vitamin $B^6$ for good health. She wants you to take the vitamin pill every day. You are not so sure it is a good idea. Who can you ask about it? (*Sample answers:* local nutritionist or dietitian, school nurse)
    c. You saw an advertisement for a personalized nutritional analysis. All you do is send a sample of hair and $15 to get a report about how nutritionally balanced you are. Where do you go for more information? (*Sample answers:* the nutrition department at a local college, the Food and Drug Administration, the American Dietetic Association)
5. **Evaluation:** Distribute Quiz Sheet 16-1 and have students complete it independently. Have students exchange papers and grade one another following your directions. Then discuss the answers as a class.

## FOLLOW-UP ACTIVITIES

1. Using Sheet 16-3, "The Reliability Detector," have small groups of students each develop a food product and a related *unreliable* TV or radio advertisement for it. Each advertisement must be made unreliable according to at least two screening questions from Sheet 16-3. Then, using tape recorders with background music and/or other equipment or techniques, have each group present its advertisement to the class. The class should identify the specific screening questions from Sheet 16-3 that determine the unreliability of each advertisement.

2. Have students make a slide presentation about false nutritional claims and present it to another class or group of parents. Have two classes interchange slide presentations.

3. Have students write to or visit one of the professional organizations that disseminate nutrition information (for example, the Food and Drug Administration, local March of Dimes, local American Heart Association, local American Diabetes Association, a food trade association), and have them request some of their printed nutrition information. Once all of the information has been received, students can set up a display in the classroom or on a hallway bulletin board to share with others.

4. Invite a speaker from one of the local associations to talk about his or her reasons for concern about proper nutrient intake or special diets.

5. Invite a guest speaker to talk about reliable and unbiased nutrition information sources and also about their professional training. Some professionals you might invite include a dietitian, a nutritionist, a nurse, or a physician.

6. Set up a debate to argue the statement: "False claims may be made about many food and nutrition products. These claims may or may not be dangerous. Food manufacturers should be allowed to market any product in whatever manner they find to be profitable. Consumers must be responsible for their own purchases."

Name ______________________________ 



# WHICH NUTRITION CLAIMS ARE RELIABLE?

**Directions:** If you feel the nutrition claim is reliable, mark it "OK." If you feel the claim is unreliable, mark it "UR."

____ 1. Vitamin C is essential if you want healthy gums!

____ 2. Bee pollen is one of the best sources of energy to make you a strong runner. One month's supply is only $5.95.

____ 3. Power Tabs,™ which contain natural vitamins and minerals, will help maximize body efficiency and energy, which is depleted by the nutritional inadequacies of overprocessed foods.

____ 4. Vitamin D will assist in the utilization of calcium by the bones, a necessary function for skeletal maintenance.

____ 5. Chocolate Energy Bars™ play a vital role as quick pick-me-ups before your athletic performance.

____ 6. Chromill GTF,™ containing the mineral chromium, is an excellent supplement to maintain youthful vitality that is lost due to chromium deficiencies.

____ 7. Meta E,™ a gelatin capsule containing Vitamin E, wheat germ oil, and lecithin, is an effective aid in minimizing the damaging effects of pollution on one's looks, health, and heart.

____ 8. If your diet is low in Vitamin A, you may have trouble seeing in dim light.

____ 9. Pregnant women should drink specially prepared vegetable juice to prevent miscarriages and infant deformities. In this way, they will receive a larger amount of necessary vitamins and minerals than from eating whole vegetables, which have become devoid of nutrients through too much handling and which contain many contaminants from chemical fertilizers and pesticides used for growth.

____ 10. Doctor J. D. Livingston, from Arlington, Virginia, has come out with a report that promotes simple food formulas as treatments for arthritis. His book, *Your Diet and Arthritis,* was written after the successful treatment of six arthritis patients.

____ 11. Vita Formula 96,™ with its secret ingredients, makes up for the nutrients you lose daily as a result of the poor food sources found in the American diet. A must for every household!

# WHICH NUTRITION CLAIMS ARE RELIABLE?

____ 12. *Food, the National Medicine* is a book by Jim Brody which gives testimony about the body's ability to ward off many diseases through different food combinations. Only $5.95.

____ 13. A decrease in calories and an increase in activity is a diet regimen recommended by many experts.

____ 14. Dr. K. J. Hilliman has launched a diet that keeps the intake of carbohydrates very low and allows you to drink as much of any beverage as you like—from soft drinks to alcoholic beverages. Many of his followers cite the diet as a success, with weight losses being very controlled. Dr. Hilliman says the medical profession is critical of him since many diabetics are following his diet. "Diabetics are required to keep their carbohydrate intake low, and following my diet is simply the way they choose to do it," says Dr. Hilliman.

____ 15. You can lose weight while you sleep, with the special Weight Away Capsule manufactured by the J. B. Pharmaceutical Company. The specially formulated capsule has been recommended by successful users and costs only $2.95 for a package of 30 (less than 10¢ a capsule).

____ 16. America's biggest problem today is overeating, especially the overconsumption of many of the foods found in supermarkets. Most of these foods, by being processed and manufactured for a long shelf life (the amount of time they stay in the market), lack the nutrients necessary for optimum body function, but retain the fats. Smart eaters know they must supplement these foods with vitamins but often do not realize which vitamins to choose. First, for optimum performance one must read the label to be sure the vitamins are organic. Second, one should make sure one is getting a good supply of B vitamins, which many multipurpose vitamins do not supply. BETA-B™ is the best source of B vitamins on the market today and has a good supply of other minerals as well. You may pay more, but isn't your health worth it?

# THE RELIABILITY DETECTOR

A nutritional claim is unreliable if the answer is "Yes" to one or more of the questions below.

1. Is fear a tactic? Are you urged to buy something you would not have otherwise bought?
2. Does the promoter downgrade normal foods as being worthless, devoid of nutrients, or dangerous to your health?
3. Does the promoter attribute most diseases to a faulty diet and state that his or her special product(s) or diet will cure your ills dramatically?
4. Does the promoter lack important credentials? Does he or she fail to have the backing of qualified nutritionists and/or professional organizations recognized for publishing credible nutrition information? Does he or she lack an earned degree in nutrition or a related field, such as physiology or human medicine?
5. Are testimonies and "case histories" rather than scientifically controlled studies used to support the claims or theories?
6. Does the promoter claim that *everyone* needs vitamin supplements to offer insurance for poor dietary habits? Are "natural" vitamins promoted over synthetic vitamins?
7. Is the promoter claiming "persecution" by the "establishment"?
8. Are magical or secret properties about certain food products or nutrients suggested?
9. Does the promoter promise quick, dramatic, and miraculous cures?
10. Does the promoter suggest that only a few foods be eaten?
11. Does the promoter promise cures for many *different* kinds of ill health with the same, or similar, food products or nutrient supplements?

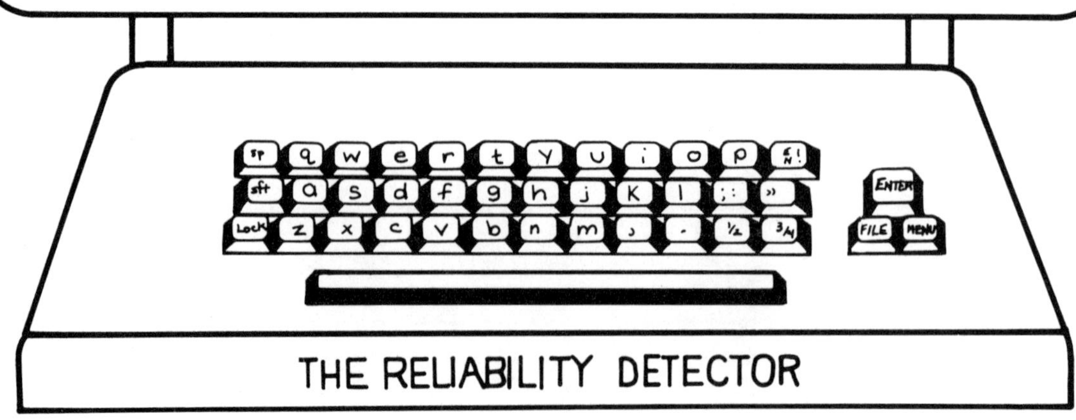

Name ______________________________ Quiz Sheet 16-1

# QUIZ
# EVALUATING NUTRITION INFORMATION

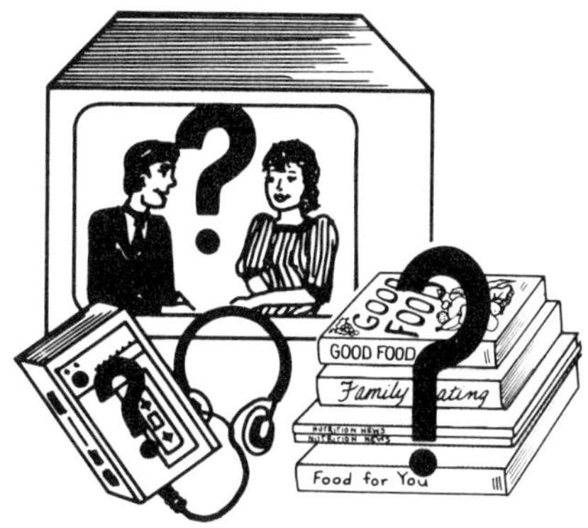


1. Read the case history below, then name two screening questions that can be used to determine if the food product's claim is unreliable or false.

   Mary Ann is overweight and has a family history of cardiovascular disease. She would like to lose weight. She therefore purchases some capsules that are advertised as helpful to those who want to lose five pounds overnight. The capsule advertisement goes on to say that this secret remedy is the envy of the medical profession and has been condemned by the profession as being ineffective.

______________________________

______________________________

____ 2. Which of the following is *not* a reliable contact for nutrition information?

   a. American Heart Association
   b. The Vitamin Discount House
   c. The American Dietetic Association
   d. Society for Nutrition Education

3. Suppose your best friend is overweight and has asked you to help find information about losing weight. Where would you go for information? List three sources.

   a. ______________________________
   b. ______________________________
   c. ______________________________

4. Someone you know has just been released from the hospital following a major heart attack. His doctor gave him a diet to follow but did not explain it very well. He asks you to help him figure it out. Where would you go to find out about his diet? List three sources.

   a. ______________________________
   b. ______________________________
   c. ______________________________

5. A friend of yours has stopped eating meat. You are afraid that your friend may not be getting enough of the proper nutrients. Where would you find information to give to your friend? List three sources.

   a. ______________________________
   b. ______________________________
   c. ______________________________

# *Unit 17: Diet and Disease: Obesity*

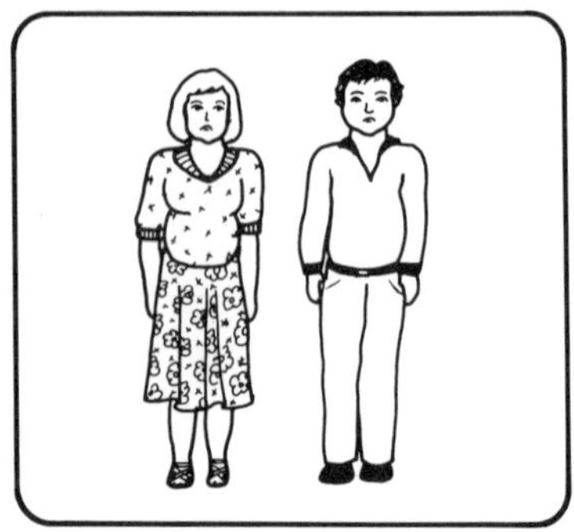

## CONCEPTS

–Obesity is a prevalent public health problem in the United States and in most affluent nations.

–Several disorders and diseases are associated with obesity.

–Obesity can put an individual at a disadvantage psychologically, physically, socially, and economically.

–The ability to differentiate between the facts and fallacies associated with weight control is critical to the success of any weight-control program.

## OBJECTIVES

–The student will be able to identify three health problems, one social problem, and one economic problem associated with obesity.

–The student will be able to apply two techniques for diagnosing obesity.

–The student will be able to evaluate criteria for a sound weight-reduction program.

## TEACHER'S UNIT INTRODUCTION

Obesity is a significant public health problem in the United States and in most other affluent nations. More than 10 percent of all school-aged children, about 15 percent of teenagers and young adults, and up to 30 percent of adults in America are considered to be obese. Obesity affects all ages, all races, and all socioeconomic classes.

*Obesity* may be defined most simply as a condition in which there is an excessive accumulation of body fat. Certain health problems (disorders and diseases) are found to appear more frequently in obese individuals. These health problems are related, in part, to the increased stress obesity places upon the heart, blood vessels, pancreas, kidneys, and skeletal structure. Obesity is a risk factor for such problems as adult-onset diabetes, arthritis, hypertension, gout, menstrual abnormalities, reproductive problems, gallbladder disease, kidney disease, heart attack, stroke, some types of cancer in females, and complications during childbirth and surgery.

Normally, the body weight of an adult female is composed of from 20 to 24 percent fat, and the body weight of an adult male is from 12 to 18 percent fat. When these figures reach from 28 to 30 percent for the female and greater than 20 percent for the male, the amount of fat is judged to be abnormally high.

According to height-weight tables, a person is considered to be obese if his or her weight is greater than 20 percent above the ideal or desirable weight for his or her height and body frame. For example, if the ideal weight for a 6-foot-tall, medium-frame man is 167 pounds, he would be considered to be obese by these standards if he weighed 201 pounds ($201 - 167 = 34$; $34 \div 167 = 20.4\%$). Because individuals between the ages of 11 and 17 have considerable variability in their growth spurts, height-weight tables for them are less accurate than tables for adults. Sheet 17-3, "What Weight Is Desirable?," in this unit is an adaptation of the commonly cited Metropolitan Life Insurance Company's "Height and Weight Tables." It lists desirable weights for heights of 18 year olds. It is important to note that some individuals can be overweight and yet not be obese (or overfat). For example, athletes who have a large amount of muscle tissue are often overweight but have very little body fat.

Obesity should be diagnosed using techniques that measure body fat such as skinfold measurements. An instrument called a *caliper* pinches a fold of skin while applying constant pressure at various places on the body in order to measure body fat. While there are several body sites on which to take skinfold measurements, one of the most common is that point located at the back of the upper arm, halfway between the elbow and the shoulder. A skinfold measurement taken at this point is referred to as a triceps skinfold measurement. The "Basic Activity" in this unit illustrates a crude but simplified way to take a triceps skinfold measurement using the thumb and forefinger instead of calipers. Of course, an accurate diagnosis requires the use of calipers by an individual trained in the techniques of taking such measurements.

For the obese individual, there are many disadvantages. In addition to the physical disadvantages mentioned above, the obese individual also finds himself or herself at a social disadvantage, which may result in what can be viewed as a "vicious circle." Sometimes the initial weight gain is caused by some type of unhappy social adjustment. This overweight state eventually results in obesity, which can, in turn, result in social rejection. This, in turn, can lead to *more* overeating, to more weight gain, and to continued or more profound rejection. Adolescents are often prime targets for this particular chain of events. Excessive weight can decrease the person's participation in many sports activities as well as in social activities. From an economic point of view, the obese individual has a difficult time obtaining employment in occupations where public impressions are important (for example, in jobs such as flight attendant, nurse, dietitian, salesperson, receptionist). Additionally, some employers are reluctant to hire persons who are obvious health risks, which thus places additional restrictions on job opportunities for the obese. The economic stability of the obese is further affected by the price of special clothing, medical expenses, and the money lost to various fad diet plans.

In order for weight gain to occur, calorie intake must exceed calorie expenditure. This is referred to as a positive energy balance. Weight gain can occur very slowly and can creep up on an unsuspecting individual. Although it takes 3,500 calories in excess of needs to produce one additional pound of fat, this calorie excess can be gradually accumulated over a long period of time. For example, ten calories (for example, one potato chip) extra every day for 350 days will lead to an additional pound of body weight at the end of one year. Similarly, 700 calories (for example, one quarter-pound hamburger with cheese and french fries) extra every day for five days will result in the same weight gain in less than one week. By the same token, for an individual to lose one pound of body fat, a state of negative energy balance must persist: the diet must provide 3,500 calories less than the body needs. Ideally, weight loss is achieved through a combination of dietary restriction and increased physical activity. A healthy rate of weight loss is one to two pounds per week.

The importance of some type of exercise in a weight-reduction program cannot be overemphasized. A program that includes physical activity as well as diet modifications has been shown to be the most successful type of weight-reduction program. Without increased physical activity, dietary restrictions will have to be more severe to accomplish the same weight-loss goal (holding time constant). In addition to directly using calories, regular physical activity helps control appetite and tones muscles. The exercise need not be tedious and strenuous. The best type of exercise is that which involves some type of individual or team sport that the dieter enjoys. That way, exercising will not be a chore. Something as simple as a brisk walk for a set amount of time each day can be quite effective. Dieters should analyze the types of activities they enjoy most. If they cannot think of any enjoyable exercises, they should start trying some out! An extensive chart listing the calorie expenditure of various activities is provided on Chart G, "Calorie Expenditure by Activity."

---

The introduction to Unit 17 and the manner in which it is presented are important because of the students' sensitivities about body image. Teenagers are preoccupied with the way they look, especially when compared to their peers. This unit encourages the students to measure themselves and, in so doing, also encourages comparisons between students. For the overweight teen, these comparisons could be shattering. The tone when presenting Unit 17 should be impersonal and nondiscriminatory. The problem of being overweight should be viewed as just that: a problem. It is not something to be taken lightly; it is not an easy problem for anyone to overcome.

## BASIC ACTIVITY

**Time Needed:** One class period

**Materials Needed:** Sheet 17-1: "What's a Good Diet?"
Sheet 17-2: "A Reason for Concern"
Sheet 17-3: "What Weight Is Desirable"
Sheet 17-4: "What Is the Truth About Weight Control?"
Quiz Sheet 17-1

1. Distribute Sheet 17-1, "What's a Good Diet?" Have students read the material and make notes about personal weight-reduction problems. Students should look specifically for health, social, and economic problems.

2. Distribute Sheet 17-2, "A Reason for Concern," and have students complete it independently. Then, as a class, discuss the problems identified by students in each category: health, social, and economic. Use the problems cited in the "Teacher's Unit Introduction" to expand each category, and make sure to identify several of the disorders and diseases associated with obesity. Students should also identify the principal cause of obesity for Barbara and should propose a general weight-reduction program for her.

3. Ask students to identify ways an individual can tell if he or she is obese. Several methods, which include the following, are available:

a. Skinfold measurements—to determine the percentage of body fat

b. Height-weight tables—to compare a person's weight with a desirable weight for a specific height and frame size

c. Mirror test—to check for excess fat by examining your naked body in the mirror

4. If you wish, students who want to can get a *rough* estimate of whether they have too much body fat by doing the "pinch test." *This part of the "Basic Activity" should be strictly optional.* If there are several overweight students in the class who may be uncomfortable with this activity, you should conduct it as a demonstration with a student volunteer. The student should

a. Roll up his or her shirt sleeves beyond the midpoint of the upper arm

b. Estimate the midpoint between the elbow and the top of the shoulder

c. Pinch and pull away the skin and fat at the midpoint, being careful not to pinch up the muscle too

Females who pinch up an inch or more and males who pinch up more than three-quarters of an inch are considered overfat.

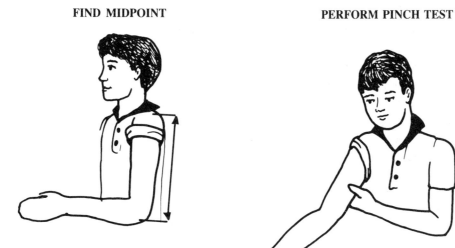

**FIND MIDPOINT**

**PERFORM PINCH TEST**

5. Distribute Sheet 17-3, "What Weight Is Desirable?," and have students find the desirable weight for an 18 year old of each student's height and frame size. (Note that the majority of the students will have a medium frame size.) Frame size can be assessed by grasping the wrist with the thumb and middle finger. If the thumb and middle finger overlap by a half inch or more, the person is considered to have a small frame. If the thumb and middle finger just touch or overlap slightly, the person is considered to have a medium frame. If the thumb and middle finger do not touch, the person is considered to have a large frame.

6. Distribute Sheet 17-4, "What Is the Truth About Weight Control?" and assign one question to each student or pair of students to answer. Give students three minutes to jot down their answers; then go over the sheet and elicit students' answers. (*See* the "Answer Key" at the end of this kit.)

7. Proceed with the "Advanced Activity" if you wish; otherwise use the quiz mentioned in step 8.

8. **Evaluation:** Distribute Quiz Sheet 17-1 and have students complete it independently. Discuss the answers as a class.

## ADVANCED ACTIVITY

**Time Needed:** One class period

**Materials Needed:** Sheets 17-5 through 17-6: "Obesity Relay Race"
Chart G: "Calorie Expenditure by Activity" *(optional)*
Quiz Sheet 17-1

1. The game "Obesity Relay Race" is designed for students who have had some exposure to all of the concepts presented in Unit 17.

2. Play the game according to the directions below:

- Copy Sheets 17-5 and 17-6, "Obesity Relay Race," and cut each sheet in half to make 4 sets of 10 questions each.
- Divide the class into 4 teams and organize them in 4 separate sections of the classroom.
- Divide the chalkboard into 4 sections numbered from 1 to 10 on which the teams will write their answers. Place the question sheet for each team on the chalkboard ledge directly below its assigned area.
- Tell each team that they will find on the chalkboard ledge a list of 10 questions to be answered in turn by each team member. At the command "Go," the first "runner" from each team will run to the board and write the answer to the first question in his or her team's chalkboard area and then will run back to the team's area of the classroom. The race will continue with each player going to the board and writing an answer in turn, until each player has answered at least one question. Since each team will most likely have more questions than players, the team should decide before the race which person(s) should go twice.

- If a teammate has difficulty answering his or her question, he or she may "pass" by leaving his or her space on the board blank. Then, once the team has completed all other questions, they may work as a unit to help that player answer the question.
- The teacher or a selected student will check each team's answers. (*See* the "Answer Key" at the end of this kit.) The first team to finish with all of the correct answers is the winner.

3. **Evaluation:** Distribute Quiz Sheet 17-1 and have students complete it independently. Discuss the answers as a class.

## FOLLOW-UP ACTIVITIES

1. Students should keep a record of *all* the activities they do and the time (minutes) spent doing each over a 24-hour period.

To determine the calories they expended, students should

- Find the calories expended per unit time for each activity on Chart G, "Calorie Expenditure by Activity"
- Multiply calories expended per unit time by the number of units spent doing the activity
- Multiply the sum total of calories expended by body weight

An example of a calculation tracing through the above steps is found on Chart G.

2. Divide the class into groups. Give each group a different case study supplying the following information:

- The obese person's present weight
- The obese person's ideal weight-height and frame size
- The total number of pounds the individual wishes to lose
- The number of calories the individual is presently consuming per day (use 2,200 if female and 2,900 if male)

Each group must then determine

- How much weight the person will lose per week.
- How many calories the person will eat per day.
- What additional activities the person will do each day; the length of time and number of calories expended must be given. Students should refer to Chart G, "Calorie Expenditure by Activity."

Further challenge could be added by having each group construct a balanced daily diet for three days that would provide the calorie limit determined above. Students should use Chart D, "Food Composition Table for Selected Nutrients," as a resource.

Name ______________________________ 

# WHAT'S A GOOD DIET?

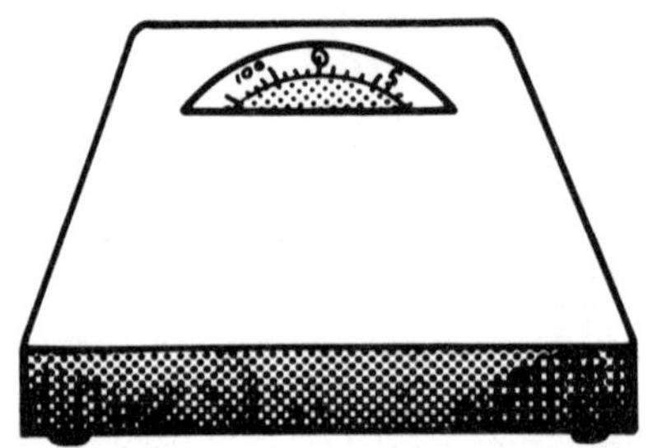

**Directions:** A lot of people are overweight. Other people are just about the right weight. If you need to lose weight, jot down your weight-reduction problems on the back of this sheet. Look specifically at your health, social, and economic problems. Then read the dieting information below. If you don't need to lose weight, share the information with someone you love. It's a matter of life and health!

Many different approaches to weight control exist. Many diets are both safe and effective. Others may pose serious health threats to the dieter or may produce little loss of stored fat. Rather than look at these diets individually, a few criteria that may be used to judge the merits of dietary approaches are listed below.

1. The diet must be lower in calories than what you are eating now to maintain your present weight.
2. The diet should be adequate in all other nutrients, except calories. Foods from the Fats-Sweets-Alcohol group should be greatly reduced. These foods are typically thought of as being "empty-calorie" foods becuase they are poor sources of protein, vitamins, and minerals. Conversely, the diet should emphasize nutrient-dense foods as well as low-calorie foods that provide bulk to the diet, such as foods in the Fruit-Vegetable group and the Bread-Cereal group.
3. The diet shouuld have a high satiety (fullness) value, meaning that small amounts of fat should be included in the diet to delay the onset of hunger pangs. Additionally, foods that are moderate to good sources of fiber should also be emphasized because they provide bulk to the diet and give the dieter a sense of being full. Use more vegetables, fruits, legumes, and whole grains to achieve this.
4. The dieter should be able to readily adjust the diet to family meals and to eating meals away from home.
5. The cost of the diet should be reasonable.
6. The diet should be one that can be used for a long period of time. The food selection should be quite varied.
7. The diet should retrain the eating habits of the dieter. This new set of eating habits can be maintained for life. While this primarily refers to the actual portions of food consumed, it is also important to point out that the obese individual may need to learn to eat more slowly in order to thoroughly taste the food. Also, the individual may need to dissociate eating from reading or watching TV and may also need to learn to use nonfood rewards.
8. The diet should point out the role physical activity plays in weight loss and maintenance.

When you begin a weight-reduction program, you may find yourself losing little or no weight at first since the body often has a tendency to replace lost fat with water. This is only temporary, however, and dieters should not be discouraged. Dieters may not see any significant weight loss for as much as a month or two, and it is important for the dieter to have support and reassurance from family, friends, or physician during this period.

Name ______________________________ Sheet 17-2

# A REASON FOR CONCERN

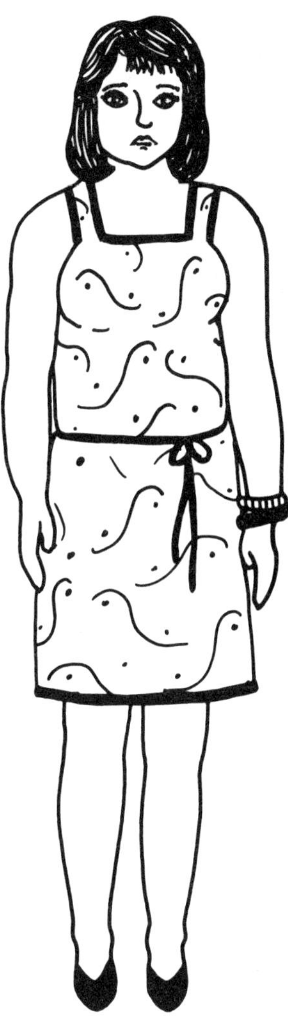

**Case History:** Barbara is 23 years old and has recently graduated from college with a degree in sales and marketing. Throughout the last two years of college, she worried about her grades and found a few courses very difficult. As a result, she studied a lot and made little time for any kind of physical activity. She also became nervous and began to eat more than usual. By the time her senior year began, she had gained about 25 pounds and had to buy a lot of new clothes because the old ones no longer fit. During her senior year, she tried to get into a new routine but found it difficult to do. She purchased special diet books and diet foods, but they just did not help much. She tried participating in some of the sports she liked, but found she was not as good as she used to be and became discouraged. She moved more slowly, got winded quickly, and was simply out of practice. Barbara became overly self-conscious about her weight and began to keep to herself. She continued to overeat and gain weight. At graduation, she weighed 30 pounds more than what she should. She began to worry about getting a job in her profession, because she realized that personal appearance is very important in making sales. She had also heard that some employers are reluctant to hire people who are considerably overweight because they are more likely to develop certain disorders and diseases.

**Directions:** Identify Barbara's current and future problems in each category below. Then, on the back of this sheet, write a general weight-reduction plan for Barbara.

HEALTH PROBLEMS: ______________________________

______________________________

______________________________

SOCIAL PROBLEMS: ______________________________

______________________________

______________________________

ECONOMIC PROBLEMS: ______________________________

______________________________

______________________________

Barbara's principal problem: ______________________________

______________________________

______________________________

# WHAT WEIGHT IS DESIRABLE?

| | Desirable Weights for 18 Year Olds* | | | | | |
|---|---|---|---|---|---|---|
| | MALES | | | FEMALES | | |
| Height in Inches Without Shoes | Small Frame | Medium Frame | Large Frame | Small Frame | Medium Frame | Large Frame |
| 56 | | | | 88 | 95 | 105 |
| 57 | | | | 91 | 97 | 107 |
| 58 | | | | 93 | 100 | 110 |
| 59 | | | | 96 | 103 | 113 |
| 60 | | | | 99 | 106 | 116 |
| 61 | 109 | 117 | 127 | 102 | 109 | 119 |
| 62 | 112 | 120 | 130 | 105 | 113 | 123 |
| 63 | 115 | 123 | 133 | 108 | 116 | 127 |
| 64 | 118 | 126 | 137 | 112 | 121 | 131 |
| 65 | 122 | 130 | 140 | 116 | 125 | 135 |
| 66 | 126 | 134 | 145 | 120 | 129 | 139 |
| 67 | 130 | 138 | 150 | 124 | 133 | 143 |
| 68 | 134 | 142 | 154 | 128 | 137 | 147 |
| 69 | 138 | 146 | 158 | 132 | 141 | 152 |
| 70 | 142 | 151 | 162 | 136 | 145 | 156 |
| 71 | 146 | 155 | 167 | | | |
| 72 | 150 | 160 | 172 | | | |
| 73 | 155 | 164 | 177 | | | |
| 74 | 159 | 169 | 182 | | | |
| 75 | 163 | 175 | 187 | | | |

*Weights given are for individuals in indoor clothing, shoes removed.

Weights adapted from Metropolitan Life Insurance Company by taking the midpoint of weight range for each frame size and subtracting 7 pounds. For individuals up to 25 years, add 1 pound for each year over 18. Individuals over 25 years of age should use the desirable weights for 25 years olds.

Adapted from "Height and Weight Tables." Courtesy of the Metropolitan Life Insurance Company, New York, NY, 1982.

Name ______________________________ Sheet 17-4

# WHAT IS THE TRUTH ABOUT WEIGHT CONTROL?

**Directions:** Read the statement you were assigned and determine if it is true (circle T) or false (circle F). On the other side of this paper, explain why you believe the answer to be true or false.

T or F 1. Obesity is due almost entirely to heredity.

T or F 2. In the experience of some people, all foods turn to fat; however, other people can continuously eat more calories than they need and never become obese.

T or F 3. Skipping meals is a good way to lose weight.

T or F 4. You can eat all you want and still lose weight if you take reducing pills.

T or F 5. Special low-calorie bread should be used in reducing diets.

T or F 6. Toast has fewer calories than bread.

T or F 7. One must not drink water when trying to lose weight.

T or F 8. Eating candy enriched with vitamins is a good way to reduce because you can satisfy your desire for sweets and still get your needed nutrients.

T or F 9. No fat should be consumed when on a diet.

T or F 10. Sugar is not as fattening as starch.

T or F 11. Fruits and high-protein foods have no calories.

T or F 12. Gelatin dessert is nonfattening.

T or F 13. Walking an extra mile a day will result in a one-pound weight loss each week.

T or F 14. Starchy foods, like potatoes and bread, are more fattening than hamburger, hot dogs, and cheddar cheese.

T or F 15. Running a mile burns more calories than walking a mile.

T or F 16. Margarine contains fewer calories than butter.

T or F 17. For reducing, eat high-protein foods for a week; for the next week, eat anything you want.

T or F 18. Grapefruit will burn up body fat.

T or F 19. It is not wise to exercise very much when trying to lose weight. This is because exercise tends to make you overeat.

T or F 20. When trying to lose weight, you should lose at least four pounds per week.

## A OBESITY RELAY RACE

1. Obesity is a condition in which there is an excessive amount of ______________________.
2. Name one economic problem associated with obesity.
3. The increase in fat levels that occurs with obesity usually corresponds to a weight that is greater than ____ percent above ideal weight.
4. A female who should weigh 130 pounds would be obese if she weighed more than ____ pounds.
5. ____ calories comprise one pound of body fat.
6. A healthy amount of weight loss is ____ to ____ pounds per week.
7. To delay the onset of hunger pangs, diets should have small amounts of ____.
8. The dieter must be retrained to learn ______________________________.
9. In addition to eating modifications, ____________ is also important in a weight-reduction program.
10. Name three diseases or disorders that an obese person is "at risk" of developing.

---

## B OBESITY RELAY RACE

1. Name three diseases or disorders that an obese person is "at risk" of developing.
2. Name one social problem associated with obesity.
3. What kind of chart is used to diagnose obesity?
4. An obese male whose desirable weight is 150 pounds has to weigh more than ____ pounds to be considered obese.
5. Another way to diagnose obesity would be to take a ____________________ measurement.
6. In planning a good diet, one should make sure that the diet is deficient in ____________ when compared to the individual's need.
7. Which is more fattening: sugar or starch?
8. Which burns more calories: walking a mile or running a mile?
9. Obesity is a condition in which there is an excessive amount of ______________________
10. Name one economic problem associated with obesity.

## C OBESITY RELAY RACE

1. Name one economic problem associated with obesity.
2. What kind of chart is used to diagnose obesity?
3. _____ calories comprise one pound of body fat.
4. In planning a good diet, one should make sure that the diet is deficient in _____________ when compared to the individual's need.
5. The dieter must be retrained to learn ________________________________________________
6. Name three diseases or disorders that an obese person is "at risk" of developing.
7. The increase in fat levels that occurs with obesity usually corresponds to a weight that is greater than _____ percent above ideal weight.
8. An obese male whose desirable weight is 150 pounds has to weigh more than _____ pounds to be considered obese.
9. A healthy amount of weight loss is _____ to _____ pounds per week.
10. Which burns more calories: walking a mile or running a mile?

---

## D OBESITY RELAY RACE

1. Name one social problem associated with obesity.
2. An obese male whose desirable weight is 150 pounds has to weigh more than _____ pounds to be considered obese.
3. In planning a good diet, one should make sure that the diet is deficient in _____________ when compared to the individual's need.
4. The increase in fat levels that occurs with obesity usually corresponds to a weight that is greater than _____ percent above ideal weight.
5. _____ calories comprise one pound of body fat.
6. To delay the onset of hunger pangs, diets should have small amounts of _________________.
7. What kind of chart is used to diagnose obesity?
8. Another way to diagnose obesity would be to take a _______________________ measurement.
9. Which is more fattening: sugar or starch?
10. A female who should weigh 130 pounds would be obese if she weighed more than _____ pounds.

# QUIZ
# DIET AND DISEASE: OBESITY

_____ 1. One is considered obese if one is greater than __________ over the ideal for one's weight and height and body frame size.

a. 5 percent c. 20 percent
b. 10 percent d. 25 percent

_____ 2. Which of the following guidelines should not be used when trying to reduce one's weight?

a. The diet should be deficient in calories compared to one's energy needs.
b. The diet should eliminate at least one of the following: carbohydrates, proteins, and fats.
c. The diet should be one that can be used over a long period of time.
d. The diet should be reasonable in cost.

_____ 3. What is the purpose of taking a skinfold measurement?

a. To measure the amount of muscle an individual has
b. To determine if an individual can run a mile
c. To measure the amount of water a person has in his or her body
d. To determine if an individual has too much body fat

_____ 4. Susan went on a diet that recommended eating the correct number of servings from each of the food groups in the "Daily Food Guide." The diet emphasized eating a small amount of fat. It also encouraged high-protein foods and grapefruit because these foods will burn off body fat directly. What is the matter with this diet?

a. It recommends eating fat.
b. It claims certain foods will burn off excess fat.
c. The Milk-Cheese group should be excluded from a good diet.
d. There is nothing wrong with this diet.

_____ 5. Obesity may result due to an excess intake of:

a. Carbohydrate, protein, and fat
b. Protein and fat
c. Fat only
d. Carbohydrate only

_____ 6. Obesity is a risk factor for:

a. Stroke c. Tuberculosis
b. Low blood pressure d. Lung cancer

7. Which disease is *not* associated with obesity?

a. Bronchitis c. Arthritis
b. Adult-onset diabetes d. Heart disease

# Unit 18: Diet and Disease: World Health Problems

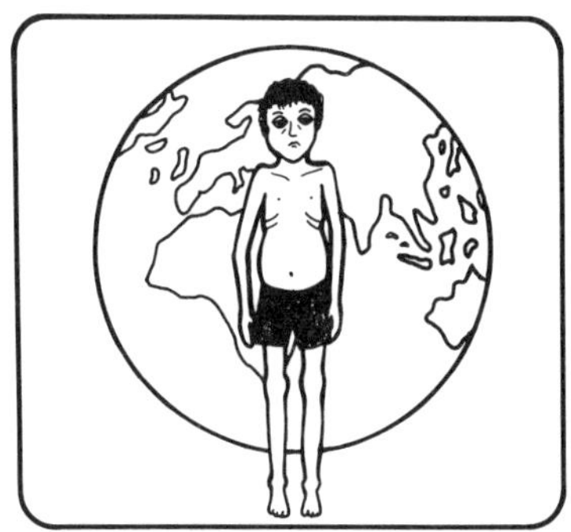

## CONCEPTS

–In developing countries, the major nutrition-related problems are the result of undernutrition.

–Compared with people who are adequately nourished, undernourished people are more likely to be fatigued, to be sick, and to die at an earlier age.

## OBJECTIVES

–The student will be able to identify public health problems caused by malnutrition.

–The student will be able to discuss the consequences of undernutrition.

## TEACHER'S UNIT INTRODUCTION

On a worldwide basis, malnutrition may be caused by overnutrition or undernutrition. The continuum shown here illustrates some health problems related to excess and deficient nutrient intakes, with death as the extreme consequence at either end. [Display the continuum on an overhead or opaque projector.]

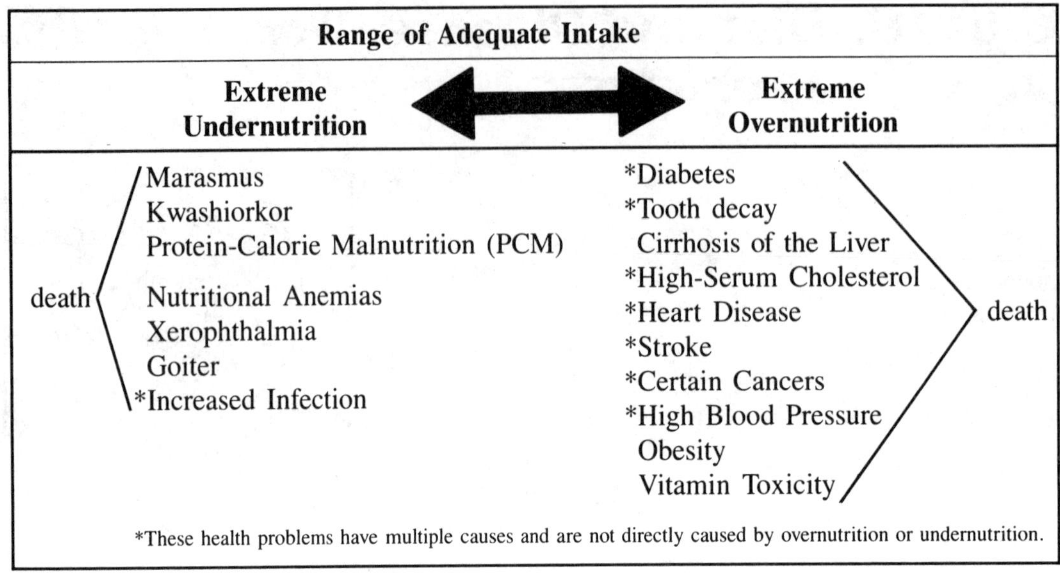


Undernutrition can be defined as a general lack of calories and/or nutrients. Any nutrient deficiency disease is classified as undernutrition. Overnutrition, on the other hand, is a group of nutrient-excess diseases in which calories and/or nutrients are overabundant in the diet. You are already acquainted with some of the health problems that are directly or indirectly related to overnutrition such as obesity, heart disease, hypertension, cirrhosis of the liver, and dental caries. Overnutrition, in the form of obesity, is known to be a direct risk factor for diabetes and is also cited as a risk factor for a few types of cancer in females. Certain constituents of the diet, including fat, fiber, and certain food additives, may also play roles in the development of certain forms of cancer, but more research is needed to ascertain these roles.

The health problems related to overnutrition, relative to those related to undernutrition, are much more prevalent in many of the developed countries of the world, such as the United States, Canada, New Zealand, Australia, the USSR, and the European nations. Interestingly, people in these countries, relative to the "developing" countries, consume about one and a half times as many calories per capita, and they also have an extremely high utilization of petroleum per capita, with six to ten times as much used.

In the developing countries (sometimes referred to as "underdeveloped" countries), health problems related to undernutrition predominate. The geographical areas most afflicted include Latin America, much of Africa, Southeast Asia, and India. Combined, they contain about half of the world's population.

The population group most affected by undernutrition is that of infants and children. This is not surprising when you consider that, per pound of body weight, the nutritional needs of this group are much greater than those of adults. The most extreme consequence of undernutrition is death. It is well documented that a chronically undernourished individual's ability to resist infection and disease, as well as his chances of survival from them, are reduced. World health statistics indicate that in developing countries about half of all young children suffer from undernutrition and that undernutrition contributes to at least half of all childhood deaths.

Let us now examine some of the more prevalent health problems existing today that are the direct result of undernutrition. These problems are referred to as deficiency disorders or deficiency diseases.

**Marasmus.** Derived from the Greek word "marasmos," meaning "wasting." This is perhaps the most extreme form of undernutrition and results from a chronic lack of calories. Put quite simply, it is caused by a chronic lack of food. The individual lives on his or her own tissues. When the fatty tissue reserves are used, muscle tissue then becomes the primary energy source. The individual appears very gaunt; the absence of fat and muscle wasting are obvious.

**Kwashiorkor.** Derived from the Ghan language of West Africa, "kwashiorkor" literally means "the sickness of the older child when the next baby is born." This disorder is the result of a lack of protein. Calories are provided in sufficient or near sufficient amounts. It most often develops in children after they are weaned from breast milk onto a diet low in protein. Edema (water retention) and skin disorders are typical.

**Protein-Calorie Malnutrition (PCM).** Sometimes referred to as "Protein-Energy Malnutrition" (PEM). This is a result of a severe deficiency of protein and calories. PCM is characterized by an increased susceptibility to infection, stunted growth, and poor mental performance if severe deprivation occurs during infancy and early childhood.

**Nutritional Anemias.** Anemia is defined as the condition in which there is a lack of red blood cells or hemoglobin in the blood. While many types of anemia can be caused by internal bleeding, infections, or parasites, nutritional anemias are caused by lack of one or more nutrients including protein, iron, folic acid, and Vitamin $B_{12}$.

**Xerophthalmia.** Blindness is the end result of this eye disorder. The condition is ultimately precipitated by a chronic lack of Vitamin A in the diet. Forerunners to xerophthalmia are night blindness and eye infections.

**Goiter.** Goiter is a condition characterized by excessive swelling in the throat region, reflecting the enlargement of the thyroid gland. The thyroid gland produces a hormone which is closely involved in regulating basal metabolism (body processes). This hormone contains iodine, an element supplied to the body through the diet. When the diet is deficient in iodine, the thyroid gland enlarges in an attempt to compensate for the lack of iodine. If the thyroid gland is permitted to grow, it may interfere with breathing. Goiter in pregnant women may lead to dwarfism and mental retardation in infants.

Just as undernutrition can lead to increased susceptibility to, and increased severity of, infection and disease, the opposite is also true: infection and disease can precipitate or add to the severity of undernutrition. For example, diarrhea and vomiting increase nutritional losses; fever and infection increase nutritional requirements; and gastrointestinal diseases interfere with the absorption of nutrients. Additionally, all may decrease nutritional intake due to poor appetite. A deficiency of one or more nutrients due to infection or disease is termed "secondary undernutrition."

The combined effects of undernutrition, infection, and disease lead to high infant mortality statistics in the developing countries. One out of every four babies dies during infancy in Bolivia and Zambia; one out of seven dies in India, and one out of ten dies in Brazil. Compare this to the United States where only 1 out of 50 dies and to Sweden where only 1 out of 90 dies.

Obviously, the direct cause of undernutrition is that individuals do not consume enough food or the proper variety of food to meet their nutritional needs. However, the reasons people do not have the proper amount or variety of food are multiple and interrelated. Listed here are some of those most critical:

1. Poverty at the family level
2. Shortages of water, fuel, fertilizer, and other resources
3. Inequitable distribution of resources within a country
4. Exponential population growth
5. Unsanitary living conditions
6. Inadequate health services
7. Natural disasters such as drought
8. Poorly developed food transport and storage systems
9. Lack of credit or price supports for local farmers
10. Extensive use of arable land by agribusiness for exportable "cash" crops such as coffee and rubber

Humanitarian efforts by individuals in developed countries to "eat lower on the food chain" and fund-raising efforts like the "Live Aid" Concert to feed starving children are certainly commendable. However, long-range solutions to the problem of undernutrition must address not only the immediate problem of an insufficient food supply, but also the social structures within each individual country that propagate malnutrition. Solutions for improving the nutritional quality of the food supply must be affordable and acceptable to the vast majority of the country's population.

---

Unit 18 could be easily dovetailed with other subject areas such as world history, geography, or current events. The subject of world hunger is one that confronts Americans nearly every day in the newspapers or on television or radio. Students should be encouraged to ponder these issues and to extend their thinking beyond the four walls of their schools or homes.

## BASIC ACTIVITY

**Time Needed:** One class period

**Materials Needed:** World map or globe
Slides or pictures of persons afflicted with the deficiency disorders or diseases referred to in "Teacher's Unit Introduction" *(optional)*

Small pins with flags or colored heads
Quiz Sheet 18-1

1. Begin this activity by defining world health problems related to nutrition and by using the information in the "Teacher's Unit Introduction." Elicit from students a definition of "overnutrition" and of "undernutrition." Have students volunteer health problems caused by overnutrition.

2. Display the "Range of Adequate Intake" continuum in the "Introduction" using an overhead or opaque projector. Review the health problems caused by extreme overnutrition. Then discuss each of the health problems caused by extreme undernutrition. Display slides or pictures of persons afflicted with each one of these diseases if such slides or pictures are available. The asterisk by each disease indicates that it has multiple causes and is not directly caused by overnutrition or undernutrition.

3. Explain to students that the focus of this unit will be on some of the most prevalent nutrition-related health problems in the developing countries, that is, on those diseases related to undernutrition. Explain that these developing countries (sometimes referred to as "underdeveloped" or "Third World" countries) contain the majority of the world's population.

4. On the world map or globe, identify the main geographic areas encompassing the developing countries (Latin America, much of Africa, Southeast Asia, India). Place small pins with flags or colored heads into each country for identification purposes.

5. To help students discover the consequences of undernutrition other than those diseases identified, read aloud the following situations. Students should independently write responses to the questions contained in each.

- Imagine that, for the next several years, the majority of people in this country have only half as many calories to eat as they do now. You are one of these people. Other than contracting one of the diseases listed, what are at least three ways this lack of calories might affect you? (*Sample answers:* I would feel hungry; I would feel deprived; I would be jealous of others who had food.)
- Pregnant women, infants, and young children will also be included in this majority of people. How might a lack of calories affect each of these population groups? (*Sample answers:* Pregnant women might have miscarriages, premature births, or low birth-weight babies. Infants might not gain weight adequately or might die if calories are severely restricted. Infants and children might cry from hunger. Young children might not develop normally; they might not learn easily.)

6. Discuss students' responses. Make sure the following consequences are addressed:

- weight loss
- mind would be preoccupied with the thought of food
- fatigue
- decreased energy and desire to learn
- decreased ability to perform well in sports
- decreased ability to perform well at work
- reduced resistance to infection and disease

- stunting of growth in children
- more babies would die (the infant mortality rate would be higher)

7. Proceed with the "Advanced Activity" if you wish; otherwise use the quiz mentioned in step 8.

8. **Evaluation:** Distribute Quiz Sheet 18-1 and have students complete it as a homework assignment. Discuss the answers in class during the next class period.

## ADVANCED ACTIVITY

**Time Needed:** One class period

**Materials Needed:** Sheets 18-1 through 18-2: "Too Little for Too Many"
Resource materials—encyclopedias, geography books, sociology books, current periodicals and newspapers

1. Distribute Sheets 18-1 through 18-2, "Too Little for Too Many," and have students read the material silently.

2. Discuss the health problems of India that are related to poor nutrition. Elicit from students their ideas as to why India has such problems and have them propose possible solutions.

3. Have small groups of students or individuals choose a developing country from those identified in the "Basic Activity." The students will research the economic, political, and social structure of the chosen country in resource materials.

4. Students will write a brief report that identifies the underlying factors that contribute to undernutrition in this country and will propose action steps toward solving the problem of undernutrition. Students should include in their reports the following information:

- the size of the population
- the size of the country
- the birth rate
- the projected population by the year 2000
- the infant mortality rate
- the average family income
- the typical diet
- the major nutritional disorders
- the cultural or religious customs related to diet
- the life expectancy in years
- the educational level
- the percentage of arable land

The data from all students' reports could be combined on a very large wall chart listing the specifics above for all countries studied.

5. Students should present their reports to the class in whatever way they wish—oral report, panel discussion, newscast, role-play, and so forth.

## FOLLOW-UP ACTIVITIES

1. Have students make collages illustrating the consequences of undernutrition and the underlying factors contributing to it in developing countries. Use the collages as springboards for discussion pertaining to strategies for decreasing worldwide undernutrition.

2. Have students research the typical diets of a few developing countries and contrast each one with the typical American diet. Discuss the differences and bring out the fact that American diets contain more protein, calories, and take considerably more energy to produce (animals must be fed to obtain animal products).

3. Have the class plan and prepare a "Hunger Awareness Dinner" for other students, teachers, or parents. A Hunger Awareness Dinner is designed to dramatically display how people throughout the world eat. According to studies of current world populations and their eating practices, one-third of the world's population typically eat a simple meal of rice and water, one-third eat a small amount of fish, a vegetable or potato, and some fruit, and the remaining eat a typical American meal of meat, potatoes, vegetable, salad, and dessert. To serve a Hunger Awareness Dinner, prepare the three types of meals. When the guests arrive, have each one select a card that designates the type of meal he or she will receive. Include at the dinner a discussion of what world hunger really means in terms of how a person feels about eating what people in the rest of the world eat.

4. If a Hunger Awareness Dinner is not feasible, have a "Mini-Hunger Awareness Experience." Prepare three types of snacks as described below and divide the class into thirds by having each student select a card that designates the type of snack he or she will receive. Offer one-third of the class the complete snack, one-third of the class part of the snack, and one-third of the class only water. Some examples of snacks are:

| Proportion of the Class Receiving the Snack | Snack |
|---|---|
| 1/3 | Peanut butter on saltines and apple juice |
| 1/3 | Saltines only |
| 1/3 | Water only |
| OR | |
| 1/3 | Oatmeal cookies or Bran muffins with milk |
| 1/3 | Milk only |
| 1/3 | Water only |

While the students are eating the snack, have them discuss how they feel and what hunger in America must be like.

5. Use news reports of famine or food supply shortages in developing countries to stimulate research and discussion of these problems.

# TOO LITTLE FOR TOO MANY

Compared to at least half of the world's population, most Americans and persons who live in developed countries live in luxury. We have clean water for drinking, cooking, bathing, and washing clothes. We have a plentiful and varied supply of food.

Often, we are guilty of wasting both water and food, or at least of using or consuming more of each than is really necessary. What about health services and disease? Most of us can see a doctor, dentist, or optometrist whenever needed. Additionally, we are healthy and have plenty of energy most of the time.

Let us take a few moments to look at a developing country that has about half of the land area of the United States (not including Alaska and Hawaii) but more than 2.5 times as many people. There are 14 main languages in this country. The life expectancy in this country is a little more than 50 years, and about 1 out of every 7 babies dies before he or she is 1 year old. The birth rate in this country is also very high. For every 1,000 people, 35 or 40 children are born each year. In 1975 alone, this country grew in size by about 17 million people!

Do you know which country is being described? Think about your studies of geography and history as we further describe this country. The average yearly income per person is estimated to be equal to about $200 (U.S.). But, as in most developing countries, there is a small segment of the population that is as well off as middle- or upper-class Americans.

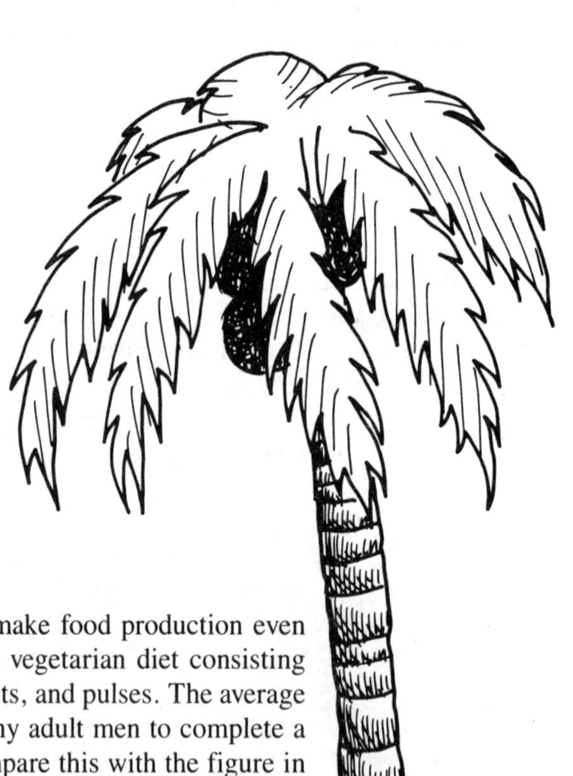

Cereal grains (wheat, rice, and millet) are the major crops in this country. Other important crops include pulses (legumes), milk, and oil seeds (groundnut, sesame, safflower, and coconut). However, the total amount of food produced is not nearly enough to meet the nutritional needs of the people. Due to poor sanitation and rodent control, rats are prevalent and consume a good deal of the wheat and rice grown. Other food production problems include shortages of agricultural land, fertilizer, fresh water, and fuel. In fact, many inhabitants have little other than dried manure to use as fuel.

Natural disasters, such as drought and soil erosion, make food production even harder. The vast majority of the people subsist on a lacto vegetarian diet consisting principally of cereals, grains, vegetables, milk, milk products, and pulses. The average daily calorie intake per person is not enough to enable many adult men to complete a full day's work. It is not quite 2,000 calories per day. (Compare this with the figure in the United States—about 3,000 calories per day.)

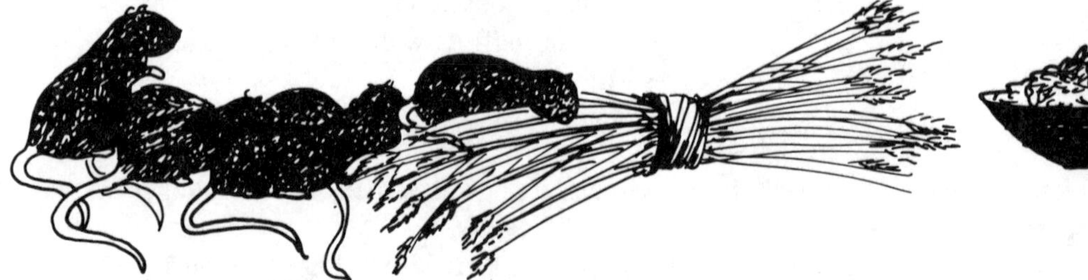

Children between the ages of six months and five years grow at a slow rate and are not as tall nor as heavy as children of the same age in developed countries such as the United States and Canada. There are two major reasons for this slow growth rate:

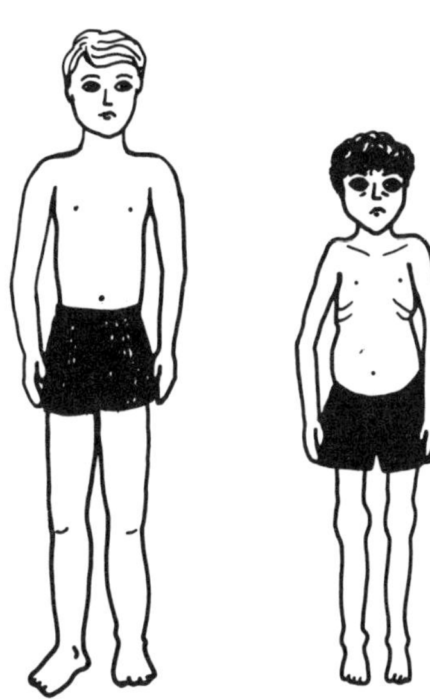

1. Their diets often do not supply enough calories and protein. In fact, the shortage is so severe in some children that they develop marasmus, kwashiorkor, or Protein-Calorie Malnutrition (PCM).
2. They have many infectious diseases such as measles, influenza, and intestinal worms, which further increase the child's need for calories and nutrients. It is not uncommon for young children to die of these diseases in this country.

In addition to slow growth, marasmus, and kwashiorkor, many children and women are reported to have anemia or to have "borderline" anemia. Also, about one out of every ten children has a Vitamin A deficiency which leads to night blindness and sometimes to eye infections or xerophthalmia. In certain parts of this country, one-quarter of the people have goiter.

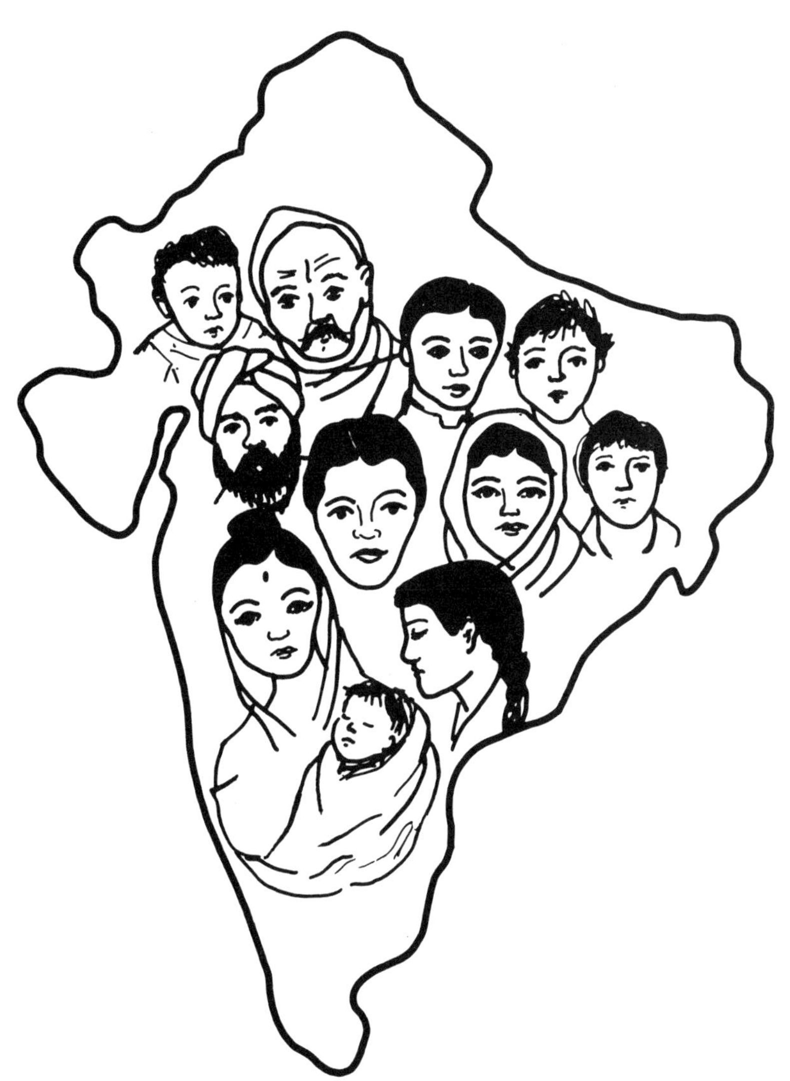

The country that has been described is *India*. Based on what you have read, what do you think causes undernutrition in India? What do you think could be done to help reduce this problem? Prepare for class discussion of these questions by writing your answers on the back of this sheet.

Name ________________________________ 

# QUIZ
# DIET AND DISEASE: WORLD HEALTH PROBLEMS

In the box below are listed several nutrition-related health problems. Five of them are major problems in some developing countries and are caused by undernutrition. Write the names of these five problems in the blanks provided.

1. ________________________________
2. ________________________________
3. ________________________________
4. ________________________________
5. ________________________________

| | |
|---|---|
| obesity | kwashiorkor |
| stroke | diabetes |
| anemia | marasmus |
| cirrhosis | colon cancer |
| xerophthalmia | goiter |
| Vitamin A toxicity | high blood pressure |

For each condition you identified above, there is at least one nutritional component lacking in the diet that is the cause of the problem. In the spaces below, write the name of each problem and the "lacking" nutritional component causing it.

6. ________________________________________________
7. ________________________________________________
8. ________________________________________________
9. ________________________________________________
10. ________________________________________________

What are three consequences (regardless of age or sex) of being undernourished for a long period of time?

11. ________________________________
12. ________________________________
13. ________________________________

14. Write a short paragraph describing a solution to the world food shortage. Imagine that you will present this solution to the United Nations General Assembly. Continue your paragraph on the back of this sheet if necessary.

________________________________________________

________________________________________________

________________________________________________

________________________________________________

# Unit 19: Dietary Guidelines for Americans

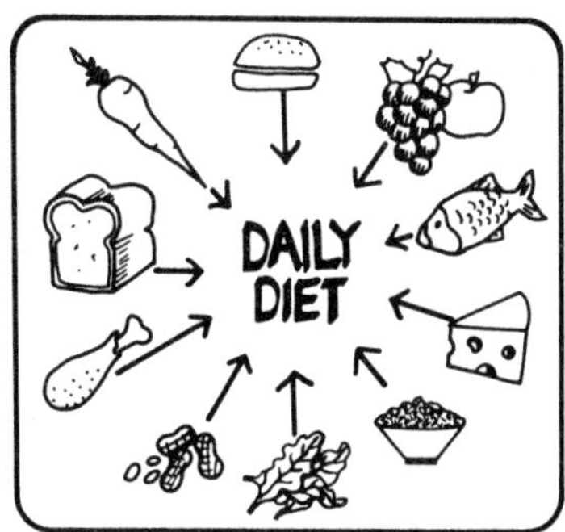


## CONCEPTS

–Many of the most prevalent health problems in the United States are diet-related. These include obesity, cardiovascular disease, hypertension, diabetes, and certain types of cancer.

–Using the Dietary Guidelines for Americans in food selection and preparation can help maintain and may even improve health.

–The Dietary Guidelines can be easily implemented in the diet.

## OBJECTIVES

–Students will be able to recognize dietary practices that contribute to major health problems in the United States.

–Students will compare the quality of food prepared from traditional recipes with food prepared from recipes that incorporate the Dietary Guidelines for Americans.

–Students will be able to recommend small changes that can be made in food selection and preparation in order to follow the Dietary Guidelines for Americans.

## TEACHER'S UNIT INTRODUCTION

Americans have become very interested in their diets as well as in the effects that their eating habits have on their health. This is not surprising, since many of the most prevalent health problems in the United States have been associated with the American diet. For instance, obesity results from taking in more calories than are needed over a period of time. Heart disease has been related to an excessive amount of cholesterol and saturated fat in the diet as well as to the consumption of an excessive amount of calories. Hypertension (high blood pressure) has strong ties to the salt content of the diet. And, colon cancer has been associated with a lack of fiber in the diet. Evidence of the awakened interest of Americans in the relationship between diet and health can be found in any health food store or bookstore, where sales for health formulas and nutritional advice are soaring. Unfortunately, much of this advice is conflicting, misleading, and sometimes totally incorrect, and leaves Americans with little direction regarding how to improve their diets. The government has recognized the confusion and has responded to the need for specific ways Americans could implement what is currently known about nutrition by issuing the Dietary Guidelines in 1980.

The Dietary Guidelines combine reliable nutrition information with dietary recommendations so that Americans can improve their food choices and preparation techniques. The Dietary Guidelines and their effects on food selection and eating behavior are shown on Sheets 19-1 and 19-2. [Display Sheets 19-1 and 19-2 on an overhead or opaque projector and read them with the class.]

Although the Dietary Guidelines were issued with Americans in mind, people in any developed nation could easily adapt them to their own habits. The diseases of developed nations are similar and could be prevented by incorporating the Dietary Guidelines into the diets of people all over the world.

You may feel as though the changes called for are radical and could be difficult to implement. Actually, small changes can be made in order to incorporate many of the Guidelines. For example, drinking skim milk instead of whole milk will lower the fat and cholesterol content in your diet as well as decrease calories. Serving fresh fruits instead of rich desserts decreases fat, sugar, and calories and increases fiber in the diet. Slight alterations of traditional recipes can also incorporate a number of the Guidelines without affecting food quality. The important principle to remember is that small changes are more likely to be continued over a long period of time than are major or radical changes. Also, small changes add up! Decreasing the fat in a recipe by just 2 tablespoons saves 200 calories. Omitting a teaspoon of salt from recipes and/or cooking decreases sodium intake by 2 grams.* These changes are not "painful" to make; that is, they do not make you feel deprived and could more easily become permanent behaviors. Unit 19 focuses on making small changes to follow the U.S. Dietary Guidelines.

---

Before beginning the "Advanced Activity" in Unit 19, students must be familiar with the Dietary Guidelines and with recipe modifications. If additional assistance or information is needed to present these activities, the local chapter of the American Heart Association or Red Cross may be helpful. Both of these organizations have courses and literature designed to help consumers make wise choices.

## BASIC ACTIVITY

**Time Needed:** Two class periods

---

*Table salt is composed of 40 percent sodium and 60 percent chloride. A high intake of sodium is linked to the incidence of high blood pressure.

**Materials Needed:** Sheet 19-1: "Scoring Your Diet"
Sheets 19-2 through 19-3: "How to Make the Dietary Guidelines Work for You"
Sheet 19-4: "Zucchini Muffins I" and "Zucchini Muffins II"
Sheet 19-5: "Coleslaw I" and "Coleslaw II"
Ingredients for recipes and disposable serving equipment
Three- by five-inch cards
Sheet 19-6: "What Did I Save with the Alternate Recipe?" (two for each student)
Quiz Sheet 19-1

### Class Period 1

1. Begin this activity by distributing Sheet 19-1, "Scoring Your Diet." Explain that this worksheet compares diets to the Dietary Guidelines for Americans rather than with the "Daily Food Guide." Simply describe the Dietary Guidelines with the information in the "Teacher's Unit Introduction."

2. Have students approximate their scores in each of the five diet-related categories on Sheet 19-1. Then have them add these individual category scores to determine their total score.

3. Conduct a large-group discussion of individual category and total scores.

4. Distribute Sheets 19-2 through 19-3, "How to Make the Dietary Guidelines Work for You." Have students read the sheets silently or review the material aloud in a group discussion. Students will already be familiar with the material through the "Teacher's Unit Introduction."

### Class Period 2

1. Divide the class into four groups. Give each group one of the following recipes: Sheet 19-4, "Zucchini Muffins I," and "Zucchini Muffins II," and Sheet 19-5, "Coleslaw I" and "Coleslaw II." Each group should prepare its assigned recipe and have it ready for tasting at the end of the period. Set up a taste-testing table so that students can sample all recipes. Each of the foods on the table should be labeled with a three- by five-inch card indicating which recipe was used.

2. Have students taste all of the prepared foods and complete the "Alternate Recipe Evaluation Sheet" on Sheet 19-5 for each one. After everyone has sampled and evaluated the foods, tally the responses to the questions listed on the evaluation worksheet.

3. Have the group that prepared "Zucchini Muffins I" join the group that prepared "Zucchini Muffins II." Do the same with the groups that prepared "Coleslaw I" and "Coleslaw II." Have the groups compare the prepared foods and any differences in quality. First, ask the following questions about "Zucchini Muffins I" and "II":

- What differences did you find when you compared "Zucchini Muffins I" and "Zucchini Muffins II" (*Answers:* "Muffins I" had less oil, less sugar, no salt, no walnuts)
- Which recipe best followed the Dietary Guidelines? (*Answer:* "Muffins I")

- Which Guidelines did the "Zucchini Muffins I" implement? (*Answers:* Guideline 3, Avoid Too Much Fat, Saturated Fat, and Cholesterol by decreasing the oil and omitting the walnuts; Guideline 5, Avoid Too Much Sugar, by decreasing the brown sugar; Guideline 6, Avoid Too Much Sodium, by cutting out the salt.)

4. Next, place on the board the information given below, which compares the two recipes. Indicate that Guideline 2, Maintain Ideal Weight, was also followed since calories were decreased with the lessened ingredients and with the omission of walnuts.

**Zucchini Muffin Comparison**

| | RECIPE I | RECIPE II | Per Muffin |
|---|---|---|---|
| eggs | 1 | 1 | |
| oil | 1/4 cup + 2 tbsp. | 1/2 cup | −20 calories |
| grated zucchini | 1 cup | 1 cup | |
| vanilla extract | 1½ tsp. | 1½ tsp. | |
| brown sugar | 3/4 cup | 1 cup | −19 calories |
| all-purpose flour | 1 cup | 1 cup | |
| whole wheat flour | 1/2 cup | 1/2 cup | |
| salt | NONE | 1/2 tsp. | [−83 mg sodium] |
| baking soda | 1/2 tsp. | 1/2 tsp. | |
| baking powder | 1/2 tsp. | 1/2 tsp. | |
| cinnamon | 1/2 tsp. | 1/2 tsp. | |
| chopped walnuts | NONE | 1/2 cup | −33 calories |
| | | | −72 calories |

"Zucchini Muffin Recipe I" contains 72 fewer calories per muffin and 83 fewer milligrams of sodium per muffin.

5. Now ask the same questions about "Coleslaw I" and "Coleslaw II":

- What differences did you find when you compared "Coleslaw I" and "Coleslaw II"? (*Answers:* "Coleslaw II" had less sugar, no salt, and no oil).
- Which recipe best followed the Dietary Guidelines? (*Answer:* "Coleslaw II")
- Which Guidelines did "Coleslaw II" implement? (*Answers:* Guideline 3, Avoid Too Much Fat, Saturated Fat, and Cholesterol because there is no oil in the recipe; Guideline 5, Avoid Too Much Sugar by decreasing the sugar; Guideline 6, Avoid Too Much Sodium because there is no salt in the recipe—garlic powder is used instead of garlic salt.)

6. Next, place on the board the information given below which compares the two coleslaw recipes. Indicate again that Guideline 2, Maintain Ideal Weight, was also followed, since calories were decreased with the lessened ingredients.

**Coleslaw Comparison**

| | RECIPE I | RECIPE II | Per Serving |
|---|---|---|---|
| sugar | 1/3 cup | 1/4 cup | −11 calories |
| garlic salt | 1/2 tsp. | NONE | [−167 mg sodium] |
| celery seed | 1/4 tsp. | 1/4 tsp. | |
| vinegar | 3 tbsp. | 3 tbsp. | |
| lemon juice | 3 tbsp. | 3 tbsp. | |
| oil | 1/4 cup | NONE | −80 calories |
| shredded cabbage | 3 cups | 3 cups | |
| chopped green pepper | 1/4 cup | 1/4 cup | |
| chopped celery | 1 stalk | 1 stalk | ———— |
| sliced green onions | 3-4 | 3-4 | −91 calories |

"Coleslaw II" contains 91 fewer calories per serving and 167 fewer milligrams of sodium per serving.

7. Emphasize that the recipes were altered to follow the Dietary Guidelines by slightly decreasing the sugar and fat and omitting the salt. Have students offer suggestions about how they could alter other recipes.

8. Proceed with the "Advanced Activity" if you wish; otherwise use the quiz mentioned in step 9.

9. **Evaluation:** Distribute Quiz Sheet 19-1 and have students complete it as a homework assignment. Discuss the answers as a class during the next class period.

## ADVANCED ACTIVITY

**Time Needed:** Two class periods

**Materials Needed:** Sheet 19-4 or 19-5 for the "Alternate Recipe Evaluation Sheet" (three copies per student)
Sheet 19-6: "What Did I Save with the Alternate Recipe?"
Three- by five-inch cards
Food composition tables (*See* "References/Resources" at the end of this kit)
Cookie recipe (for example, oatmeal cookie recipe)
Cookie ingredients and disposable serving plates
Quiz Sheet 19-1

**Class Period 1**

1. Introduce this activity by briefly reviewing the Dietary Guidelines. Explain to the students that simple modifications of traditional recipes can be made that adhere to the Dietary Guidelines. Explain to the students that they will alter a cookie recipe in this activity.

2. Divide the class into five groups. Give each group a copy of a cookie recipe (oatmeal cookie recipe works well).

- Group #1 should make the traditional recipe.
- Group #2 should decrease the sugar by approximately 1/4 cup.
- Group #3 should decrease the fat by approximately 2 tablespoons.
- Group #4 should omit the salt.
- Group #5 should decrease the sugar, decrease the fat, and omit the salt.

3. Each group should place samples of its cookies on the taste-testing table and label them on three- by five-inch cards according to what was decreased or omitted.

4. Distribute three copies of the "Alternate Recipe Evaluation Sheet," to each student and have them complete independent evaluations of all samples.

5. After everyone has sampled and evaluated the foods, tally the responses to the questions listed on the "Alternate Recipe Evaluation Sheet."

**Class Period 2**

1. Have students compute the calories and/or sodium they saved by altering the cookie recipe.

2. Display the "Zucchini Muffin" comparison in the "Basic Activity" on the chalkboard or on an overhead projector, as an example. You might explain it as follows:

In the traditional Recipe II, 1/2 cup of oil was used, which contains 963 calories. In Recipe I, 1/4 cup plus 2 tablespoons of oil were used, an amount which contains 722 calories. By finding the difference in calories and dividing by the number of servings (12), we can find how many calories were saved per muffin. (963 − 722 = 241; 241 ÷ 12 = 20 calories fewer per muffin.) Continue this explanation with the brown sugar, walnuts, and salt. The figures you need are:

| | | | |
|---|---|---|---|
| brown sugar | 1 cup | = | 820 calories |
| walnuts | 1/2 cup | = | 390 calories |
| salt | tsp. | = | 1,000 milligrams sodium |

3. Distribute Sheet 19-6 "What Did I Save with the Alternate Recipe? " and food composition tables. Each group should calculate the total number of calories in one cookie of the traditional recipe by adding the calories of all ingredients and dividing by the number of cookies made (the number will be constant for each group).

- Group #2 should calculate the calories saved by decreasing the sugar.
- Group #3 should calculate the calories saved by decreasing the fat.
- Group #4 should calculate the amount of sodium saved by omitting the salt.

- Group #5 should calculate the calories saved by decreasing fat and sugar and the amount of sodium saved by omitting the salt.

Have students record their calculations on Sheet 19-6.

4. Compare the results of each group. Discuss other recipes that students could alter and discuss the ways they could alter them.

5. **Evaluation:** Distribute Quiz Sheet 19-1 and have students complete it as a homework assignment. Discuss the answers as a class during the next class period.

## FOLLOW-UP ACTIVITIES

1. Have the class devise a menu for an entire meal. Divide the class into groups. Each group should apply one of the Dietary Guidelines to the menu. For example, one group could concentrate on fat, another on sugar, and another on sodium. The altered menus should be evaluated in terms of calories or sodium saved.

2. Have students visit a supermarket and record the types of processed foods that follow the Dietary Guidelines for Americans. Dietetic foods should not be included.

3. Do a values-voting activity to point out that often the way we eat does not relate to a lack of knowledge but often relates to not having positive attitudes. As you read aloud each statement listed below, students should vote to agree (arms up), disagree (arms down), or remain undecided (arms folded). As students vote, call on a few volunteers to support their vote. Ask: Why do you feel the way you do? There are no right or wrong answers, but try to point out which attitudes are positive and why.

- I feel the foods I eat now will affect my future.
- I do not have time to think about nutrition.
- For a snack, juice is no substitute for a soft drink.
- A proper diet is a major factor in preventing disease.
- If I am not overweight, I do not have to worry about nutrition.
- I think exercising is boring.
- Even if I take vitamins, I feel I should be concerned about the food I eat.
- I would take a candy bar instead of an apple anytime.
- I do not have time to eat a nutritious diet.
- If I exercise regularly, I will have better control of my appetite.
- I do not have to worry about nutrition if I drink milk.
- I know what I should eat, but I often eat things that are not nutritious.
- I do not need to be concerned about nutrition if my doctor says I am healthy.
- Dinner is not complete without meat.
- Fruit is just no substitute for cake, pie, and cookies.
- I do not have time to exercise.

4. Discuss the economics of preventing nutrition-related disorders and diseases versus having them and treating them. For example, there are no costs associated with preventing

obesity. In fact, dollars spent for food might actually be saved by not overeating. Consider, however, the costs of having and treating obesity: (1) having to buy new clothes because present ones do not fit; (2) spending extra money to purchase special food supplements in order to follow a "fad" diet; (3) spending money to join exercise clubs; (4) increasing the risk of developing diabetes, heart disease, and high blood pressure, all of which have considerable medical costs associated with them. Another example might be tooth decay. One can find a variety of low-sugar snacks at the same or less cost than that of high-sugar snacks. Additionally, the expenditures for a toothbrush, tooth paste, and dental floss are minimal compared to the cost of fillings, pulling teeth, or false teeth.

5. Have students interview health professionals, such as physicians, dentists, nurses, nutritionists, dietitions, and others. Find out how many of these people have heard about the Dietary Guidelines for Americans and whether they personally adhere to these guidelines. If the professionals are willing, have them record their dietary intake for one day. Then have the students analyze their diets to see if they meet the Dietary Guidelines for Americans. Discuss food habits and why they are difficult to change, even for professionals.

6. Have students analyze their school lunch menu to see if it adheres to the Dietary Guidelines for Americans.

7. Have students select one of the Dietary Guidelines for Americans and investigate it. Have them find information that describes why these dietary changes might help reduce nutrition-related diseases. Have them report these findings to the class or prepare a written report.

8. Stage a mock Congressional hearing during which the acceptance or rejection of the Dietary Guidelines for Americans is debated. Have several students represent senators who are opposed to the guidelines, several who are proponents of the guidelines, and several who are uncommitted. Also have some students represent various lobbying groups such as the meat industry, the consumer industry, the dairy industry, the fruit and vegetable industry, consumer advocates, physicians, nutritionists, and other health-care providers and government officials. Appoint one student to preside as committee chairperson. Allow students time to investigate and prepare their arguments and opinions. Following the hearing, have students write a report of the mock Congressional hearing in a newspaper news article format as an evaluation.

**Name** ______________________________ **Sheet 19-1**

# SCORING YOUR DIET

**Directions:** Determine where your dietary habits fall in each category below by giving yourself a score of 1 to 5. Then add your score in each category to find your diet's TOTAL SCORE.

| SCORE | 1 | 2 | 3 | 4 | 5 |
|---|---|---|---|---|---|
| Body Weight | Ideal weight | Ideal weight | Ideal weight | 10-19 pounds excess | 20 or more pounds excess |
| Fat, Saturated fat, and Cholesterol Intake | Very rare use of solid fats; rare use of meat, eggs, or cheese; nonfat milk only | Occasional use of animal or solid fats; lean meat, eggs, or cheese 7 times/week; nonfat milk only | Some animal or solid fats, meat, eggs, or cheese 7-14 times/week, whole milk rarely—nonfat milk primarily | Frequent use of animal or solid fats; meat, eggs, cheese 14-21 times/week; whole milk only | Use only animal or solid fats; meat, eggs, or cheese more than 21 times/week; whole milk only |
| Fiber and Starch Intake | Average daily intake of 4+ servings fruits/vegetables; 4+ servings whole-grain products; 1+ serving legumes/seeds/nuts | Average daily intake of 4 servings fruits/vegetables; 4 servings whole-grain products; 1/2 serving legumes/seeds/nuts | Average daily intake of 4 servings fruits/vegetables; 4 servings whole-grain products; frequent use of legumes/seeds/nuts | Average daily intake of <3 servings fruits/vegetables; <3 servings whole-grain products; frequent use of refried products; rare use of legumes/seeds/nuts | Rare use of fruits/vegetables; rare use of whole-grain products; never use legumes/seeds/nuts |
| Refined Sugar Intake | No sweeteners (sugar, honey, syrup) at table; no sweetened foods (canned fruits and vegetables, fruit drinks, baked goods); no highly sweetened foods (candy, soft drinks, cookies) | No sweeteners at table; sweetened foods 7 times/week; rare use of highly sweetened foods | No sweeteners at table; sweetened foods 7-14 times/week; occasional use of highly sweetened foods | Frequent use of sweeteners at table; frequent use of sweetened foods (21 times/week), frequent use of highly sweetened foods | Frequent use of sweeteners at table; sweetened foods more than 21 times/week, daily use of highly sweetened foods |
| Salt Intake | No salt added in cooking or at table; no condiments; no pickled foods, no cured meats; use salt-free or low-sodium products and prepared foods | No salt added at table; little salt added in cooking; rare use of highly salted foods, convenience foods, or condiments | Some salt in cooking; little or no salt added at table; occasional use of highly salted foods and condiments | Frequent use of salt at table; salt always used in cooking; frequent use of highly salted foods and condiments | Salt added to foods before tasting; salt always used in cooking; daily use of highly salted foods, convenience foods, or condiments |

YOUR TOTAL SCORE: __________

SCORING SYSTEM:
- *5 or below..... You're on a therapeutic diet—you have special dietary needs!
- *6 to 10........ You're on a special diet. You still need some special diet treatment!
- 11 to 15........ You're right on target with the Dietary Guidelines.
- 16 to 20........ You're trying, but watch out! Review the Dietary Guidelines for Americans.
- 21 to 25........ You're heading for trouble!! (Did you ever hear of the Dietary Guidelines for Americans?)

*Scores below 10 should occur only for individuals on special or therapeutic diets for the treatment of disease; such regimens are not recommended for normal nutrition.

# HOW TO MAKE THE DIETARY GUIDELINES WORK FOR YOU

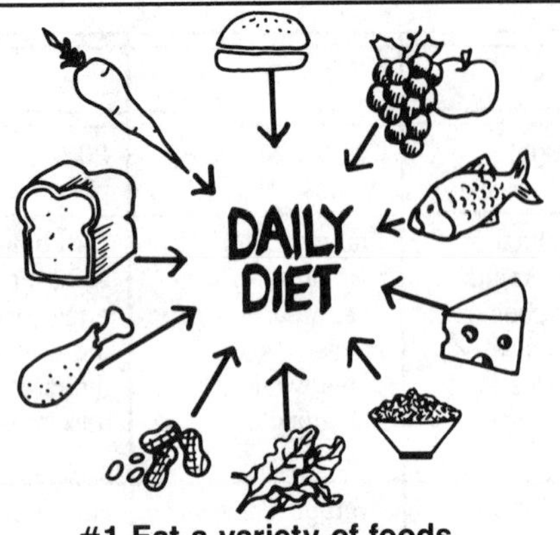


**#1 Eat a variety of foods.**

Eat a variety of foods every day, including some fruits; vegetables; whole-grain and enriched breads, cereals, and grain products; milk, cheese, and yogurt; poultry, fish, eggs, and meat; and dry beans, beans, and nuts.

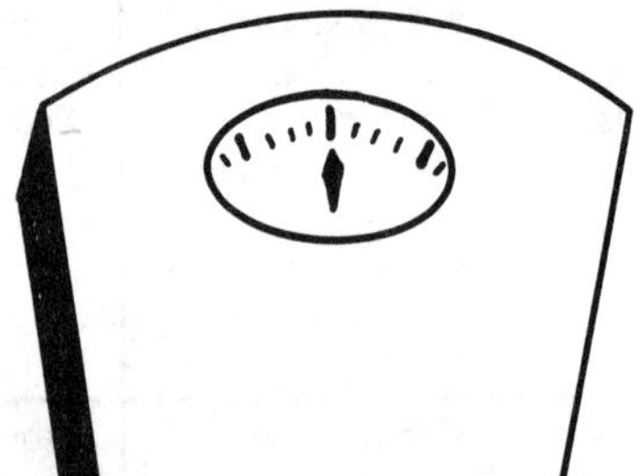

**#2 Maintain ideal weight.**

If you need to lose weight, do so slowly by increasing physical activity and by eating less fat, fatty foods, sugar, and sweets. If eating habits need to be improved, eat slowly, eat smaller portions, and avoid "seconds."

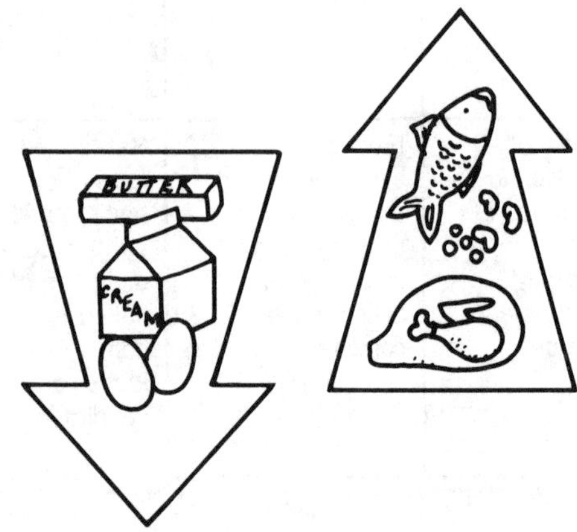


**#3 Avoid too much fat, saturated fat, and cholesterol.**

Limit your intake of butter, cream, hydrogenated margarine, and shortenings; eat less organ meats (liver) and eggs; choose fish, poultry, dry peas and beans, and lean meat for your protein sources; trim excess fat off meats; broil, bake, and boil rather than fry foods; read labels carefully to check for the types and amounts of fat in food.

| | |
|---|---|
|  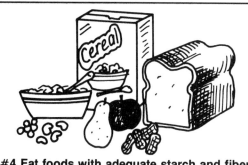  **#4 Eat foods with adequate starch and fiber.** | Select foods that are good sources of fiber and starch, including whole-grain breads and cereals, fruits and vegetables, beans, peas, and nuts. |
| 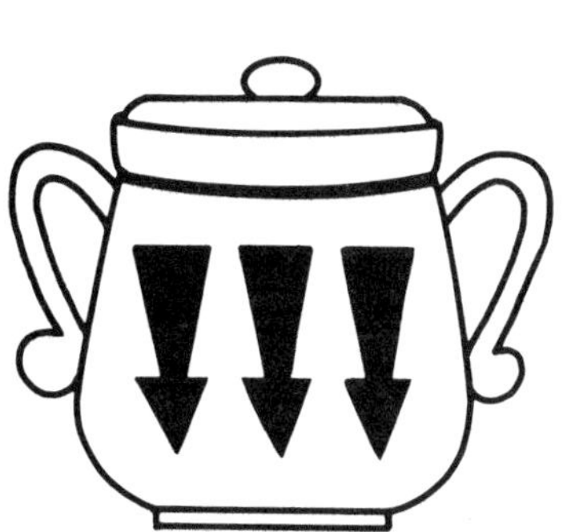 **#5 Avoid too much sugar.** | Eat less of all sugars, including white, brown, and raw sugar, honey and syrups; eat less of foods containing those sugars, including candy, soft drinks, ice cream, cakes, and cookies; choose fresh fruits or fruits packed in juice or light syrup rather than in heavy syrup; read food labels for clues on the amount of sugar in them—look for other names for sugar such as sucrose, glucose, maltose, dextrose, lactose, corn sweeteners, or syrups. |
| 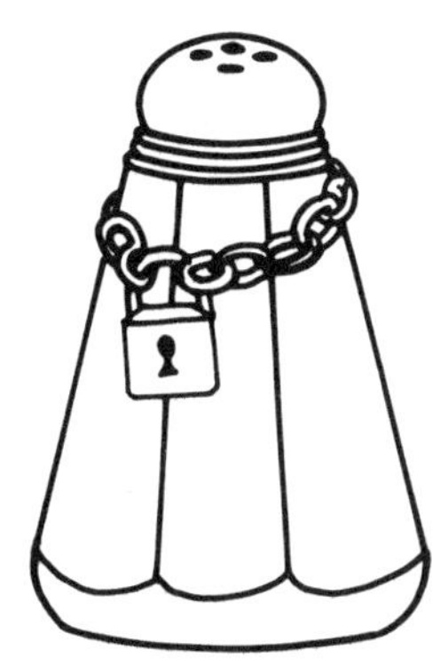 **#6 Avoid too much sodium.** | Add little or no salt to food at the table and add only small amounts in cooking; learn to enjoy the tastes of unsalted foods; cut down on your intake of salty foods such as pretzels, potato chips, salted popcorn, salted nuts, condiments (garlic salt, MSG, steak sauce, soy sauce), pickled foods, and cured meats. Read food labels carefully to check for the sodium content of food, especially of processed foods. |
| 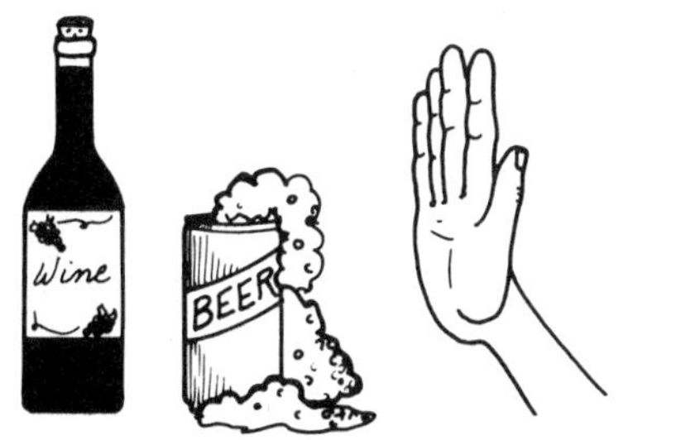  **#7 If you drink alcohol, do so in moderation.** | When you are of drinking age, offer nonalcoholic drinks at parties and limit your intake of alcohol. |

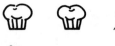

## Zucchini Muffins I

Makes 12 muffins

| | | | |
|---|---|---|---|
| egg | 1 | all-purpose flour | 1 cup |
| oil | 1/4 cup + 2 tablespoons | whole wheat flour | 1/2 cup |
| grated zucchini | 1 cup | baking soda | 1/2 teaspoon |
| vanilla extract | 1½ teaspoons | baking powder | 1/2 teaspoon |
| brown sugar | 3/4 cup | cinnamon | 1/2 teaspoon |

1. Preheat oven to 350°.
2. Grease 12 muffin cups or line with paper baking cups.
3. Mix together egg and oil. Add zucchini and vanilla and stir until blended. Set aside.
4. Combine brown sugar, flours, baking soda, baking powder, and cinnamon in a large bowl.
5. Add wet ingredients to dry ingredients and stir only until dry ingredients are moistened.
6. Fill muffin cups 2/3 full.
7. Bake 15-20 minutes or until toothpick inserted comes out clean.

## Zucchini Muffins II

Makes 12 muffins

| | | | |
|---|---|---|---|
| egg | 1 | all-purpose flour | 1 cup |
| oil | 1/2 cup | whole wheat flour | 1/2 cup |
| grated zucchini | 1 cup | salt | 1/2 teaspoon |
| vanilla extract | 1½ teaspoons | baking soda | 1/2 teaspoon |
| brown sugar | 1 cup | baking powder | 1/2 teaspoon |
| | | cinnamon | 1/2 teaspoon |
| | | chopped walnuts | 1/2 cup |

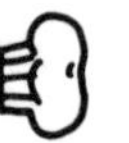

1. Preheat oven to 350°.
2. Grease 12 muffin cups or line with paper baking cups.
3. Mix together egg and oil. Add zucchini and vanilla and stir until blended. Set aside.
4. Combine brown sugar, flours, baking soda, baking powder, and cinnamon in a large bowl.
5. Add wet ingredients to dry ingredients and stir only until dry ingredients are moistened.
6. Fill muffin cups 2/3 full.
7. Bake 15-20 minutes or until toothpick inserted comes out clean.

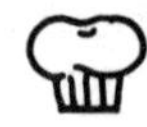

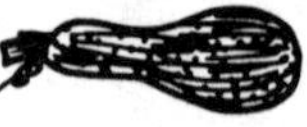

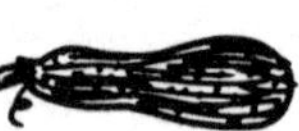

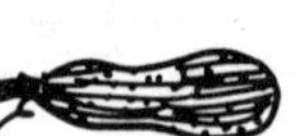

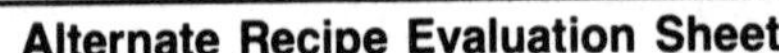

### Alternate Recipe Evaluation Sheet

Name of food tasted ______________________

Circle one answer for each question.

| | | | | | |
|---|---|---|---|---|---|
| How did it taste? (circle one) | Excellent | Very good | Good | Fair | Poor |
| How would you rate the appearance of the food? | Excellent | Very good | Good | Fair | Poor |
| How would you rate the aroma of the food? | Excellent | Very good | Good | Fair | Poor |
| How would you rate the texture of the food? | Excellent | Very good | Good | Fair | Poor |
| How would you rate the overall *quality* of the food? | Excellent | Very good | Good | Fair | Poor |

## Coleslaw I

Makes 6 1/2-cup servings

| | | | |
|---|---|---|---|
| sugar | 1/3 cup | cabbage, shredded | 3 cups (1/2 medium head) |
| garlic salt | 1/2 teaspoon | green pepper, chopped | 1/4 cup |
| celery seed | 1/4 teaspoon | celery, chopped | 1 stalk |
| vinegar | 3 tablespoons | green onions, sliced | 3 to 4 |
| lemon juice | 3 tablespoons | | |
| oil | 1/4 cup | | |

1. In a large bowl, combine sugar, garlic salt, celery seed, vinegar, lemon juice, and oil.
2. Add cabbage, green pepper, celery, and onions. Toss lightly.
3. Chill.

## Coleslaw II

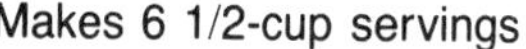

Makes 6 1/2-cup servings

| | | | |
|---|---|---|---|
| sugar | 1/4 cup | cabbage, shredded | 3 cups (1/2 medium head) |
| garlic powder | 1/2 teaspoon | green pepper, chopped | 1/4 cup |
| celery seed | 1/4 teaspoon | celery, chopped | 1 stalk |
| vinegar | 3 tablespoons | green onions, sliced | 3 to 4 |
| lemon juice | 3 tablespoons | | |

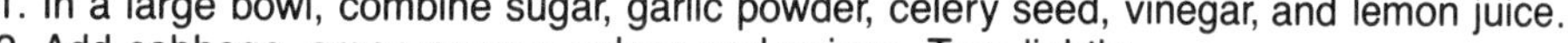

1. In a large bowl, combine sugar, garlic powder, celery seed, vinegar, and lemon juice.
2. Add cabbage, green pepper, celery, and onions. Toss lightly.
3. Chill.

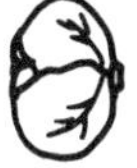

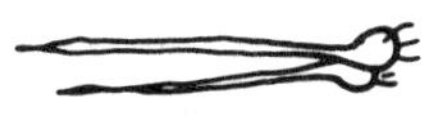

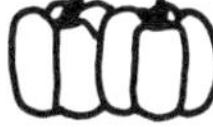

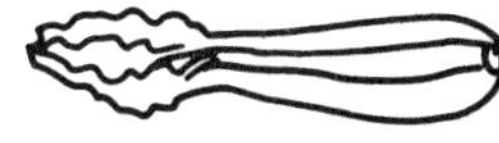

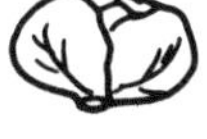

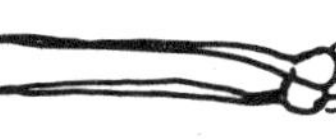

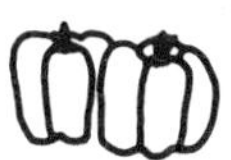

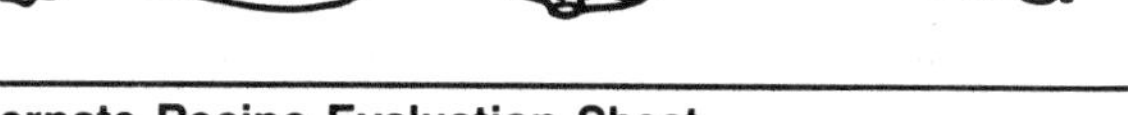

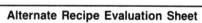

**Alternate Recipe Evaluation Sheet**

Name of food tasted ______________________________

Circle one answer for each question.

| | | | | | |
|---|---|---|---|---|---|
| How did it taste? (circle one) | Excellent | Very good | Good | Fair | Poor |
| How would you rate the appearance of the food? | Excellent | Very good | Good | Fair | Poor |
| How would you rate the aroma of the food? | Excellent | Very good | Good | Fair | Poor |
| How would you rate the texture of the food? | Excellent | Very good | Good | Fair | Poor |
| How would you rate the overall *quality* of the food? | Excellent | Very good | Good | Fair | Poor |

Name ____________________ 

# WHAT DID I SAVE WITH THE ALTERNATE RECIPE?

| Ingredients | Amount |
|---|---|
| | |

Ingredients altered: ____________________

**Group 1: Traditional recipe**

1. ____________________
Total calories in original recipe

**Group 2: Decreased sugar**

| | | | | |
|---|---|---|---|---|
| ____________ | − | ____________ | = | ____________ |
| Calories from sugar in original recipe | | Calories from sugar in altered recipe | | Calories saved from decreased sugar |
| ____________ | ÷ | ____________ | = | ____________ |
| Calories saved from decreased sugar | | No. of cookies in recipe | | Calories saved per cookie |

**Group 3: Decreased fat**

| | | | | |
|---|---|---|---|---|
| ____________ | − | ____________ | = | ____________ |
| Calories from fat in original recipe | | Calories from fat in altered recipe | | Calories saved from decreased fat |
| ____________ | ÷ | ____________ | = | ____________ |
| Calories saved from decreased fat | | No. of cookies in recipe | | Calories saved per cookie |

**Group 4: No salt**

| | | | | |
|---|---|---|---|---|
| ____________ mg. | ÷ | ____________ | = | ____________ mg. |
| Sodium from salt deleted from original recipe | | No. of cookies in altered recipe | | Sodium decreased per cookie |

**Group 5: Decreased sugar, fat, and no salt**

| | | | | |
|---|---|---|---|---|
| ____________ | − | ____________ | = | ____________ |
| Total calories in original recipe | | Total calories in altered recipe | | Calories saved |
| ____________ | ÷ | ____________ | = | ____________ |
| Calories saved | | No. of cookies in recipe | | Calories saved per cookie |
| ____________ mg. | ÷ | ____________ | = | ____________ mg. |
| Total sodium from salt deleted in original recipe | | No. of cookies in recipe | | Sodium decreased per cookie |

Name ____________________ 

# QUIZ
# DIETARY GUIDELINES FOR AMERICANS

1. The Dietary Guidelines for Americans call for changes in the eating habits of Americans. List at least five of the seven guidelines. For each guideline, state one way you can include it in your daily eating habits.

a. ____________________

b. ____________________

c. ____________________

d. ____________________

e. ____________________

_____ 2. Which of these will help you follow the Dietary Guidelines?

- a. Eat fewer fruits
- b. Eat more butter and eggs
- c. Eat lowfat dairy products
- d. Eat more meat

_____ 3. The Dietary Guidelines suggest that Americans should be:

- a. Underweight
- b. Overweight
- c. Eating less starch
- d. Eating more fiber

_____ 4. To follow the Dietary Guidelines for Americans you could:

- a. Eat fewer beans, nuts, and seeds
- b. Eat more whole-grain breads and cereals
- c. Eat fewer fruits and vegetables
- d. Eat more eggs and cheese

5. The Dietary Guidelines are designed to help improve the diet of Americans. Name several health problems that may be reduced if Americans follow these guidelines.

____________________

____________________

____________________

____________________

# Unit 20: Designing a National Nutrition Policy

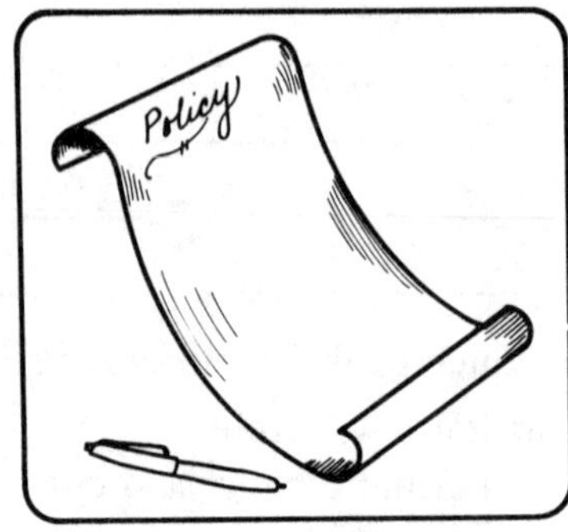


## CONCEPTS

–A national nutrition policy could provide direction to legislators for programs aimed at preserving the nutritional health of the people.

–The U.S. Dietary Guidelines for Americans represent a major step toward a national nutrition policy.

## OBJECTIVES

–Students will be able to describe the issues involved in developing a national nutrition policy.

–Students will be able to describe legislation that will be required if the Dietary Guidelines are to become part of a national nutrition policy.

–Students will be able to predict the impact that legislation for promoting the Dietary Guidelines would have on agriculture, food processing, and food purchasing.

## TEACHER'S UNIT INTRODUCTION

The United States has been moving toward a national nutrition policy since the 1940s when the School Lunch Program was initiated and standards for enrichment and fortification were developed. During the 1960s, the U.S. government became more interested in the dietary status of Americans. This interest resulted in several national nutrition surveys designed to determine if Americans were consuming an adequate diet. To alleviate the nutrition problems identified in the surveys, programs in addition to the School Lunch Program were established in the 1970s. These programs include the Special Supplemental

Food Program for Women, Infants, and Children (WIC), the Congregate Meals Program for the Elderly, and nutrition labeling.

The malnutrition identified in the surveys during the 1970s continues to exist in the United States today. Another equally serious problem that has surfaced is overconsumption. Six of the ten leading causes of death in the United States (coronary heart disease, some forms of cancer, cerebrovascular disease (stroke), diabetes, arteriosclerosis, and cirrhosis of the liver) are associated with excessive intake of some substances in the diet such as fat and cholesterol. Further, it was found that 30 percent of all Americans are obese, and obesity is directly related to increased morbidity and mortality from diabetes, hypertension, and coronary heart disease. The high incidence of these diet-related diseases may be due to changes in dietary patterns and changes in the American food supply. For example, Americans eat more processed foods, more fat and sugar, and less carbohydrate (other than sugar) than they did at the turn of the century.

In response to the high incidence of diet-related diseases in this country, the U.S. Department of Agriculture (USDA) and the Department of Health and Human Services (formerly the Department of Health, Education, and Welfare) issued a set of seven recommendations called the Dietary Guidelines for Americans. These guidelines are generally consistent with other scientific and government recommendations. The Dietary Guidelines for healthy persons of all ages are:

1. Eat a variety of food.
2. Maintain ideal weight.
3. Avoid too much fat, saturated fat, and cholesterol.
4. Eat foods with adequate starch and fiber.
5. Avoid too much sugar.
6. Avoid too much sodium.
7. If you drink alcohol, do so in moderation.

A criticism of these guidelines is that the definitions of "too much," "adequate," and "moderation" are left to the interpretation of the consumer. The consumer is required to decide on a personal definition of these terms.

The Dietary Guidelines are not a guarantee of good health. They are advice for maintaining health through a proper diet and for making informed food choices.

The Dietary Guidelines have created a heated controversy in industry and in the scientific community. Generally, the scientific community does not agree with the evidence used to develop the Dietary Guidelines. In addition, many industries, especially the meat and egg industries, fear the financial consequences of a reduction in the consumption of meat, some of which is high in fat, and of eggs, which are high in cholesterol. Despite such problems and the national debate sparked by the Dietary Guidelines, policymakers cannot ignore the health risks associated with overconsumption.

There is general agreement in government agencies, the scientific community, and industry that government policies should encourage production of food in sufficient quantity and quality to provide a nutritionally adequate diet for everyone. Disagreement centers on how to define a "nutritionally adequate diet" and on what action should be taken by the government to implement the policy.

A nutritional policy, or any policy for that matter, is a framework designed to provide direction for actions. For example, a restaurant's policy may be that only those in formal attire may eat there. If an individual wearing shorts and sneakers wants to enter the restaurant, appropriate action will be taken to enforce the policy. Notice that the policy does not specify what specific steps will be taken to implement it. The policy merely gives a general direction for action.

To formulate a policy, a problem must first be identified. Second, the problem must be analyzed for possible solutions. Third, key decision makers must take an interest in the problem and create a policy to address it.

The Dietary Guidelines could form the basis of a national nutrition policy; yet, there are many obstacles to be overcome. Our knowledge concerning the nature, severity, and consequences of overconsumption is not complete. Policy decisions involve not only our scientific knowledge but also financial and political considerations, as well as emotions, moral, ethical, and religious beliefs. Many decision makers are not interested in the problem of overconsumption. Many more are pressured by the interests of the food industry and other powerful lobbies. Further, the political party in power determines where priorities lie, what programs receive funding, and how much funding is allocated.

Many feel, however, that the government has an obligation to inform its citizens and to help people improve their eating habits. A national nutrition policy would be a step toward accomplishing this. There are segments of the population that support the development of a national nutrition policy. General public opinion backing such a policy can influence its progress.

---

Unit 19 described the Dietary Guidelines in detail. The Dietary Guidelines should be understood by all students before embarking on this unit. The emphasis in Unit 19 was to illustrate the idea that certain changes in an individual's diet could have a long-lasting impact on health. The emphasis in this unit is on a discussion of how the Dietary Guidelines might be a cornerstone of a national nutrition policy. The issues in this unit are not personal or individual; they revolve around the decision-making experience for the good of the nation. The students are required to take a look at a variety of viewpoints, not only their own.

## BASIC ACTIVITY

**Time Needed:** One class period

**Materials Needed:** Quiz Sheet 20-1

1. Divide the class into seven groups. Write the seven Dietary Guidelines on the chalkboard. Assign one guideline to each group.

2. Announce that the groups should imagine that the United States government has just adopted a national nutrition policy and the Dietary Guidelines are a part of the new policy.

Each group represents legislators who must develop three laws to support the particular guideline assigned to their group. It may be helpful to give examples of legislation for each Dietary Guideline before the class breaks into groups. Examples are given below:

A. **Eat a Variety of Foods.**
Sample Legislation—Fast-food restaurants are required to include a salad bar in their operations. The salad bar must have at least one food source of Vitamin A and one food source of Vitamin C.
Schools are required to teach in home economics classes a unit on how to increase variety in the diet through ethnic foods.

B. **Maintain Ideal Weight.**
Sample Legislation—Insurance companies are required to give persons of ideal body weight discounts on insurance policies.
Corporations will receive a tax break if exercise facilities are available for employee use.
Physical fitness classes are required for children in grades K-12.

C. **Avoid too Much Fat, Saturated Fat, and Cholesterol.**
Sample Legislation—The USDA is required to change its grading system of meats. "Prime" will mean a lean piece of beef rather than a heavily marbled piece.
All foods are required to list their total fat, saturated fat, and cholesterol content per serving on the label.

D. **Eat Foods with Adequate Starch and Fiber.**
Sample Legislation—School lunches will receive government subsidies only if whole wheat bread is on the menu each day.
Government subsidies will help to reduce the cost to the consumer of fresh fruits and vegetables.

E. **Avoid too Much Sugar.**
Sample Legislation—Presweetened cereals are banned.
Advertising of candy and soft drinks is limited during prime-time television.

F. **Avoid too Much Sodium.**
Sample Legislation—The FDA will require food companies to reduce the salt (a major source of sodium) in snack foods (pretzels, potato chips) by one-half.
The USDA will require school lunches to limit their use of processed foods such as condensed soups and processed meats, which are high in sodium.

G. **If You Drink Alcohol, Do So in Moderation.**
Sample Legislation—The government will impose a heavy tax on distilled spirits.
Federal programs will be developed to educate women about the dangers of alcohol ingestion during pregnancy.
Stiff fines and mandatory jail sentences will be levied against drunk drivers.

3. Allow adequate time for brainstorming and the formulation of formally written laws.

4. When the groups are finished, a spokesperson from each group should present the newly developed legislation. A discussion should follow each presentation. The following questions may be helpful:

- What kind of opposition would the new legislation face?
- Would any group (for example, the dairy industry, meat industry, or others) be particularly hurt by it?
- What groups would benefit from the legislation?
- What unintended consequences might the new legislation have?

5. After the discussion, have the class vote on the legislation.
6. Proceed with the "Advanced Activity" if you wish; otherwise use the quiz mentioned in step 7.
7. **Evaluation:** Distribute Quiz Sheet 20-1 and have students complete it independently. Discuss the answers as a class.

## ADVANCED ACTIVITY

**Time Needed:** Two class periods

**Materials Needed:** Library resources

### Class Period 1

1. Ask the class to imagine that the United States is considering the adoption of the Dietary Guidelines as a major part of a national nutrition policy.
2. Divide the class into seven groups. Each group represents the following committees:
The Nutrition Committee
The Agriculture Committee
The Cattlemen Committee
The Food Company Committee
The Economic Committee
The Consumer Committee
The Judges
Make sure there are an odd number of judges.
3. Each committee should prepare a short speech *either* for or against the Guidelines. Arguments should be based on real data derived from library research. A spokesperson from each committee should be chosen. The Judges should inform themselves on as many aspects of the issue as possible by speaking with committee members and discussing various aspects among themselves.

### Class Period 2

1. A date should be set for a "hearing." At the hearing, each committee spokesperson should present a committee speech either for or against the Guidelines.
2. At the end of all of the speeches, each committee should have ten minutes to prepare a short rebuttal (if necessary) to any of the speeches made. The rebuttals can then be given.
3. Next, the Judges should meet, discuss the issues presented, and vote.
4. Regardless of the outcome, initiate a discussion that addresses the following:

- What are your reactions to this process?
- What problems did you face in developing your speeches and rebuttals?
- (To the Judges)—What pressures did you feel when you were making your decisions (that is, peer pressure, friendship ties, emotions)?
- How do you think this process relates to what happens on a national level?
- How many of you were satisfied with the outcome?
- What actions would you take if not satisfied?

## FOLLOW-UP ACTIVITIES

1. Have students draw up menus that follow the Dietary Guidelines.
2. Have students visit the grocery store and record items that do not follow the Dietary Guidelines. For example, condensed soups are high in salt and, therefore, high in sodium.
3. Have students make a display for the school which illustrates the Dietary Guidelines.
4. Invite a senator or congressman to discuss his or her opinion of the U.S. Dietary Guidelines. Invite industry representatives to discuss the effects of the U.S. Guidelines. Invite a nutritionist to discuss the U.S. Dietary Guidelines. Alternatively, have students interview community resource people and report back to the class.
5. Encourage students to write a policy that adheres to the Dietary Guidelines and that could be incorporated into your School Lunch Program. If possible, have students present the policy at a school board meeting or to the food service director.

Name ______________________________ Quiz Sheet 20-1

# QUIZ
# DESIGNING A NATIONAL NUTRITION POLICY

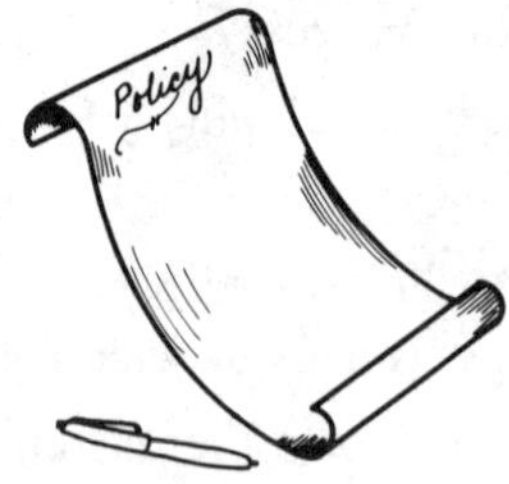


____ 1. The best term to describe a policy is:

a. Law
b. Framework
c. Budget
d. Claim

____ 2. The Dietary Guidelines were created by:

a. The United States Department of Agriculture and The Department of Health and Human Services
b. The Food and Drug Administration and The Federal Trade Commission
c. The National Academy of Sciences and The Food and Nutrition Board
d. The Surgeon General and The National Research Council

3. List 2 possible barriers to policy formation.

a. ______________________________

b. ______________________________

4. Steven wants to develop a policy of banning presweetened cereals. What should be his first steps in developing the policy?

______________________________

______________________________

______________________________

______________________________

____ 5. Which law might be proposed if the Dietary Guidelines are adopted as U.S. government guidelines?

a. The FTC would ban commercials that advertise candy.
b. The FDA would ban food companies from canning fruit.
c. Hot dogs and ham could only be served for lunch at restaurants.
d. Food labels would warn pregnant women about caffeine content.

____ 6. Which group would probably be the most supportive of legislation promoting the Dietary Guidelines?

a. Produce Marketing Association
b. National Livestock and Meat Board
c. National Food Processors Association
d. National Dairy Council

# APPENDICES

*Reproducible Student Charts and Tables*
*References/Resources*
*Answer Keys for Units 1-20*

# RECOMMENDED DIETARY ALLOWANCES[a]

| | Age (years) | Weight (kg) | Weight (lb) | Height (cm) | Height (in) | Protein (g) | Fat-Soluble Vitamins: Vitamin A (μg RE)[b] | Vitamin D (μg)[c] | Vitamin E (mg α-TE)[d] | Water-Soluble Vitamins: Vitamin C (mg) | Thiamin (mg) | Riboflavin (mg) |
|---|---|---|---|---|---|---|---|---|---|---|---|---|
| **Infants** | 0.0–0.5 | 6 | 13 | 60 | 24 | kg × 2.2 | 420 | 10 | 3 | 35 | 0.3 | 0.4 |
| | 0.5–1.0 | 9 | 20 | 71 | 28 | kg × 2.0 | 400 | 10 | 4 | 35 | 0.5 | 0.6 |
| **Children** | 1–3 | 13 | 29 | 90 | 35 | 23 | 400 | 10 | 5 | 45 | 0.7 | 0.8 |
| | 4–6 | 20 | 44 | 112 | 44 | 30 | 500 | 10 | 6 | 45 | 0.9 | 1.0 |
| | 7–10 | 28 | 62 | 132 | 52 | 34 | 700 | 10 | 7 | 45 | 1.2 | 1.4 |
| **Males** | 11–14 | 45 | 99 | 157 | 62 | 45 | 1,000 | 10 | 8 | 50 | 1.4 | 1.6 |
| | 15–18 | 66 | 145 | 176 | 69 | 56 | 1,000 | 10 | 10 | 60 | 1.4 | 1.7 |
| | 19–22 | 70 | 154 | 177 | 70 | 56 | 1,000 | 7.5 | 10 | 60 | 1.5 | 1.7 |
| | 23–50 | 70 | 154 | 178 | 70 | 56 | 1,000 | 5 | 10 | 60 | 1.4 | 1.6 |
| | 51+ | 70 | 154 | 178 | 70 | 56 | 1,000 | 5 | 10 | 60 | 1.2 | 1.4 |
| **Females** | 11–14 | 46 | 101 | 157 | 62 | 46 | 800 | 10 | 8 | 50 | 1.1 | 1.3 |
| | 15–18 | 55 | 120 | 163 | 64 | 46 | 800 | 10 | 8 | 60 | 1.1 | 1.3 |
| | 19–22 | 55 | 120 | 163 | 64 | 44 | 800 | 7.5 | 8 | 60 | 1.1 | 1.3 |
| | 23–50 | 55 | 120 | 163 | 64 | 44 | 800 | 5 | 8 | 60 | 1.0 | 1.2 |
| | 51+ | 55 | 120 | 163 | 64 | 44 | 800 | 5 | 8 | 60 | 1.0 | 1.2 |
| **Pregnant** | | | | | | +30 | +200 | +5 | +2 | +20 | +0.4 | +0.3 |
| **Lactating** | | | | | | +20 | +400 | +5 | +3 | +40 | +0.5 | +0.5 |

# RECOMMENDED DIETARY ALLOWANCES[a]

| | Niacin (mg NE)[e] | Vitamin $B_6$ (mg) | Folacin (μg)[c] | Vitamin $B_{12}$ (μg)[g] | Minerals Calcium (mg) | Phosphorus (mg) | Magnesium (mg) | Iron (mg)[h] | Zinc (mg) | Iodine (μg) |
|---|---|---|---|---|---|---|---|---|---|---|
| **Infants** | 6 | 0.3 | 30 | 0.5 | 360 | 240 | 50 | 10 | 3 | 40 |
| | 8 | 0.6 | 45 | 1.5 | 540 | 360 | 70 | 15 | 5 | 50 |
| **Children** | 9 | 0.9 | 100 | 2.0 | 800 | 800 | 150 | 15 | 10 | 70 |
| | 11 | 1.3 | 200 | 2.5 | 800 | 800 | 200 | 10 | 10 | 90 |
| | 16 | 1.6 | 300 | 3.0 | 800 | 800 | 250 | 10 | 10 | 120 |
| **Males** | 18 | 1.8 | 400 | 3.0 | 1,200 | 1,200 | 350 | 18 | 15 | 150 |
| | 18 | 2.0 | 400 | 3.0 | 1,200 | 1,200 | 400 | 18 | 15 | 150 |
| | 19 | 2.2 | 400 | 3.0 | 800 | 800 | 350 | 10 | 15 | 150 |
| | 18 | 2.2 | 400 | 3.0 | 800 | 800 | 350 | 10 | 15 | 150 |
| | 16 | 2.2 | 400 | 3.0 | 800 | 800 | 350 | 10 | 15 | 150 |
| **Females** | 15 | 1.8 | 400 | 3.0 | 1,200 | 1,200 | 300 | 18 | 15 | 150 |
| | 14 | 2.0 | 400 | 3.0 | 1,200 | 1,200 | 300 | 18 | 15 | 150 |
| | 14 | 2.0 | 400 | 3.0 | 800 | 800 | 300 | 18 | 15 | 150 |
| | 13 | 2.0 | 400 | 3.0 | 800 | 800 | 300 | 18 | 15 | 150 |
| | 13 | 2.0 | 400 | 3.0 | 800 | 800 | 300 | 10 | 15 | 150 |
| **Pregnant** | +2 | +0.6 | +400 | +1.0 | +400 | +400 | +150 | *h* | +5 | +25 |
| **Lactating** | +5 | +0.5 | +100 | +1.0 | +400 | +400 | +150 | *h* | +10 | +50 |

[a]Adapted from *Recommended Dietary Allowances*, 1980. Washington, D.C.: National Academy Press, with permission. The allowances are intended to provide for individual variations among most normal persons as they live in the United States under usual environmental stresses. Diets should be based on a variety of common foods in order to provide other nutrients for which human requirements have been less well defined.

[b]Retinol equivalents. 1 retinol equivalent = 1 μg retinol or 6 μg beta-carotene.

[c]As cholecalciferol. 10 μg cholecalciferol = 400 IUs of Vitamin D.

[d]α-tocopherol equivalents. 1 mg d-αtocopherol = 1 α-TE.

[e]1 NE (niacin equivalent) is equal to 1 mg of niacin or 60 mg. of dietary tryptophan.

[f]The folacin allowances refer to dietary sources as determined by Lactobacillus casei assay after treatment with enzymes (conjugases) to make polyglutamyl forms of the vitamin available to the test organism.

[g]The recommended dietary allowances for Vitamin $B_{12}$ in infants in based on average concentration (as recommended by the American Academy of Pediatrics) and consideration of other factors, such as intestinal absorption.

[h]The increased requirement during pregnancy cannot be met by the iron content of habitual American diets nor by the existing iron stores of many women; therefore the use of 30–60 mg of supplemental iron is recommended. Iron needs during lactation are not substantially different from those of nonpregnant women, but continued supplementation of the mother for 2–3 months after parturition is advisable in order to replenish stores depleted by pregnancy.

# DAILY FOOD GUIDE*

| FRUIT-VEGETABLE | BREAD-CEREAL | MILK-CHEESE | MEAT-POULTRY-FISH-BEANS | FATS-SWEETS-ALCOHOL |
|---|---|---|---|---|
| | | **HOW MANY SERVINGS?** | | |
| Four Basic Servings Daily | Four Basic Servings Daily | Basic Servings Daily:<br>*child under 9 2–3 servings<br>*child 9–12 3 servings<br>*teen 4 servings<br>*adult 2 servings<br>*pregnant women 3 servings<br>*nursing women 4 servings | Two Basic Servings Daily | In general, the number of calories you need determines the amount of these "extra" foods you can eat. It's a good idea to concentrate first on the calorie-plus-nutrients foods provided in the other groups. |
| | | **WHICH FOODS?** | | |
| All fruits and vegetables. Include one good Vitamin C source each day. Also frequently use deep-yellow or dark-green vegetables (for Vitamin A) and unpeeled fruits and vegetables and those with edible seeds, such as berries (for fiber). | Select only whole-grain and enriched products. (But include *some* whole-grain bread or cereal, for sure!) Include breads, biscuits, muffins, waffles, pancakes, cereals, pasta, rice, barley, rolled oats, and bulgur. | All types of milk and milk products, including whole, skim, low fat, evaporated, and nonfat dried milks, buttermilk, yogurt, cheese, ice cream, and foods prepared with milk such as puddings or cream soups. | Includes beef, veal, lamb, pork, poultry, fish, shellfish, organ meats, dried peas, soybeans, lentils, eggs, sesame seeds, sunflower seeds, nuts, peanuts, and peanut butter. | Includes butter, margarine, mayonnaise, salad dressings and other fats and oils; candy, sugar, jams, jellies, and syrups; soft drinks and other highly-sugared drinks; alcoholic beverages such as wine, beer, and liquor. Also included are refined but unenriched breads, pastries, and other grain products. |
| | | **WHAT'S A SERVING?** | | |
| Count ½ cup as a serving or a typical portion such as one orange, half a grapefruit or cantaloupe, juice of one lemon, a wedge of lettuce, a bowl of salad, or one medium potato. | Count as one serving 1 slice of bread, ½ to ¾ cup of cooked cereal, cornmeal, grits, pasta, or rice; or 1 oz. of ready-to-eat cereal. | Count an 8 oz. cup of milk as a serving. Equivalent amounts of calcium (but different amounts of calories) are found in the following: 1 cup yogurt, 1½ oz. hard cheese, 1½ cups ice milk or ice cream, or 2 cups of cottage cheese. | Count 2–3 oz. of lean, cooked meat, poultry, or fish without bones as a serving. One egg, ½ to ¾ cup cooked dried beans, dried peas, soybeans, or lentils, 2 Tbsp. peanut butter, or ¼ to ½ cup nuts or seeds count as 1 oz. of meat, poultry, or fish. | No serving sizes have been defined because a basic number of servings is not suggested for this group. Use these foods in moderation. |
| | | **WHAT'S IN IT FOR YOU?** | | |
| Carbohydrates, fiber, Vitamins A and C. Dark-green vegetables are valued for riboflavin, folacin (B vitamins), iron, and magnesium. Certain greens provide calcium. Nearly all fruits and vegetables are low in fat and none contain cholesterol. | Carbohydrates, proteins, B vitamins, iron. Whole-grain products also provide magnesium, folacin (B vitamin), and fiber. | Calcium, riboflavin, protein, vitamins A, $B_6$, and $B_{12}$. Milk products also provide Vitamin D when fortified with this vitamin. Fortified lowfat or skim milk products have the same nutrients as whole-milk products but fewer calories. | Protein, B vitamins, iron, phosphorous. Some of these foods also provide zinc, Vitamin A, and magnesium. Foods of animal origin (except fish) are relatively high in cholesterol and saturated fats. Seeds and fish are relatively high in unsaturated fats. | These foods, with the exception of vegetable oils, provide mainly calories. Vegetable oils generally provide Vitamin E and essential fatty acids. Sweets and alcohol provide mainly calories without other essential nutrients. |

*Adapted from *Food*, Home and Garden Bulletin Number 228, 1979. Washington, D.C.: U.S. Department of Agriculture.

# KEY NUTRIENTS IN FOOD*

| FAT-SOLUBLE VITAMINS | IMPORTANT FUNCTIONS | IMPORTANT SOURCES |
|---|---|---|
| Vitamin A | Helps keep skin clear and smooth<br>Helps keep mucous membranes firm and resistant to infection<br>Promotes normal vision in dim light<br>Helps promote bone growth | Liver, egg yolk<br>Dark-green and orange vegetables<br>Yellowish-pink fruits such as cantaloupe or peaches<br>Butter, margarine, milk, cream, hard cheese, ice cream |
| Vitamin D (The Sunshine Vitamin) | Assists the body's utilization of calcium and phosphorus in building bones and teeth | Vitamin D-fortified milk<br>Fish liver oils<br>(Sunshine on skin) |
| Vitamin E | Protects cell membranes from damage<br>Prevents oxidation (destruction) of fats in the body and in food | Meat (especially liver), eggs, vegetable oils<br>Green leafy vegetables<br>Whole-grain cereals, wheat germ |
| Vitamin K | Maintains normal clotting of the blood | Pork, liver, egg yolk<br>Green leafy vegetables, cauliflower<br>(Synthesized by bacteria in the intestines) |
| **WATER-SOLUBLE VITAMINS** | **IMPORTANT FUNCTIONS** | **IMPORTANT SOURCES** |
| Thiamin (Vitamin $B_1$) | Helps promote normal appetite and digestion<br>Helps keep nervous system healthy and prevents irritability<br>Helps body release energy from carbohydrates and fats in food | Meat (especially pork), fish, poultry<br>Eggs<br>Enriched or whole-grain breads and cereals<br>Dried beans and peas<br>Potatoes, broccoli, green leafy vegetables |

**Adapted from M. Martin,* The Great Vitamin Mystery. *1968. Rosemont, IL: National Dairy Council.*

Chart C-2

| WATER-SOLUBLE VITAMINS, cont. | IMPORTANT FUNCTIONS | IMPORTANT SOURCES |
|---|---|---|
| Riboflavin (Vitamin $B_2$) | Helps cells use oxygen<br>Helps keep skin, tongue, and lips normal<br>Helps prevent scaly, greasy skin around mouth and nose<br>Helps body release energy from carbohydrates and fats in food | Milk and milk products<br>Meat (especially liver and kidney), fish, poultry, and eggs<br>Green leafy vegetables, broccoli |
| Niacin | Helps keep nervous system healthy<br>Helps keep skin, mouth, tongue, and digestive tract in healthy condition<br>Helps cells use other nutrients<br>Helps body release energy from carbohydrates and fats in food | Peanut butter<br>Meat (especially liver), fish, poultry<br>Milk and eggs (high in tryptophan)<br>Enriched or whole-grain breads and cereals<br>Dried beans and peas |
| Pyridoxine (Vitamin $B_6$) | Helps nervous system tissues function normally<br>Plays a role in red blood cell regeneration<br>Involved in the metabolism of amino acids, fats, and carbohydrates | Liver, pork, ham, salmon<br>Soybeans and lima beans<br>Bananas<br>Yeast<br>Whole-grain cereals<br>Egg yolks<br>Vegetables |
| Folacin (Folic Acid) | Helps cure (and prevent) megaloblastic anemia<br>Helps enzyme and other biochemical systems function normally | Green leafy vegetables, lima beans, broccoli<br>Liver, kidney<br>Whole-grain cereals<br>Dried beans and peas |
| Cobalamin (Vitamin $B_{12}$) | Protects against the development of pernicious anemia<br>Maintains healthy nerves | Eggs, fish, liver, kidney, other meats<br>Milk and milk products |

**Chart C-3**

| WATER-SOLUBLE VITAMINS, cont. | IMPORTANT FUNCTIONS | IMPORTANT SOURCES |
|---|---|---|
| Ascorbic Acid (Vitamin C) | Helps make cementing materials that hold body cells together<br>Helps make walls of blood vessels firm<br>Helps in healing wounds and broken bones<br>Helps body resist infections<br>Helps tissues such as gums and teeth stay healthy | Citrus fruits (orange, grapefruit, lemon, lime)<br>Strawberries, cantaloupe, melons<br>Tomatoes<br>Green peppers, broccoli<br>Green leafy vegetables, cabbage<br>Potatoes |
| **ENERGY NUTRIENTS** | **IMPORTANT FUNCTIONS** | **IMPORTANT SOURCES** |
| Proteins | Builds and repairs all tissues such as muscle, blood, and bone<br>Helps form antibodies to fight infection<br>Helps produce enzymes and hormones<br>Supplies energy | Lean meat, fish, seafood, poultry, eggs<br>Milk, cheese, yogurt<br>Dried beans and peas, other legumes<br>Peanut butter, peanuts, other nuts, seeds<br>Breads and cereals |
| Carbohydrates (Sugar, Starch, and Fiber) | Supplies energy<br>Carries other nutrients present in foods<br>Provides fiber which assists in the elimination of body wastes | Breads and cereals<br>Potatoes, lima beans, corn<br>Dried beans and peas<br>Dried fruits, sweetened fruits<br>Sugar, syrup, jelly, jam, honey |
| Fats | Supplies large amounts of energy in a small amount of food<br>Supplies essential fatty acids<br>Carries fat-soluble vitamins A, D, E, K | Butter, margarine, shortenings<br>Salad oils and dressings<br>Fatty meats like bacon<br>Marbling in meats<br>Butterfat in milk and cream<br>Nuts and seeds |

**Chart C-4**

| MINERALS | IMPORTANT FUNCTIONS | IMPORTANT SOURCES |
|---|---|---|
| Calcium | Helps build bones and teeth<br>Helps blood to clot<br>Helps muscles, nerves, and heart to work<br>Helps regulate the use of other minerals in the body | Milk and milk products (low amounts in cottage cheese)<br>Dark-green leafy vegetables<br>Salmon, sardines, and other fish with edible bones<br>Tofu (soybean curd), soybeans, other legumes |
| Phosphorus | Helps build bones and teeth<br>Helps regulate many internal activities of the body | Liver, fish, poultry, eggs<br>Milk and milk products<br>Whole-grain cereals<br>Nuts |
| Iron | Combines with protein to make hemoglobin, the red substance in the blood that carries oxygen to the cells | Lean meat (especially liver, kidney), poultry, oysters<br>Dried beans and peas, other legumes<br>Dark-green leafy vegetables<br>Prunes, raisins, dried apricots<br>Fortified, enriched, or whole-grain breads and cereals<br>Molasses |
| Iodine | Helps the thyroid gland control the rate at which the body uses energy | Seafood, plants grown in soil near salt water, iodized salt |
| Water | Important in all cells and body fluids<br>Regulates body temperature<br>Transports nutrients to cells and carries wastes away | Water<br>Beverages such as juice or milk<br>Soups<br>Fruits and vegetables |

# FOOD COMPOSITION TABLE FOR SELECTED NUTRIENTS[a]

| Food and Amount | Gm | Calories | %[b] | Protein | Vitamin A | Vitamin C | Thiamin | Riboflavin | Niacin | Calcium | Iron |
|---|---|---|---|---|---|---|---|---|---|---|---|
| | | | | Percentages of U.S. RDA | | | | | | | |
| Almonds, in shell—½ cup | 39 | 120 | 5 | 6 | * | * | 3 | 11 | 5 | 5 | 5 |
| Apple, fresh—1 | 138 | 80 | 3 | * | 3 | 9 | 3 | 2 | 1 | 1 | 1 |
| Apple pie—1/7 of 9″ diameter | 135 | 400 | 16 | 5 | 4 | 5 | 10 | 5 | 6 | 1 | 6 |
| Applesauce, sweetened, ½ cup | 128 | 115 | 5 | * | 1 | 2 | 2 | 1 | * | 1 | 4 |
| Apricots: | | | | | | | | | | | |
| dried—½ cup | 65 | 170 | 7 | 5 | 142 | 13 | * | 6 | 11 | 4 | 20 |
| fresh—3 | 108 | 55 | 2 | 3 | 57 | 18 | 3 | 3 | 3 | * | 3 |
| Asparagus—½ cup | 90 | 20 | * | 3 | 16 | 39 | 10 | 10 | 6 | 2 | 3 |
| Avocado—½ | 114 | 190 | 8 | 4 | 7 | 27 | 9 | 14 | 9 | 1 | 4 |
| Bacon—2 slices | 15 | 90 | 4 | 10 | * | * | 5 | 3 | 4 | * | 3 |
| Bagel, egg—1 | 55 | 165 | 7 | 9 | * | * | 9 | 6 | 6 | * | 7 |
| Baked beans, with pork—¾ cup | 178 | 220 | 17 | 24 | 5 | 6 | 10 | 3 | 5 | 10 | 18 |
| Banana—1 | 119 | 100 | 4 | 2 | 5 | 20 | 4 | 4 | 4 | * | 1 |
| Beans, dried, then cooked—½ cup | 128 | 115 | 5 | 11 | * | * | 4 | 3 | 4 | 4 | 13 |
| Bean sprouts, cooked—½ cup | 63 | 20 | * | 3 | * | 6 | 4 | 4 | 2 | 1 | 3 |
| Beef pot pie—4¼″ diameter | 227 | 560 | 22 | 35 | 37 | 11 | 17 | 16 | 23 | 3 | 23 |
| Beet greens, cooked—½ cup | 73 | 15 | * | 2 | 74 | 18 | 3 | 6 | 1 | 7 | 8 |
| Beets, cooked—½ cup | 85 | 30 | * | 1 | * | 9 | 2 | 2 | 1 | 1 | 2 |
| Biscuit—1, 2½″ diameter | 40 | 155 | 6 | 5 | 1 | * | 7 | 5 | 4 | 5 | 4 |
| Blueberries, fresh—½ cup | 73 | 45 | 2 | * | 1 | 17 | 1 | 3 | 2 | 1 | 4 |
| Bologna—1 slice, 1 oz. | 28 | 85 | 3 | 8 | * | * | 3 | 4 | 4 | * | 3 |
| Bread, enriched: | | | | | | | | | | | |
| cracked wheat—1 slice | 25 | 65 | 3 | 3 | * | * | 2 | 1 | 4 | 2 | 2 |
| Italian–1 slice | 30 | 85 | 3 | 4 | * | * | 6 | 4 | 4 | 1 | 4 |
| rye (light)—1 slice | 25 | 60 | 2 | 4 | * | * | 3 | 1 | 4 | 2 | 2 |
| white—1 slice | 25 | 70 | 3 | 3 | * | * | 4 | 3 | 3 | 2 | 4 |
| whole wheat—1 slice | 23 | 55 | 2 | 4 | * | * | 4 | 2 | 3 | 2 | 3 |
| Broccoli, cooked—½ cup | 78 | 20 | * | 4 | 39 | 116 | 5 | 9 | 3 | 7 | 3 |
| Butter—1 Tbsp. | 14 | 100 | 4 | * | 9 | * | * | * | * | * | * |
| Cabbage, cooked—½ cup | 73 | 15 | * | 1 | 2 | 40 | 2 | 2 | 1 | 3 | 1 |
| Cake: | | | | | | | | | | | |
| devils food, with chocolate icing—1 piece | 92 | 350 | 14 | 6 | 8 | * | 2 | 4 | 1 | 5 | 4 |
| yellow, with chocolate icing —1 piece | 125 | 465 | 19 | 7 | 10 | * | 6 | 7 | 4 | 5 | 6 |
| yellow, without icing—1 piece | 85 | 320 | 13 | 8 | 9 | * | 8 | 7 | 4 | 6 | 5 |
| Candy: | | | | | | | | | | | |
| caramels, plain—1 square | 10 | 40 | 2 | 1 | * | * | * | 1 | * | 2 | 1 |
| chocolate bar—1 oz. | 28 | 150 | 6 | 3 | 2 | 1 | 1 | 6 | * | 7 | 2 |
| gumdrops, starch jelly pieces—1 average | 2 | 10 | * | * | * | * | * | * | * | * | * |
| hard—1 average ball | 5 | 20 | * | * | * | * | * | * | * | * | 1 |
| peanut bar—1 oz. | 28 | 145 | 6 | 8 | * | * | 8 | 1 | 13 | 1 | 3 |
| peanut brittle—1 oz. | 28 | 120 | 5 | 3 | * | * | 3 | 1 | 5 | 1 | 4 |
| Cantaloupe—¼, 5″ diameter | 133 | 40 | 2 | 1 | 90 | 73 | 4 | 2 | 4 | 2 | 3 |
| Carrot, raw—1 medium | 81 | 35 | 1 | 1 | 178 | 11 | 3 | 2 | 2 | 3 | 3 |
| Cauliflower, cooked—½ cup | 68 | 15 | * | 2 | 1 | 62 | 4 | 3 | 2 | 1 | 3 |
| Celery—1 stalk | 40 | 5 | * | 1 | 2 | 6 | 1 | 1 | 1 | 2 | 1 |

[a]*Nutrients in Foods.* Leveille, G. A., Zabik, M. E., and Morgan, K. J. The Nutrition Guild, Cambridge, MA, 1983.

[b]Percent of 2,500 calories.

[c]For more precise information refer to package label of specific cereal.

*None or less than one percent.

| Food and Amount | Gm | Calories | %[b] | Protein | Vitamin A | Vitamin C | Thiamin | Riboflavin | Niacin | Calcium | Iron |
|---|---|---|---|---|---|---|---|---|---|---|---|
| | | | | | Percentages of U.S. RDA | | | | | | |
| Cereal, ready-to-eat: | | | | | | | | | | | |
| enriched[c]—1 oz. | 28 | 110 | 4 | 3 | * | * | 25 | 25 | 25 | 1 | 13 |
| fortified[c]—1 oz. | 28 | 110 | 4 | 5 | 100 | 100 | 100 | 100 | 100 | 4 | 100 |
| Cheese: | | | | | | | | | | | |
| American—1 slice, 1 oz. | 28 | 95 | 4 | 12 | 5 | * | * | 7 | * | 16 | * |
| Parmesan, grated—1 Tbsp. | 5 | 25 | 1 | 5 | 1 | * | * | 1 | * | 7 | * |
| Chicken, roasted | | | | | | | | | | | |
| breast, ½ | 98 | 195 | 8 | 65 | 2 | * | 5 | 7 | 62 | 1 | 6 |
| drumstick, 1 | 52 | 110 | 4 | 31 | 1 | * | 2 | 7 | 16 | 1 | 4 |
| Chicken livers, chopped 1 cup | 140 | 220 | 9 | 76 | 458 | 36 | 14 | 144 | 32 | 2 | 66 |
| Chicken pie—1 average | 302 | 705 | 28 | 61 | 94 | 34 | 23 | 18 | 59 | 5 | 20 |
| Chili con carne w/beans—1 cup | 230 | 305 | 12 | 36 | 3 | * | 5 | 16 | 28 | 8 | 33 |
| Chocolate chip cookie—1 | 12 | 60 | 2 | 1 | * | * | 1 | 1 | 1 | * | 1 |
| Cocoa, instant powder—1 Tbsp. | 7 | 30 | 1 | 1 | * | * | * | 2 | * | 2 | 1 |
| Corn, canned—½ cup | 83 | 70 | 3 | 3 | 6 | 6 | 2 | 2 | 4 | * | 2 |
| Cornbread—1 piece | 42 | 110 | 4 | 4 | 4 | * | 3 | 4 | 2 | 4 | 2 |
| Corn grits, enriched—½ oz. dry (½ cup prepared) | 123 | 60 | 3 | 2 | 2 | * | 3 | 2 | 2 | * | 2 |
| Crackers: | | | | | | | | | | | |
| animal—11 pieces | 29 | 125 | 5 | 3 | 1 | * | 1 | 2 | * | 2 | 1 |
| butter rounds—9 pieces | 30 | 150 | 6 | 3 | * | * | 8 | 6 | 6 | 4 | 5 |
| saltines—10 pieces | 28 | 120 | 5 | 4 | * | * | * | 1 | 1 | 1 | 2 |
| Creamed beef on toast—⅔ cup/slice | 158 | 280 | 11 | 39 | 8 | 2 | 8 | 19 | 11 | 13 | 16 |
| Cupcake: | | | | | | | | | | | |
| yellow, with chocolate icing—1 average | 46 | 185 | 7 | 3 | 4 | * | 2 | 3 | 2 | 2 | 2 |
| yellow, without icing—1 average | 33 | 130 | 5 | 3 | 4 | * | 3 | 3 | 2 | 2 | 2 |
| Doughnut, cake, plain—1 | 42 | 165 | 7 | 3 | 1 | * | 5 | 4 | 3 | 2 | 3 |
| Egg: | | | | | | | | | | | |
| plain—1 | 51 | 80 | 3 | 14 | 5 | * | 3 | 9 | * | 3 | 6 |
| scrambled, with butter—1 | 64 | 95 | 4 | 13 | 6 | * | 3 | 9 | * | 5 | 5 |
| Flounder, fillet, baked, with butter—2 oz. | 56 | 115 | 5 | 37 | * | 2 | 3 | 3 | 7 | 1 | 4 |
| Fruit Cocktail—½ cup | 128 | 100 | 4 | 1 | 4 | 4 | 2 | 1 | 3 | 1 | 3 |
| Gelatin (Jell-O)—½ cup | 120 | 70 | 3 | 3 | * | * | * | * | * | * | * |
| Gingerbread, homemade—1 piece | 76 | 275 | 11 | 5 | 1 | 3 | 7 | 6 | 5 | 13 | 23 |
| Graham crackers—4 pieces | 28 | 110 | 4 | 3 | * | * | 1 | 4 | 2 | 1 | 2 |
| Grapefruit—½ | 98 | 40 | 2 | 1 | 2 | 62 | 3 | 1 | 1 | 2 | 2 |
| Grapefruit juice, fresh—4 oz. | 123 | 50 | 2 | 1 | 2 | 78 | 3 | 1 | 1 | 1 | 1 |
| Grape juice—4 oz. | 127 | 85 | 3 | * | * | * | 3 | 2 | 1 | 1 | 2 |
| Grape juice drink, enriched–8 oz. | 247 | 110 | 4 | * | * | 133 | * | * | * | * | * |
| Grapes, fresh–½ cup | 80 | 55 | 2 | 1 | 2 | 5 | 3 | 1 | 1 | 1 | 2 |
| Green beans, fresh, cooked—½ cup | 63 | 15 | * | 2 | 7 | 13 | 3 | 3 | 2 | 3 | 2 |
| Hamburger, no roll—1 | 85 | 245 | 10 | 46 | 1 | * | 5 | 11 | 23 | 1 | 15 |
| Hot dog, no roll—1 | 44 | 135 | 5 | 12 | * | * | 4 | 5 | 6 | * | 4 |
| Ice cream, regular—⅔ cup | 89 | 180 | 7 | 7 | 7 | * | 2 | 13 | * | 12 | * |
| Jams and preserves—1 Tbsp. | 20 | 55 | 2 | * | * | 1 | * | * | * | * | 1 |
| Ketchup—1 Tbsp. | 15 | 15 | * | 1 | 4 | 4 | 1 | 1 | 1 | 0 | 1 |

[a]*Nutrients in Foods.* Leveille, G. A., Zabik, M. E., and Morgan, K. J. The Nutrition Guild, Cambridge, MA, 1983.

[b]Percent of 2,500 calories.

[c]For more precise information refer to package label of specific cereal.

*None or less than one percent.

| Food and Amount | Gm | Calories | %[b] | Protein | Vitamin A | Vitamin C | Thiamin | Riboflavin | Niacin | Calcium | Iron |
|---|---|---|---|---|---|---|---|---|---|---|---|
| | | | | Percentages of U.S. RDA | | | | | | | |
| Lamb chop—2½ oz. | 71 | 255 | 10 | 35 | * | * | 6 | 10 | 18 | 1 | 5 |
| Lemonade—8 oz. | 248 | 110 | 4 | 1 | 1 | 146 | 4 | 5 | 4 | 1 | 3 |
| Lettuce, iceberg—½ cup | 28 | 5 | * | * | 2 | 3 | 1 | 1 | * | 1 | 1 |
| Liver, beef—3 oz. | 85 | 195 | 8 | 50 | 908 | 38 | 15 | 210 | 70 | 1 | 42 |
| Macaroni, cooked—½ cup | 70 | 80 | 3 | 4 | * | * | 7 | 3 | 4 | 1 | 4 |
| Macaroni and cheese, prepared from mix—¾ cup | 156 | 290 | 12 | 17 | 11 | * | 18 | 12 | 10 | 11 | * |
| Maple syrup—1 Tbsp. | 19 | 50 | 2 | * | * | * | * | * | * | * | * |
| Margarine—1 Tbsp. | 14 | 100 | 4 | * | 9 | * | * | * | * | * | * |
| Milk, fluid: | | | | | | | | | | | |
| chocolate, 2% butterfat—8 oz. | 250 | 180 | 7 | 18 | 10 | 4 | 5 | 24 | 2 | 29 | 3 |
| evaporated—8 oz. | 244 | 330 | 13 | 37 | 12 | 8 | 7 | 45 | 2 | 64 | 3 |
| nonfat dry, powder—⅓ cup | 23 | 80 | 3 | 18 | 11 | 2 | 6 | 23 | 1 | 28 | * |
| skim—8 oz. | 245 | 85 | 3 | 19 | 10 | 4 | 5 | 20 | 1 | 30 | 1 |
| 2% butterfat—8 oz. | 244 | 125 | 5 | 18 | 10 | 4 | 5 | 23 | 1 | 30 | 1 |
| whole—8 oz. | 244 | 160 | 6 | 18 | 7 | 6 | 5 | 23 | 1 | 29 | 1 |
| Noodles, enriched, cooked—½ cup | 80 | 100 | 4 | 7 | 1 | * | 8 | 4 | 5 | 1 | 7 |
| Oatmeal, cooked—½ cup | 123 | 67 | 3 | 4 | * | 0 | 7 | 1 | 1 | 1 | 4 |
| Ocean perch: | | | | | | | | | | | |
| breaded, fried—2½ oz. | 70 | 160 | 6 | 30 | * | * | 5 | 5 | 6 | 2 | 5 |
| broiled, 2½ oz. | 65 | 60 | 2 | 27 | * | * | 4 | 4 | 6 | 2 | 5 |
| Onions, raw—½ cup | 85 | 30 | 1 | 2 | 1 | 14 | 2 | 2 | 1 | 2 | 2 |
| Orange, fresh—1 | 131 | 65 | 3 | 2 | 5 | 109 | 9 | 3 | 3 | 5 | 3 |
| Orange juice, fresh—4 oz. | 123 | 55 | 2 | 1 | 5 | 103 | 7 | 2 | 3 | 1 | 1 |
| Oysters, raw—6 | 90 | 60 | 2 | 18 | 6 | * | 6 | 12 | 12 | 6 | 30 |
| Pancakes—1, 4″ diameter | 27 | 60 | 2 | 3 | 1 | * | 3 | 4 | 1 | 6 | 2 |
| Papaya—¼ average | 114 | 50 | 2 | 1 | 40 | 28 | 2 | 1 | 1 | 3 | 3 |
| Peach: | | | | | | | | | | | |
| canned, water packed—½ cup | 122 | 40 | 2 | 1 | 11 | 6 | 1 | 2 | 4 | 1 | 2 |
| fresh-1 | 100 | 40 | 2 | 1 | 27 | 12 | 1 | 3 | 5 | 1 | 3 |
| Peanut butter—1 Tbsp. | 15 | 90 | 4 | 6 | * | * | 1 | 1 | 12 | 1 | 2 |
| Peanuts: | | | | | | | | | | | |
| in shell—10 | 18 | 70 | 3 | 10 | * | * | * | * | 10 | * | * |
| salted—¼ cup | 36 | 210 | 8 | 14 | * | * | 8 | 3 | 31 | 3 | 4 |
| Pear, fresh—1 | 164 | 100 | 4 | 2 | 1 | 11 | 2 | 4 | 1 | 1 | 3 |
| Peas, fresh, cooked—½ cup | 80 | 60 | 2 | 7 | 9 | 27 | 15 | 5 | 9 | 2 | 8 |
| Pepper, green, raw—1 | 164 | 35 | 1 | 3 | 14 | 350 | 9 | 8 | 4 | 2 | 6 |
| Pineapple, water pack—1 slice | 58 | 25 | 1 | * | 1 | 7 | 3 | 1 | 1 | 1 | 1 |
| Pizza with cheese—⅐ of 10″ diameter | 57 | 140 | 6 | 8 | 5 | 6 | 7 | 8 | 5 | 9 | 5 |
| Plum, fresh—1 | 28 | 20 | * | * | 2 | 2 | 1 | 1 | 1 | * | 1 |
| Popcorn, plain—1 cup | 12 | 45 | 2 | 2 | * | * | * | 1 | 1 | * | 2 |
| Pork chop—3 oz. | 85 | 330 | 13 | 47 | * | * | 54 | 14 | 25 | 1 | 16 |
| Potato: | | | | | | | | | | | |
| baked—1 | 165 | 145 | 6 | 6 | * | 52 | 10 | 4 | 13 | 1 | 6 |
| chips—14 | 28 | 160 | 6 | 2 | * | 8 | 4 | 1 | 7 | 1 | 3 |
| french fries—½ cup | 55 | 150 | 6 | 4 | * | 19 | 5 | 3 | 9 | 1 | 4 |
| Pretzels, thin sticks—47 pieces | 28 | 110 | 4 | 4 | * | * | * | 1 | 1 | 1 | 2 |
| Prune juice—4 oz. | 128 | 100 | 4 | 1 | * | 4 | 1 | 1 | 3 | 2 | 29 |
| Prunes–10 medium | 96 | 240 | 10 | * | 30 | 10 | 10 | 10 | 10 | 10 | 20 |
| Pudding, chocolate, prepared from mix—½ cup | 144 | 155 | 6 | 19 | 3 | 3 | 2 | 12 | 1 | 15 | * |
| Pumpkin pie—⅐ of 9″ diameter | 135 | 290 | 12 | 12 | 49 | 4 | 8 | 13 | 5 | 11 | 7 |

[a]*Nutrients in Foods.* Leveille, G. A., Zabik, M. E., and Morgan, K. J. The Nutrition Guild, Cambridge, MA, 1983.

[b]Percent of 2,500 calories.

[c]For more precise information refer to package label of specific cereal.

*None or less than one percent.

| Food and Amount | Gm | Calories | %[b] | Protein | Vitamin A | Vitamin C | Thiamin | Riboflavin | Niacin | Calcium | Iron |
|---|---|---|---|---|---|---|---|---|---|---|---|
| | | | | Percentages of U.S. RDA | | | | | | | |
| Pumpkin seeds, hulled—1/4 cup | 35 | 195 | 8 | 16 | 1 | 1 | 6 | 4 | 4 | 2 | 22 |
| Raisins—1/4 cup | 42 | 125 | 5 | 2 | * | 1 | 4 | 1 | 1 | 2 | 5 |
| Rice, enriched—1/2 cup | 103 | 110 | 4 | 3 | * | * | 8 | 4 | 5 | 1 | 5 |
| Roast beef—3 oz. | 85 | 365 | 15 | 37 | * | * | 3 | 7 | 15 | 1 | 12 |
| Roll: | | | | | | | | | | | |
| hamburger—1 | 40 | 120 | 5 | 5 | * | * | 8 | 4 | 7 | 3 | 4 |
| hard—1 medium | 25 | 80 | 3 | 4 | * | * | 4 | 3 | 3 | 1 | 3 |
| Salad oil—1 Tbsp. | 14 | 120 | 5 | * | * | * | * | * | * | * | * |
| Shrimp, cooked—1/2 cup | 55 | 65 | 3 | 30 | 1 | * | * | 1 | 5 | 6 | 10 |
| Sloppy Joe—3/4 cup | 187 | 205 | 8 | 26 | 10 | 26 | 8 | 10 | 15 | 8 | 12 |
| Sodas: | | | | | | | | | | | |
| club—12 oz. | 356 | * | * | * | * | * | * | * | * | * | * |
| cola type—12 oz. | 370 | 145 | 6 | * | * | * | * | * | * | * | * |
| cream—12 oz. | 371 | 160 | 6 | * | * | * | * | * | * | * | * |
| fruit-flavored—12 oz. | 372 | 170 | 7 | * | * | * | * | * | * | * | * |
| root beer—12 oz. | 370 | 150 | 6 | * | * | * | * | * | * | * | * |
| Soup, canned: | | | | | | | | | | | |
| chicken noodle—1 cup | 241 | 75 | 3 | 6 | 14 | * | 3 | 4 | 7 | 2 | 4 |
| cream of chicken, prepared with water—1 cup | 244 | 120 | 5 | 5 | 11 | * | 2 | 4 | 4 | 3 | 3 |
| vegetarian vegetable—1 cup | 241 | 70 | 3 | 3 | 60 | 2 | 3 | 3 | 5 | 2 | 6 |
| Soup, dehydrated: | | | | | | | | | | | |
| beef noodle—1 cup | 251 | 40 | 2 | 3 | * | 2 | 8 | 3 | 4 | 1 | 2 |
| chicken noodle—1 cup | 252 | 55 | 2 | 5 | 1 | * | 5 | 3 | 4 | 3 | 3 |
| Spaghetti with meatballs and tomato sauce—1 cup | 248 | 330 | 13 | 41 | 32 | 37 | 17 | 18 | 20 | 12 | 21 |
| Spinach, cooked—1/2 cup | 90 | 20 | * | 4 | 146 | 42 | 4 | 7 | 2 | 8 | 11 |
| Steak—3 oz. | 85 | 330 | 13 | 43 | 1 | * | 3 | 9 | 20 | 1 | 14 |
| Strawberries, whole—1/2 cup | 75 | 30 | 1 | 1 | 1 | 73 | 2 | 3 | 2 | 2 | 4 |
| Stuffed pepper, beef–1 average | 185 | 320 | 13 | 43 | 29 | 277 | 13 | 20 | 18 | 15 | 18 |
| Sugar: | | | | | | | | | | | |
| brown—1 Tbsp. | 14 | 50 | 2 | * | * | * | * | * | * | 1 | 3 |
| white, granulated—1 Tbsp. | 12 | 45 | 2 | * | * | * | * | * | * | * | * |
| Sunflower seeds, hulled—1/4 cup | 38 | 215 | 9 | 14 | 5 | * | 50 | 5 | 10 | 5 | 15 |
| Sweet potato, baked—1 | 146 | 205 | 8 | 5 | 237 | 54 | 9 | 6 | 5 | 6 | 7 |
| Tangerine—1 | 86 | 40 | 2 | 1 | 7 | 44 | 3 | 1 | 0 | 2 | 2 |
| Tomato: | | | | | | | | | | | |
| canned, juice—4 oz. | 122 | 25 | 1 | 2 | 20 | 33 | 4 | 2 | 5 | 1 | 6 |
| fresh—1 medium | 123 | 30 | 1 | 2 | 22 | 47 | 5 | 3 | 4 | 2 | 3 |
| Tuna, cannedin oil, drained—1/2 cup | 80 | 160 | 6 | 51 | 1 | * | 3 | 6 | 48 | 1 | 8 |
| Turkey: | | | | | | | | | | | |
| dark meat—3 oz. | 85 | 155 | 6 | 52 | * | * | 3 | 12 | 14 | 2 | 11 |
| white meat—3 oz. | 85 | 140 | 6 | 54 | * | * | 2 | 7 | 27 | 2 | 8 |
| Turnip greens, cooked—1/2 cup | 73 | 15 | * | 3 | 91 | 83 | 7 | 10 | 2 | 13 | 4 |
| Turnips, cooked—1/2 cup | 78 | 20 | * | 1 | * | 28 | 2 | 2 | 1 | 3 | 2 |
| Veal roast—3 oz. | 85 | 200 | 8 | 53 | * | * | 4 | 13 | 23 | 1 | 15 |
| Watermelon, fresh—1 piece | 426 | 140 | 6 | 5 | 50 | 70 | 30 | 8 | 4 | 3 | 4 |
| Yogurt: | | | | | | | | | | | |
| skim milk—1 cup | 227 | 125 | 5 | 29 | * | 3 | 6 | 31 | 1 | 45 | 1 |
| whole milk—1 cup | 227 | 140 | 6 | 18 | 6 | 2 | 3 | 19 | 1 | 28 | 1 |

[a]*Nutrients in Foods*. Leveille, G. A., Zabik, M. E., and Morgan, K. J. The Nutrition Guild, Cambridge, MA, 1983.

[b]Percent of 2,500 calories.

[c]For more precise information refer to package label of specific cereal.

*None or less than one percent.

Name ____________________ Chart E-1

# DIETARY CALCULATION CHART

| Name of Food and Amount Eaten | Calories | Protein (gms) | Vitamin A (IUs)*[1] | Vitamin C (mgs) | Thiamin (mgs) | Riboflavin (mgs) | Niacin (mgs) | Calcium (mgs) | Iron (mgs) |
|---|---|---|---|---|---|---|---|---|---|
| Milk-Cheese Group: | | | | | | | | | |
| Subtotal: | | | | | | | | | |
| Meat-Poultry-Fish-Beans Group: | | | | | | | | | |
| Subtotal: | | | | | | | | | |
| Fruit-Vegetable Group: | | | | | | | | | |
| Subtotal: | | | | | | | | | |

*IUs stands for International Units which are standard units of measurement. A similar measurement, Retinol Equivalent (RE), may replace IUs. To convert IUs to RE divide IUs by 5.

[1]To convert RDA for vitamin A to IU, multiply µgRE by 5.
To convert RDA for vitamin D to IU, multiply µg by 40.

Name ______________________________ Chart E-2

# DIETARY CALCULATION CHART

| Name of Food and Amount Eaten | Calories | Protein (gms) | Vitamin A (IUs)*[1] | Vitamin C (mgs) | Thiamin (mgs) | Riboflavin (mgs) | Niacin (mgs) | Calcium (mgs) | Iron (mgs) |
|---|---|---|---|---|---|---|---|---|---|
| Bread-Cereal Group: | | | | | | | | | |
| Subtotal: | | | | | | | | | |
| Fats-Sweets-Alcohol Group: | | | | | | | | | |
| Subtotal: | | | | | | | | | |
| Grand Total: | | | | | | | | | |
| Recommended Dietary Allowance: | | | | | | | | | |
| Difference (+ or − RDA) | | | | | | | | | |

*IUs stands for International Units which are standard units of measurement. A similar measurement, Retinol Equivalent (RE), may replace IUs. To convert IUs to RE divide IUs by 5.

[1]To convert RDA for vitamin A to IU, multiply μgRE by 5.
To convert RDA for vitamin D to IU, multiply μg by 40.

# HEIGHT/WEIGHT AND RECOMMENDED ENERGY INTAKE*

| Age and Sex Group | Weight | | Height | | Energy | |
|---|---|---|---|---|---|---|
| | kg. | lb. | cm. | in. | needs in calories | range in calories |
| infants | | | | | | |
| 0.0–0.5 year | 6 | 13 | 60 | 24 | kg. × 115 | 95– 145 |
| 0.5–1.0 year | 9 | 20 | 71 | 28 | kg. × 105 | 80– 135 |
| children | | | | | | |
| 1–3 years | 13 | 29 | 90 | 35 | 1,300 | 900–1,800 |
| 4–6 years | 20 | 44 | 112 | 44 | 1,700 | 1,300–2,300 |
| 7–10 years | 28 | 62 | 132 | 52 | 2,400 | 1,650–3,300 |
| males | | | | | | |
| 11–14 years | 45 | 99 | 157 | 62 | 2,700 | 2,000–3,700 |
| 15–18 years | 66 | 145 | 176 | 69 | 2,800 | 2,100–3,900 |
| 19–22 years | 70 | 154 | 177 | 70 | 2,900 | 2,500–3,300 |
| 23–50 years | 70 | 154 | 178 | 70 | 2,700 | 2,300–3,100 |
| 51–75 years | 70 | 154 | 178 | 70 | 2,400 | 2,000–2,800 |
| 76+ years | 70 | 154 | 178 | 70 | 2,050 | 1,650–2,450 |
| females | | | | | | |
| 11–14 years | 46 | 101 | 157 | 62 | 2,200 | 1,500–3,000 |
| 15–18 years | 55 | 120 | 163 | 64 | 2,100 | 1,200–3,000 |
| 19–22 years | 55 | 120 | 163 | 64 | 2,100 | 1,700–2,500 |
| 23–50 years | 55 | 120 | 163 | 64 | 2,000 | 1,600–2,400 |
| 51–75 years | 55 | 120 | 163 | 64 | 1,800 | 1,400–2,200 |
| 76+ years | 55 | 120 | 163 | 64 | 1,600 | 1,200–2,000 |
| pregnancy | | | | | +300 | |
| lactation | | | | | +500 | |

*Adapted from *Recommended Dietary Allowances,* 1980. Washington, D.C.: National Academy Press, with permission.

The data in this table have been assembled from the observed median heights and weights of children, together with desirable weights for adults for mean heights of men (70 inches) and women (64 inches) between the ages of eighteen and thirty-four years as surveyed in the U.S. population data (DHEW/NCHS).

Energy allowances for the young adults are for men and women doing light work. The allowances for the two older groups represent mean energy needs over these age spans, allowing for a 2% decrease in basal (resting) metabolic rate per decade and a reduction in activity of 200 calories per day for men and women between fifty-one and seventy-five years: 500 calories for men over seventy-five years; and 400 calories for women over seventy-five. The customary range of daily energy output is shown for adults in the range column and is based on a variation in energy needs of ±400 calories at any one age, emphasizing the wide range of energy intakes appropriate for any group of people.

Energy allowances for children through age eighteen are based on median energy intakes of children of these ages followed in longitudinal growth studies. Ranges are in the 10th and 90th percentiles of energy intake to indicate range of energy consumption among children of these ages.

# CALORIE EXPENDITURE BY ACTIVITY

**Directions:** This table shows the number of calories burned per pound of body weight. To calculate your energy expenditures, multiply the appropriate figure on the chart by your body weight in pounds. If you spent more or less time in any activity, you will need to adjust your calculations as shown in the example.

**EXAMPLE:**

You weigh 100 pounds and spend 30 minutes doing class work:

(0.3 calories/pound) × 100 pounds = 30 calories

Your friend weighs 100 pounds and spends 15 minutes doing class work:

(0.3 calories/pound ÷ 2) × 100 pounds = 15 calories

| Daily Activities | Calories Burned Per Pound* 30 min. | 60 min. |
|---|---|---|
| Brick Laying | 3.4 | 6.8 |
| Calisthenics | 1.0 | 2.0 |
| Car Repairs | 0.8 | 1.6 |
| Carpentry or Farm Chores | 0.8 | 1.6 |
| Chopping Wood | 1.4 | 2.8 |
| Class Work | 0.3 | 0.6 |
| Conversing | 0.4 | 0.8 |
| Dancing | 1.0 | 2.0 |
| Dressing or Showering | 0.6 | 1.2 |
| Driving | 0.6 | 1.2 |
| Eating | 0.3 | 0.6 |
| Gardening and Weeding | 1.2 | 2.4 |
| House Painting or Metal Working | 0.7 | 1.4 |
| Housework | 0.8 | 1.6 |
| Motorcycling | 0.7 | 1.4 |
| Mountain Climbing | 2.0 | 4.0 |
| Mowing Grass | 0.8 | 1.6 |
| Office Work | 0.6 | 1.2 |
| Personal Care | 0.9 | 1.8 |
| Pick and Shovel Work | 1.3 | 2.6 |
| Resting in Bed | 0.2 | 0.4 |
| Sawing Wood | 1.6 | 3.2 |
| Shoveling Snow | 1.5 | 3.0 |
| Sleeping | 0.2 | 0.4 |
| Standing–no activity | 0.3 | 0.6 |
| Standing–light activity | 0.5 | 1.0 |
| Walking (3 mph) | 1.0 | 2.0 |
| Walking–downstairs | 1.3 | 2.6 |
| Walking–upstairs | 3.4 | 6.8 |
| Watching TV | 0.2 | 0.4 |
| Working in Yard | 0.7 | 1.4 |
| Writing | 1.0 | 2.0 |

| Sports Activities | Calories Burned Per Pound* 30 min. | 60 min. |
|---|---|---|
| Archery | 1.0 | 2.0 |
| Badminton or Volleyball | 1.1 | 2.2 |
| Baseball | 1.0 | 2.0 |
| Basketball | 1.4 | 2.8 |
| Bicycling on level (10 mph) | 1.6 | 3.2 |
| Bowling | 1.3 | 2.6 |
| Canoeing | 1.4 | 2.8 |
| Fencing | 1.0 | 2.0 |
| Football | 1.7 | 3.4 |
| Golf | 1.1 | 2.2 |
| Handball | 1.9 | 3.8 |
| Horseback Riding | 1.4 | 2.8 |
| Ping Pong | 0.8 | 1.6 |
| Rowing | 1.0 | 2.0 |
| Running (6 mph) | 2.5 | 5.0 |
| Sailing | 0.6 | 1.2 |
| Skating | 2.0 | 4.0 |
| Skiing | 1.9 | 3.8 |
| Soccer | 1.8 | 3.6 |
| Squash | 2.1 | 4.2 |
| Swimming | 1.4 | 2.8 |
| Tennis | 1.9 | 3.8 |
| Water skiing | 1.5 | 3.0 |
| Wrestling, Judo, or Karate | 2.6 | 5.2 |

*Figures include calories spent for basal metabolism and digestion of food.

# References/Resources

## FOOD AND NUTRITION INFORMATION AND EDUCATION RESOURCES CENTER

What is FNIC?

FNIC is an information center that serves people who are interested in human nutrition, food service management, and food technology.

What does FNIC do?

The Center acquires and lends books, journal articles, and audiovisual materials that deal with foods and nutrition. The AV collection includes films, filmstrips, slides, audiocassettes, videocassettes, posters, charts, games, and transparencies. The Center's collection ranges from children's materials through professional resources.*

Who uses FNIC?

FNIC serves many kinds of users, including school administrators, food service managers, teachers, and nutritionists.

What is FNIC's lending policy?

- You may borrow an unlimited number of books for a period of one month.
- You may borrow up to three audiovisual items at a time, for a period of two weeks. (Do not order them more than one month ahead of the date on which they will be used.)
- There is no charge for any of the materials.

How do I reach the Center?

| | |
|---|---|
| Street Address: | 10301 Baltimore Boulevard<br>Beltsville, MD 20705 |
| Mailing Address: | FNIC<br>National Agricultural Library<br>Room 304<br>Beltsville, MD 20705 |
| Telephone: | (301) 344-3719 (24-hour telephone monitor) |
| Office Hours: | Monday-Friday 8:00 A.M. to 4:30 P.M. |

*Many of the references and resources in this kit are available through FNIC.

## FOOD COMPOSITION TABLES

Nutritive Value of Foods—*Home and Garden Bulletin #72.* U.S. Department of Agriculture. Superintendent of Documents, U.S. Government Printing Office, Washington, DC, 20402, 1981. $4.50.

*Food Values of Portions Commonly Used.* Pennington, J. A., and Church, H. N. Harper & Row, New York, 1984. $7.64.

"Nutritive Value of American Foods in Common Units" *Agricultural Handbook #456.* U.S. Department of Agriculture. Superintendent of Documents, U.S. Government Printing Office, Washington, DC, 20402, 1981. $8.50.

*Handbook of the Nutritional Content of Foods.* Watt, B. K., and Merrill, A. L. Dover Publications, Inc., New York, 1975. $5.50.

## RELIABLE SOURCES OF NUTRITION INFORMATION

American College of Nutrition (ACN)
100 Manhattan Ave. #1606
Union City, NJ 07087
(201) 866-3518

The American Dietetic Association (ADA)
430 North Michigan Ave.
Chicago, IL 60611
(312) 280-5000

The American Heart Association (AHA)
7320 Greenville Ave.
Dallas, TX 75231
(214) 750-5300

Center for Science in the Public Interest (CSPI)
1755 S. St., NW
Washington, DC 20009
(202) 332-9110

The Children's Foundation (CF)
1420 New York Ave., NW
Suite 800
Washington, DC 20005
(202) 347-3300

Community Nutrition Institute (CNI)
1146 10th St., NW
Washington, DC 20036
(202) 833-1730

Environmental Nutrition
52 Riverside Dr., 15th Floor
New York, NY 10024

Food and Drug Administration (FDA)
U.S. Dept. of Health and Human Services
5600 Fishers Lane
Rockville, MD 20857

Food and Nutrition Service (FNS)
U.S. Department of Agriculture
Washington, DC 20250

Food Research and Action Center (FRAC)
2011 I St., NW
Washington, DC 20006
(202) 452-8250

National Dairy Council (NDC)
6300 N. River Rd.
Rosemont, IL 60018
(312) 696-1020

National Nutrition Consortium (NNC)
24 Third St., NE, Suite 200
Washington, DC 20002
(202) 547-4819

The Nutrition Foundation
888 17th St., NW
Washington, DC 20006
(202) 872-0778

The Society for Nutrition Education (SNE)
1736 Franklin St.
Oakland, CA 94612
(415) 444-7133

## SOFTWARE*

**APPLE PIE**

- From DDA
- $229.95
- Apple II+, IIe (48K), DOS 3.3, Radio Shack TRS-80 Model III or IV, one disk drive.

This package includes the programs: YOU ARE WHAT YOU EAT!, JUMPING JACK FLASH!, GREASE, SALTY DOG, MUNCHIES, SWEET TOOTH, and FOOD FOR THOUGHT. Programs may be purchased separately. Descriptions and prices of each program follow.

**YOU ARE WHAT YOU EAT!**

- From DDA
- $79.95
- Apple II+, IIe (48K), DOS 3.3, Radio Shack TRS-80 Model III or IV, one disk drive; printer optional.

This program analyzes a meal or an entire day's diet and will produce a printout of the analysis. The analysis includes ideas for improving the diet or meal; total calorie, sodium, and cholesterol intake; and a bar graph which illustrates how close the diet comes to meeting the RDA for protein and 7 vitamins and minerals.

**JUMPING JACK FLASH!**

- From DDA
- $34.95, includes instruction booklet.
- Apple II+, IIe (48K), DOS 3.3, Radio Shack TRS-80 Model II/IV one disk drive; printer optional.

This program helps students to examine the number of calories they expend when working, playing, and resting. It can be used with YOU ARE WHAT YOU EAT! to teach energy balance and weight control concepts. Designed for junior and senior high students and the general public.

**GREASE**

- From DDA
- $27.95, includes instruction booklet, student worksheets.
- Apple II+, IIe (48K), DOS 3.3, Radio Shack TRS-80 Model III/IV, one disk drive.

This is a program about fat, cholesterol, and their association with heart disease. Students can determine the amount of fat in a meal or diet. They can also learn about fat in fast foods by ordering a meal from one of three fast-food restaurant chains. The amount of fat in a food is translated into an equivalent number of teaspoons. Designed for junior and senior high students and the general public.

**SALTY DOG**

- From DDA
- $27.95.
- Apple II+, IIe (48K), DOS 3.3, Radio Shack TRS-80 Model III/IV, one disk drive.

This program examines the role of sodium in the diet, including sodium's effect on blood pressure. Bar graphs are used to compare the amount of salt found in foods. Students can analyze a meal or a day's diet to determine its sodium content, and can learn to identify food having high levels of sodium by playing the computer game SODIUM SLEUTH.

**MUNCHIES**

- From DDA
- $34.95, includes instruction card.
- Apple II+, IIe (48K), DOS 3.3, Radio Shack TRS-80 Model III/IV, one disk drive.

This program is designed to help junior and senior high students make wiser snack choices. Students can examine the nutrient profile of a wide array of popular snacks and can compare the nutrient profiles of snacks.

**SWEET TOOTH**

- From DDA
- $27.95.
- Apple II+, IIe (48K), DOS 3.3, Radio Shack TRS-80 Model III or IV, one disk drive.

This program answers questions frequently asked about sugar. Students learn to recognize "hidden" sources of sugar by playing the computer game CUBE CITY. This game graphically illustrates the amount of sugar in food by comparing it to sugar cubes.

**FOOD FOR THOUGHT**

- From DDA
- $34.95, includes instruction card.
- Apple II+, IIe (48K), DOS 3.3, Radio Shack TRS-80 Model III/IV, one disk drive.

This program is a "test your I.Q." type game. There are seven categories of questions and two difficulty levels (novice and expert). A series of questions about the selected topic is asked. The computer indicates whether the correct answer was selected and then explains the answer. Designed for junior and senior high students and the general public.

**EAT SMART NUTRITION COMPUTER PROGRAM**

- 1981. From The Pillsbury Company, M/S 3286, Pillsbury Center, Minneapolis, MN 55402.
- $19.75, includes 5¼" diskette, 25-page teacher's manual, 30 copies of worksheets and pamphlets, 4 activity sheet masters.
- Apple II+, IIe, or III (48K), disk drive; monitor, printer (optional).

An economical, easy-to-use program for junior high and high school students as well as adults, this software analyzes an individual's diet for one day. The program was designed to create awareness of key nutrients in the diet and of ways to improve diets through individual food choices. A concise food worksheet enables users to code and input food items for analysis as percent Recommended Dietary Allowances (RDAs) for eight nutrients in six age/sex categories. Total sodium, cholesterol, and percent calories from fat are also listed in the analysis. The description of calories as percent RDA, both on-line and in the documentation, is somewhat confusing because total calories are listed rather than percentages. The program is easy to follow if the user's guide supplements the on-line instructions.

With a data base of 136 representative foods, the scope of the program is limited. Other foods can be coded by using a substitution list in the kit. Analysis includes three meals (up to 9 items each) and three snack periods. The program provides analysis of individual food items, three meals, and combined snacks, as well as the total intake. Dietary recommendations are generated in response to the levels of nutrients and calories in the analysis. Recommendations are generally accurate and seem appropriate for the intended audience.

Significant features of this kit are the worksheets and follow-up activities. Educationally sound, these activities seem interesting and likely to enhance learning.

Because it is capable of rapidly providing practical, accurate information at health fairs, the program has potential to arouse interest in nutrition. Used with the related activities, it could also involve users in improving their food habits.

(Reviewed by: Ruth McNabb Dow, Ph.D., R.D., Associate Professor, School of Home Economics, Eastern Illinois University, Charleston, IL 61920.)

**EATING MACHINE**

- Thorne, B. S., 1982. From Muse Software, 347 N. Charles St., Baltimore, MD 21201.
- $49.95, includes 5¼" diskette, 3-page instruction guide, 65-page user's manual.
- Apple II+ or IIe (48K), disk drive; monitor, printer (optional).

As you examine the "consequences" of the foods you choose in your diet by comparing a day's food selection with the RDA and U.S. Dietary Goals, you will find this program entertaining, as well as educational.

Viewing the display monitor, users choose a daily menu from 500 foods listed in 11 food categories. Standard serving sizes are offered for easy input. After the user selects the day's menu, the program provides feedback, including extensive graphics. Total calories, protein, vitamins A and C, calcium, iron and sodium intake are compared to the RDA using bar graphs, sound enhancement, and a smiling or frowning face. If the user's nutrient intake is within the RDA range, the computer displays a smile. If the intake is above the range in calories or sodium, a frown appears. A bar graph also illustrates the percentage of calories provided by protein, carbohydrates, fats, and alcohol.

A short instruction guide contains enough information to run the program; the user's manual provides additional instructions for altering the data base, analyzing a recipe, and storing personal files. Program weaknesses, although noted in the manual, relate more to a new user than to the program's design. Because the new user is unfamiliar with the way in which foods are listed in the 11 food categories, initially data entry will be time consuming.

Students and adults will find the program's graphics helpful in understanding the importance of proper food selection.

(Reviewed by: Pam Boyce, Program Leader, Family Living Education, Michigan State University, Cooperative Extension Service, 103 Human Ecology Building, East Lansing, MI 48824.)

**EATS**

- Byrd-Bredbenner, C., 1981. From Pennsylvania State University, Nutrition Education Center, University Park, PA. 16802.
- $75.00; includes 5½" diskette, 59-page user's guide, 7-page factsheet.
- Apple II+ or IIe (48K), disk drive; monitor, printer (optional).

This program is designed to help teens and adults become more aware of the composition and nutritional adequacy of their diets. The program quickly analyzes reported dietary intake for one day. It then prints total calories and sodium; percent of calories from protein, fat, and carbohydrate; and percent of the RDA for selected nutrients. For nutrients in short supply (less than ⅔ RDA), the program reports a few of their functions and sources. However, the printout does not include a listing of the foods entered, so it is not easy to check for errors in data entry.

Once the program is loaded, even the novice should be able to use it and make corrections with ease. The user's manual gives clear directions and conveniently arranges foods both alphabetically and by food group. Estimating portion size to enter may occasionally pose a problem, especially for those weak in the use of decimals. Because about 700 foods are coded and the sodium intake is reported to the nearest hundredth of a milligram, the user might wrongly assume that the results are highly accurate. In fact, the data base includes only 90 different food groups; items similar in nutrient content have been grouped together via the coding system. However, provided the users are told that the results are rough estimates, the output is sufficiently accurate for nutrition education purposes. The information presented in the printout and the fact sheet is basically sound, although not always easily understood by the lay person.

This program is likely to appeal to people who are curious about how their diet stacks up and what they might do to make it better. The program can be used independently, but having a nutritionist available to answer questions is recommended.

(Reviewed by: Carol West Suitor, M.S., R.D., Assistant Director of Education, Frances Stern Nutrition Center, New England Medical Center, 171 Harrison Ave., Boston, MA 02111.)

**FAST FOOD MICRO-GUIDE**

- Schrank, J., 1983. From The Learning Seed, 21250 N. Andover, Kildeer, IL 60047.
- $36.00, includes 5¼" diskette, 10-page user's guide.
- Apple II (48K), disk drive; TRS-80 Model III (48K), disk drive, monitor, printer (optional).

This program analyzes the nutrient content of meals eaten in nine fast-food restaurants. The nutritional analysis would interest anyone who eats at these restaurants on a regular basis, such as high school students or people who travel and frequent these establishments. The nutritional analysis is provided for each meal selected at the chosen restaurant and includes: total calories; percentage of calories from fat; grams of protein; percentages of the RDA for vitamins A and C, B vitamins (riboflavin, thiamin, niacin), calcium, and iron; and milligrams of sodium. The program also provides statements regarding the adequacy of the intake. An example of one of the statements is, "Your meal is good in vitamin B but is lacking in vitamin A, C. You can get additional vitamin A, C from carrots, eggs, dairy products and fresh vegetables, citrus fruits, tomatoes, potatoes, dark-green vegetables." Because the program does not specify which foods on the list provide a particular nutrient, individuals with limited nutrition knowledge may be misled.

The program meets its objective of analyzing the nutritional content of a meal consumed at a fast-food restaurant. Overall, the program is easy to use despite the lack of documentation. However, there is no capability to store the data or make corrections during data entry, which can be frustrating for the user. The analysis is rapid and offers the user immediate feedback. The appearance of the printout is monotonous with varying-length one-line statements, some with words hyphenated incorrectly. The analysis provided appears to be valid, and I recommend this program as a supplement to other more complete diet/nutrient analysis software.

(Reviewed by: Janet H. Gannon, M.S., R.D., Nutritionist/Project Manager, Capital Systems Group, Inc., 11301 Rockville Pike, Kensington, MD 20895.)

**GRAB A BYTE**

- 1983. From the National Dairy Council, 6300 N. River Road, Rosemont, IL 60018.
- $40, includes 5¼" diskette, 8-page instructor's guide, 8-page user's guide.
- Apple II+ (48K) or IIe (64K), DOS 3.3, disk drive; monitor, printer (optional).

Developed for use with seventh through ninth-grade students, GRAB-A-BYTE uses three programs in an educational game format to review and reinforce previously taught nutrition concepts. GRAB-A-GRAPE, the first program, begins with the student selecting four categories of questions from the following: fast foods, food facts, food and sport, food basics, weight control, and body building. The student picks the desired category and level of difficulty, and is provided an answer for which he or she must choose the correct question. Depending on its difficulty, each question is assigned a score of one to three points. Incorrect responses are fully explained, and correct ones reinforced. Styled after the popular TV quiz show "Jeopardy," this program impressed me as an innovative and effective way of teaching nutrition.

The second program, NUTRITION SLEUTH, invites the student to become "Inspector Good Diet," and try to solve four nutrition mysteries—each a case in which a teenager's diet is low in a certain nutrient. Similar to the game Hangman, the object is to spell the name of the deficient nutrient by guessing one letter at a time. Wrong guesses elicit up to three clues. Depending on how readily the mystery is solved, the program confers ratings of "Flatfoot," "Detective," or "Super Sleuth." I found this game enjoyable, but a bit too short—a few more mysteries would, I am sure, be well-received by teachers and students alike.

HAVE-A-BYTE, the final program allows students to construct a meal of up to eight foods that is analyzed for calories and eight nutrients. The program presents the analysis in terms of "percent of daily needs" for the appropriate age/sex group. If desired, the students can try to improve the meal's nutritional value by adding or deleting foods, or they can select an entirely different meal for comparison. If a printer is available, printouts of the calorie and nutrient profile of each meal further enhance the educational worth of this program. Unfortunately, the program does not provide the percent of calories from fat, protein, and carbohydrate. Additional teacher information to guide interpretation of the table of "percent of daily needs" would also have been valuable. However, neither of these omissions seriously detracts from the overall usefulness of this program.

An instructor's guide lists several "suggestions for success," and provides a helpful chart that identifies activities in *Food . . . Your Choice Level 4,* that teach the content covered in this set of three programs. Other Dairy Council resources are also identified. A user's guide provides detailed descriptions of each program and contains the 90-item food list that is used with HAVE-A-BYTE.

The three programs show how sound nutrition information and effective educational approaches can be brought together with the creative application of microcomputer technology to yield excellent results.

(Reviewed by: James Krebs-Smith, M.P.H., R.D., Instructor, Nutrition Program, The Pennsylvania State University, University Park, PA 16802.)

**NUTRITION SIMULATION**

- Anderson, C., and M. Johnson, 1983. From EMC Publishing, Changing Times Education Service, 300 York Avenue, St. Paul, MN 55101.
- \$55.00, includes 5¼″ diskette, 26-page teacher's guide; \$80.00, includes same items with back-up disk.
- Apple II+ or IIe (48K), DOS 3.3, disk drive; monitor.

This simulation provides an opportunity to practice the basic skills of meal management with nutritional and economic concerns in mind. In the first of the three parts of the program, the user goes on the shopping spree with a specific amount of money and a list of 95 foods to choose from. In the second section the user plans menus for three days. The third section provides the user with an evaluation of the food choices in terms of cost, calories, and nutritional quality.

The evaluation compares grocery expenses to a twenty-dollar daily limit. The program also compares the calculated calorie intake to a rough estimate of calorie needs based on values for ideal weight and activity level. The number of servings eaten from each of the Five Food Groups is compared to suggested intakes.

The simulation can be done for any or all seasons, with food prices varying accordingly. To make the program realistic, the developers have included "freebie" food sampling, special holiday needs, unexpected eating opportunities, and unplanned purchases. The price lists can be updated by the teacher.

Although the program does not discuss specific nutrients, it does stress the effects of the method of preparation on the caloric value of a food. Some basic information concerning the Five Food Groups is given at the beginning of the simulation; however, the teacher needs to further clarify the program's use. The accompanying guide should be read carefully and used to orient a user during the first time through the program. The short version takes about an hour for the novice user; the long version may take three or more hours to complete. The program allows the user to save work to continue at a later time. This simulation provides a thorough test of basic food purchasing and meal planning skills.

(Reviewed by: Joan A. Yuhas, Ph.D., R.D., Assistant Professor, School of Home Economics, Ohio University, Athens, OH 45701.)

**NUTRITION TUTORIAL**

- Anderson, C., 1983.From EMC Publishing, 300 York Ave., St. Paul, MN 55101.
- \$55, includes 5¼″ diskette, 12-page user's guide; \$80, includes same items with back-up disk.
- Apple II+ or IIe (48K), DOS 3.3, disk drive; monitor (color preferred).

The program objectives are to teach the basic food groups, recommended food group servings, definitions of nutrition terms, functions and sources of selected nutrients, relationship of calories to activity level, nutrition labeling, and menu planning considerations. In an interactive, user-friendly style, the program teaches very basic concepts at a level appropriate for junior high, high school, or adult audiences with limited previous exposure to nutrition. The use of color graphics and sound enhances the user's experience.

The menu-driven program allows the user to focus on specific program units: food groups, serving sizes, nutrients and calories, nutrition labeling, and menu planning. Within each unit, blocks of instructional material are followed by mastery exercises with varied response formats. The use of case studies and sample menus provides practical application of concepts and stimulates decision-making. Program analysis of user's food intake by food groups personalizes the program and may increase user interest. Documentation provides useful ideas for application and follow-up activities.

Units on food groups and serving sizes are the best developed. The program provides minimal information on selected nutrients and calories; and nutrition labeling and menu planning units are limited in scope. Some concepts such as "healthful" versus "not healthful" snacks and "high" versus "low" calorie foods need follow-up explanations to avoid possible misunderstandings. A noticeable inaccuracy is the statement that as people grow older, they need fewer servings from the dairy group.

The program's educational design is sound and stimulating, and the visual design is excellent. However, without content corrections or supplemental information a user might seriously misunderstand some of the program's messages.

(Reviewed by: Martha S. Brown, Ph.D., R.D., Associate Professor, School of Home Economics, Eastern Illinois University, Charleston, IL 61920.)

**NUTRITION VOLUME 1**

- 1982. From Minnesota Educational Computing Consortium, 3490 Lexington Ave., N., St. Paul, MN 55112.
- $37, includes 5¼″ disk, 53-page user's guide.
- Apple II+ or IIe (48K), disk drive; monitor.

This program provides a nutrient analysis of a one-day food intake. It draws on a data base of 598 foods that are coded before using the software. The analyzed information is compared with the 1980 RDA. Some of the program objectives are: (1) to list foods that are key sources of selected nutrients; (2) to determine whether eating patterns need to be changed; (3) to identify basic nutrients and their functions; (4) to classify foods according to the Four Food Groups; and (5) to develop acceptable criteria for food selection. The target audiences are high school students and adults.

The program analyzes the following nutrients: calories, protein, carbohydrate, fat, Vitamin A, Vitamin C, calcium, and iron. If an individual is low in a nutrient, the amount (in mg or IU) is displayed. The program indicates the additional amount of each nutrient needed to meet the RDA and provides a list of food sources of nutrients.

Users indicate serving size in terms of a reference serving size (e.g., 1.0, .5, 1.25, etc.). The program is easy to use because the food list is arranged alphabetically, and it utilizes a wide variety of common foods. It does not attempt to analyze fast foods, but it does list some snack foods by brand names.

The software package meets its stated objectives, both with the computer program as well as with the student materials included in the user's booklet. This program is designed for beginning nutrition students. Although limited in number, the nutrients analyzed are sufficient for students at this level.

The documentation is complete and includes introductory materials, lesson ideas, data base information, follow-up ideas for students, and instructions for using the Apple computer and printer. The documentation is complete, easy to read, appropriate for the audience, accurate, and well-done.

One of the program's unusual features is a listing of the five foods from the intake that provided the greatest number of calories. This program, by nutrition professionals, is well-done and should help free the beginning nutrition student from the struggle with lengthy computations.

(Reviewed by: Nancy Dillon, Owner, Strictly Software, 4321 N. 39th St., Phoenix, AZ 85018.)

**NUTRITION VOLUME 2**

- 1982. From Minnesota Educational Computing Consortium, 3490 Lexington Ave., N., St. Paul, MN 55112.
- $37.00, includes 5¼″ program diskette, 5¼″ back-up diskette (limited usage), 53-page support manual.
- Apple II+ or IIe (48K), disk drive; monitor.

Junior high and high school students as well as adults can use this two-program package as an effective aid for analyzing the composition of food intake in relation to their body processes and activities. "Lean" estimates and evaluates an individual's calorie intake and energy expenditure for 1–3 days. A limited statement of deficiencies is given for other nutrients. The program is designed to help individuals compare their weight with established weight ranges for age, sex, height, and body structure; and to set a weight goal. The program also analyzes the diet and activities to see whether the goals are being met. "Recipe" determines how specific foods meet caloric and nutrient needs of an individual. This program indicates how a food or foods meet the RDA for calories, protein, carbohydrate, fat, iron, calcium, riboflavin, thiamin, niacin, Vitamin A, and Vitamin C for individuals in various age and size groups.

The foods list is workable but somewhat limited (432 foods); it contains no fast-food or packaged items and few combination dishes. Although somewhat difficult for secondary students to understand without an explanation, the graphs of the nutrient totals are usuable once students comprehend what is being illustrated. The printed analysis is complete, but its format requires considerable paper, which can be costly.

A well-written support manual gives excellent background information, goals, sample runs, technical information, and seven useful student handouts. The strengths outweigh the weaknesses, and for the price the program is a good one.

(Reviewed by: Kathleen S. Willson, B.S., M.A., Instructor, Home and Family Life Education, Cascade Junior High, 610 Riverview Dr., N.E., Auburn, WA 98002.)

---

*Reviews from the *Journal of Nutrition Education* 16(2):80–110, 1984.

# REFERENCES/RESOURCES FOR UNITS 1–20

## UNIT 1—METABOLISM: CALORIES IN, CALORIES OUT

### Books

*Nutrition: An Inquiry into the Issues.* Long, P. and Shannon, B. Prentice-Hall, Inc., Englewood Cliffs, NJ 07632, 1983. $24.95.

*Nutrition Concepts and Controversies.* Hamilton, E. M. and Whitney, E. West Publishing Company, P.O. Box 64526, 50 W. Kellogg Blvd., St. Paul, MN 55164-0526, 1985. $20.95.

*Nutrition, Weight Control and Exercise.* Katch, F. I. and McArdle, W. D. Lea & Febiger, 600 S. Washington Square, Philadelphia, PA, 1983. $18.50.

### Booklets

"Calories & Weight: The USDA Pocket Guide." Superintendent of Documents, U.S. Government Printing Office, Washington, DC 20402, 1981. $3.75.

"Energy Balance Throughout the Life Cycle," *Diary Council Digest,* Volume 51, Number 4, National Dairy Council, 6300 N. River Road, Rosemont, IL 60018, 1980. Free.

"Food 2." The American Dietetic Association, P.O. Box 91403, Chicago, IL 60693, 1982. $5.00.

## UNIT 2—METABOLISM: BALANCING ENERGY INPUT AND ENERGY OUTPUT

### Books

*Introductory Nutrition.* Guthrie, H. A. The C. V. Mosby Company, St. Louis, MO, 1983. $23.95.

*Understanding Nutrition.* Whitney, E. N. and Hamilton, E. M. West Publishing Company, P.O. Box 64526, 50 W. Kellogg Blvd., St. Paul, MN 55164-0526, 1984. $24.95.

### Booklets

"Calories & Weight: The USDA Pocket Guide." Superintendent of Documents, U.S. Government Printing Office, Washington, DC 20402, 1981. $3.75.

"Your Calorie Catalog." National Dairy Council, 6300 N. River Road, Rosemont, IL 60018, 1983. $ .25.

### Audiovisual

*Energy—Our Food and Our Needs.* AV Resource Center, 8 Research Park, Cornell University, Ithaca, NY 14850, 1984. Set of 64 slides, illustrated script, study guide. $30.00. (rental $12.00).

## UNIT 3—HOW FOOD PATTERNS DEVELOP

### Books

*American Cooking.* Brown, D. *Food of the World,* Time-Life Series, Alexandria, VA, 1968. $16.95.

*American Cooking: Southern Style.* Walter, E. and the Editors of Time-Life Books. Time-Life Books, New York, NY, 1971. $19.95.

*Betty Crocker's International Cookbook.* General Mills, Random House, Inc., 400 Hahn Road, Westminster, MD 21157, 1980. $14.95.

*Fascinating Foods.* McDevitt, M. A. The Interstate Printers and Publishers, Inc., 19–27 N. Jackson Street, Danville, IL 61832-0549, 1979. Text $5.00; Teacher's Manual $7.50; Tests $3.50.

*Food and People.* Lowenberg, M., et al. John Wiley & Sons, New York, NY 10158, 1979. $30.95.

*Food and Your Future.* White, R. B. Prentice-Hall, Inc., Englewood Cliffs, NJ 07632, 1979. $21.28.

*Food for Today.* Kowtaluk, H. and Kopan, A. O. Chas A. Bennett Company, Inc., Peoria, IL, 1977. Text ed. $19.96; Student Guide $3.96.

*Food: Where Nutrition, Politics and Culture Meet—An Activities Guide for Teachers.* Katz, D. and Goodwin, M. T. Center for Science in the Public Interest, 1755 S Street, NW, Washington, DC 20009, 1976. $5.50.

*Slumps, Grunts and Snickerdoodles—What Colonial America Ate and Why.* Pearl, L. Houghton Mifflin, Two Park St., Boston, MA 02108, 1975. $8.95.

### Audiovisual

*Nutrition for Teenagers Only.* Pleasantville Media, Box 415, Pleasantville, NY 10570, 1984. 3 filmstrips, 3 cassettes, teacher's guide. $139.00.

## UNIT 4—ANALYZING YOUR FOOD INTAKE

### Books

*Food and People.* Lowenberg, M., et al. John Wiley & Sons, New York, NY, 1979. $30.95.

*Looking In: Exploring One's Personal Health Values.* Read, D. A. Prentice-Hall, Inc., Englewood Cliffs, NJ 07632, 1977. $13.95.

*Nutrition, Behavior and Change.* Gifft, H. H., Washban, M. B., and Harrison, G. G. Prentice-Hall, Inc., Englewood Cliffs, NJ 07632, 1972. $24.95.

### Booklets

"Research on the Effects of Television Advertising on Children, A Review of the Literature and Recommendations for Future Research." Adler, R. P., et al. National Science Foundation, 1800 G Street, NW, Rm. 537, Washington, DC 20550, 1978. Free.

### Audiovisuals.

*It's as Easy as Selling Candy to a Baby.* Mass Media Ministries, 2116 N. Charles St., Baltimore, MD 21218, 1977. Film, 16mm, color, sound, 11 minutes. $25.00 rental.

*Nutrition for Young People: You Are What You Eat.* Guidance Associates, Inc., Communications Park, Box 3000, Mount Kisco, NY 10549, 1983. 6 filmstrips, 6 tape cassettes, teacher's guide. $199.50.

*Seeing Through Commercials: A Children's Guide to TV Advertising.* Barr Films, Box 5667, Pasadena, CA 91107, 1976. Film, 16mm, color, 15 minutes. $300.00 (rental $30.00).

## UNIT 5—THE VEGETARIAN WAY OF LIFE

### Books

*Diet for a Small Planet.* Lappe, F. M. Ballantine Books, New York, NY, 1975. Spiral binding, $7.95; paper, $2.75.

*Going Vegetarian: A Guide for Teenagers.* Fretz, S. William Morrow & Co., New York, NY, 1983. $11.50.

*Laurel's Kitchen: A Handbook for Vegetarian Cookery and Nutrition.* Robertson, L., Flinders, C., and Godfrey, B. Bantam Books, New York, NY, 1978. $4.95.

*Moosewood Cookbook.* Katzen, M. Ten Speed Press, Berkeley, CA, 1977. $12.95.

### Booklets

"The Creative Eater's Handbook: Better Nutrition Through Vegetarian Eating." Pemberton, C. and Brown, M. Publications Dept., American Heart Association, Box 5157, Oakland, CA 94605, 1983. $1.00 (1–24 copies); $ .50 (24 or more copies).

"Vegetarianism." The Nutrition Education Center. The Pennsylvania State University, Benedict House, University Park, PA 16802, 1981. Single copy free.

"A Vegetarian's Guide." The Nutrition Education Center. The Pennsylvania State University, Benedict House, University Park, PA 16802, 1981. Single copy free.

### Audiovisuals

*Basic Food Groups Vegetarian.* Professional Health Media Services, Box 922, Loma Linda, CA 92354, 1981. Poster. $2.95.

*Diet for a Small Planet.* Bullfrog Films, Oley, PA 19547, 1973. Film, 16mm, color, 28 minutes, $425.00 (rental $45.00).

*Vegetarianism in a Nutshell.* Polished Apple, 3742 Seahorn Drive, Malibu, CA 90265, 1976. Filmstrip/audiocassette, 14 minutes. $49.75.

*The Vegetarian Unit.* Professional Health Media Services, Box 922, Loma Linda, CA 92354, 1981. Poster. $3.95.

## UNIT 6—NUTRITION FOR THE EXPECTANT MOTHER

### Books

*Living Nutrition.* Stare, F. J. and McWilliams, M. John Wiley & Sons, 605 Third Ave., New York, NY 10158, 1984. $23.95.

*Nutrition During the Life Cycle.* Alford, B. B. and Bogle, M. L. Prentice-Hall, Inc., Englewood Cliffs, NJ 07632, 1982. $27.95.

*Nutrition During Pregnancy and Lactation.* Worthington-Roberts, V. S., Vermeersch, J. and Williams, S. R. C. V. Mosby Company, St. Louis, MO, 1981. $15.95.

*Nutrition for Those with Special Needs: Lesson Plans and Handouts.* Distribution Center, 7 Research Park, Cornell University, Ithaca, NY 14850, 1982. $16.00.

*Pickles and Ice Cream: The Complete Guide to Nutrition During Pregnancy.* Hess, M. A. and Hunt, A. E. Dell Publishing Co., Inc., One Dag Hammarskjold Plaza, 245 E. 47th Street, New York, NY 10017, 1985. $6.95.

### Booklets

"Adolescent Pregnancy: Leaders Alert Bulletin #30." March of Dimes, 1275 Mamaroneck Ave., White Plains, NY 10605, 1979. Free.

"Food for the Teenager During and After Pregnancy." Superintendent of Documents, Government Printing Office, Washington, DC 20402, 1982. $4.50 each; $90.00/100.

"Food and You...Partners in Growth During Pregnancy." National Dairy Council, 6300 N. River Road, Rosemont, IL 60018, 1979. $ .25.

"Munch." Wisconsin Department of Health and Social Services, Document Sales Office, 202 S. Thornton Ave., Madison, WI 53702, 1977. Comic book. $1.00.

"Pregnant? Before You Drink, Think!" March of Dimes, 1275 Mamaroneck Ave., White Plains, NY 10605, 1979. Free.

"Pregnancy and Nutrition." NNECH, Society for Nutrition Education, 2140 Shattuck Ave., Suite 1110, Berkeley, CA 94704, 1975. $21.50.

"Working with Pregnant Teenagers: A Guide for Nutrition Educators." Superintendent of Documents, Government Printing Office, Washington, DC 20402, 1981. $2.00.

### Audiovisuals

*Be Good to Your Baby Before It's Born.* March of Dimes—local chapter, 1984. Set of 6 posters. Free.

EFNEP Audiocassette Programs: *#1—Before the Baby Is Born* (Weight Gain, Morning Sickness, Indigestion, Vitamins); *#2—Before the Baby Is Born* (Breast-feeding and Bottle-feeding); *#6—Before the Baby Is Born* (Nutrient Needs). Media Services Audio-Visual Resource Center, 8 Research Park, Cornell University, Ithaca, NY 14850, 1982. Audio programs on cassette tapes, scripts, supplementary handouts. $12.00 per program (specify program number and title).

*Great Expectations.* Society for Nutrition Education, 1736 Franklin St., Suite 900, Oakland, CA 94612, 1975. Film, 16mm, color. $370.00.

*Inside My Mom.* March of Dimes, Box 2000, White Plains, NY 10602, 1975. Filmstrip or slides, 75 frames, audiocassette, teaching guide, 8 minutes. $10.00 filmstrip; $15.00 slides (free rental from local chapter).

*Nutrition During Pregnancy.* Randell, J. S. and Olson, C. M. Distribution Center, 7 Research Park, Cornell University, Ithaca, NY 14850, 1981. Flipchart, $11.50; slides and cassette, $18.00.

*Prenatal Nutrition Wall Chart.* Vitamin Information Bureau, 664 N. Michigan Avenue, Chicago, IL 60611, 1976. $3.00.

### Other Sources of Information

March of Dimes, local chapter, for free booklets, posters, and other resources.

State Health Department, regional office, for free handouts, posters, and other resources.

## UNIT 7—NUTRITION FOR INFANTS AND CHILDREN

### Books

*Jane Brody's Nutrition Book.* Brody, J. Bantam Books, New York, NY, 1981. $7.95.

*Living Nutrition.* Stare, F. and McWilliams, M. John Wiley & Sons, 605 Third Ave., New York, NY 10158, 1984. $23.95.

*No-Nonsense Nutrition for Your Baby's First Year.* Heslin, J., Natow, A. B. and Raren, B. C. Van Nostrand Reinhold Co., VNR Order Processing, 7625 Empire Dr., Florence, KY 41042, 1978. $9.95.

*Nutrition During the Life Cycle.* Alford, B. B. and Bogle, M. L. Prentice-Hall, Inc., Englewood Cliffs, NJ 07632, 1982. $27.95.

*Nutrition in Infancy and Childhood.* Pipes, P. L. C. V. Mosby Company, 11830 Westline Industrial Dr., St. Louis, MO 63146, 1981. $13.95.

*Nutrition in Pregnancy and Lactation.* Worthington-Roberts, V. S. Vermeersch, J., and Williams, S. R. C. V. Mosby Company, St. Louis, MO, 1981. $15.95.

*The Womanly Art of Breastfeeding.* LaLeche League International. New American Library, 120 Woodbine St., Bergenfield, NJ 07621, 1983. $7.95.

### Booklets

"Nutrition for those with Special Needs: Lesson Plans and Handouts." Distribution Center, 7 Research Park, Cornell University, Ithaca, NY 14850, 1982. $6.00.

"What Shall I Feed My Baby: A Month-By-Month Guide." Superintendent of Documents, Government Printing Office, Washington, DC 20402, 1981. $4.25.

### Audiovisuals

EFNEP Audio Cassette Programs: *#3—Feeding 2- 3- 4-Year-Old Children and Starting Babies on Solid Food.* Media Services Audio-Visual Resource Center, 8 Research Park, Cornell University, Ithaca, NY 14850, 1982. Two audio programs on 1 cassette tape, scripts, supplementary handouts. $12.00 per program (specify number and titles).

*Feeding Your Baby.* Distribution Center, 7 Research Park, Cornell University, Ithaca, NY, 1977. Flipchart, $11.50. Slide set, $20.00.

*First Foods.* Society for Nutrition Education, 1736 Franklin St., Suite 900, Oakland, CA 94612, 1978. Film, 14 minutes.

*Food to Grow On: Nutrition from Newborn through Teens.* Tupperware Educational Services, P.O. Box 2353, Orlando, FL, 1977. Set of 3 filmstrips/audiocassettes, 12 minutes each $14.50. 16mm, $330; ¾″ videocassette, $305; rental, $35.00.

*Healthy Mother, Healthy Baby.* Alfred Higgins Productions, Inc., 9100 Sunset Blvd., Los Angeles, CA 90069, 1975. Film, 16 minutes. Purchase $320; rental $32.

## UNIT 8—NUTRITION FOR ADOLESCENTS, ADULTS, AND THE AGED

### Books

*Am I Obligated to Be Well-Nourished? An Instructional Module.* Byrd-Bredbenner, C. and Mayer, S. Home Economics Education Program, Division of Occupational and Vocational Studies. The Pennsylvania State University, University Park, PA 16802, 1981. $6.75.

*The Art of Starvation: A Story of Anorexia and Survival.* Macleod, S. Schocken Books, New York, NY, 1982. $12.95.

*The Golden Cage: The Enigma of Anorexia Nervosa.* Bruch, H. Random House, Inc., 1400 Hahn Road, New York, NY 10022, 1979. $3.95.

*The Health Robbers.* Barret, S. Charles Scribner's Sons, New York, NY, 1981. $13.95.

*Introductory Nutrition.* Guthrie, H. A. The C. V. Mosby Co., St. Louis, MO, 1983. $23.95.

*Jane Brody's Nutrition Book.* Brody, J. Bantam Books, New York, NY, 1981. $7.95.

*Living Nutrition.* Stare, F. and McWilliams, M. John Wiley & Sons, 605 Third Ave., New York, NY 10158, 1984. $23.95.

*Nutrition During the Life Cycle.* Alford, B. B. and Bogle, M. L. Prentice-Hall, Inc., Englewood Cliffs, NJ 07632, 1982. $27.95.

*Nutrition in Adolescence.* Mahan, L. K. and Rees, J. M. C. V. Mosby Company, Westline Industrial Dr., St. Louis, MO 63146, 1978. $22.95.

*The Psychology of Eating Disorders: A Lesson Plan for Grades 7–12.* National Anorexic Aid Society, Inc., 550 S. Cleveland Avenue, Suite F, Westerville, OH 43081, 1984. $95.00.

*Rating the Diets.* Berland, T. The New American Library, Inc., New York, NY, 1980. $3.95.

### Booklets

"Experts Weigh Reducing Potions." Superintendent of Documents, Government Printing Office, Washington, DC 20402, 1980.

"Fad Diet Frauds." The Nutrition Education Center. The Pennsylvania State University, Benedict House, University Park, PA 16802, 1981. Single copy free.

"Popular Diets: How They Rate." Los Angeles District—California Dietetic Association, P.O. Box 3506, Santa Monica, CA 90403, 1982. $4.75.

### Audiovisuals

*Dangerous Dieting: The Wrong Way to Lose Weight.* Pleasantville Media, Box 415, Pleasantville, NY 10570, 1984. 3 filmstrips, 3 cassettes, teacher's guide. $145.00.

*Fad Diet Circus.* Sterling Educational Films, 241 E. 34th Street, New York, NY, 1975. Film, 16mm, color, 15 minutes. $275.00.

*Food to Live On: Nutrition from the Twenties through the Nineties.* Tupperware Educational Services, Dept. EFC80, P.O. Box 2353, Orlando, FL 32802, 1978. Set of 3 filmstrips, audiocassettes, 13 minutes each. $19.95.

*Help Yourself to Better Health.* Society for Nutrition Education, 1736 Franklin St., Suite 900, Oakland, CA 94612, 1976. Film, 16mm, 16 minutes, $330.00, cassette (rental, $35.00).

*Rate the Diets.* Hoffman-LaRoche, Inc., 100 Delawanna Ave., Clifton, NJ 07014. Posters. Free.

### Other Sources of Information

Anorexia Nervosa and Related Eating Disorders, Inc., P.O. Box 5102, Eugene, OR 97405.

American Anorexia/Bulimia Association, Inc., 133 Cedar Lane, Teaneck, NJ 07666.

Consumer Communications Staff Food and Drug Administration, Rockville, MD 20852.

National Anorexic Aid Society, Inc., 550 S. Cleveland Ave., Suite F, Westerville, OH 43081.

National Association of Anorexia Nervosa and Associated Disorders, Box 271, Highland Park, IL 60035.

## UNIT 9—INTERPRETING INGREDIENT LABELS: NUTRITIVE FOOD ADDITIVES

## UNIT 10—INTERPRETING INGREDIENT LABELS: COSMETIC FOOD ADDITIVES

### Books

*The Changing American Diet.* Jacobson, M. F. and Brewster, L. Center for Science in the Public Interest, 1755 S Street, NW, Washington, DC 20009. $2.50.

*Eat Your Heart Out: How Food Profi:eers Victimize the Consumer.* Hightower, T. Random House, Inc., 400 Hahn Road, Westminster, MD 21157, 1976. $4.95.

*Eater's Digest.* Center for Science in the Public Interest, 1755 S Street, NW, Washington, DC 20009, 1982. $5.00.

*The Food Additives Book.* Gortner, W. A. and Freydberg, N. Bantam Books, Inc., 666 Fifth Ave., New York, NY, 10019, 1982. $9.95.

*Food Science and Nutrition: Current Issues & Answers.* Clydesdale, F. Prentice-Hall, Inc., Englewood Cliffs, NJ 07632, 1979. $22.95.

*Food: Where Nutrition, Politics and Culture Meet—An Activities Guide for Teachers.* Katz, D. and Goodwin M. T. Center for Science in the Public Interest, 1755 S Street, NW, Washington, DC 20009, 1976. $5.50.

*Processed Foods and the Consumer: Additives, Labeling, Standards & Nutrition.* University of Minnesota Press, 2037 University Ave., SE, Minneapolis, MN 55414, 1975. $8.95.

### Booklets

"More Than You Ever Thought You Would Know About Food Additives." Food and Drug Administration, Office of Consumer Affairs, HFE-88, 5600 Fishers Lane, Rockville, MD, 1982. Single copy free.

"Nutrition Labeling: Tools for Its Use." Superintendent of Documents, Government Printing Office, NW, Washington, DC 20402, 1975. $4.75.

### Audiovisuals

*Chemical Cuisine.* Center for Science in the Public Interest, 1755 S Street, NW, Washington, DC 20009, 1978. Poster $3.00.

*Eat, Drink and Be Wary.* Churchill Films, 662 N. Robertson Blvd., Los Angeles, CA 90069-9990, 1975. Film, 21 minutes, color, 16mm. $365.00.

*Eat Real Food/Avoid Artificial Coloring.* Center for Science in the Public Interest, 1755 S Street, NW, Washington, DC 20009, 1979. Poster. $3.00.

*Food Additives—Help or Hazard.* Macmillan, Inc. ATTN: Order Dept., Front and Brown Streets, Riverside, NJ 08075, 1982. Filmstrip, audiocassette, 12 minutes, wallchart. $68.00.

*Nutrition, Food and the Consumer—Group I & II.* Clearvue, Inc., 5711 N. Millwake Ave., Chicago, IL 60646. No date. Each group 4 filmstrips, 4 cassettes, teachers guide. $85.00, both groups $145.00.

*Read the Label, Set a Better Table.* Food and Drug Administration, 5600 Fishers Lane, Rockville, MD, 1976. Film, 16mm, 10 minutes. $130 purchase.

## UNIT 11—GETTING THE MOST FOR YOUR FOOD DOLLAR

### Books

*American Whole Foods Cuisine.* Goldbeck, N. and Goldbeck, D. New American Library, New York, NY, 1983. $8.95.

*Eat Your Heart Out: How Food Profiteers Victimize the Consumer.* Hightower, J. Random House, Inc., New York, NY, 1976. $4.95.

*Focus on Food.* Peck, L. B., Moragne, L., Sickler, M. S. and Washington, E. O. McGraw-Hill Book Co., Inc., New York, NY, 1974. $19.60.

*The Food Sleuth Handbook.* Friday, S. K. and Hurwitz, H. S. Atheneum Publishers, New York, NY, 1982.

*Keep It Simple.* Burrow, M. Simon & Schuster, Inc., New York, NY, 1982. $7.95.

*Laurel's Kitchen Bread Book: A Guide to Whole-Grain Breadmaking.* Robertson, L. Flinders, C. and Godfrey, B. Random House, Inc., New York, NY, 1984. $19.95.

*The Supermarket Handbook: Access to Whole Foods.* Goldbeck, N. and Goldbeck, D. The New American Library, New York, NY, 1974. $5.95.

### Audiovisuals

*Advanced Grocery Shopping.* The Learning Seed, 21250 N. Andover Road, Kildeer, IL 60047, 1983. 2 filmstrips, teacher reference, activity guide. $65.00.

*The Consumer and the Supermarket.* Barr Films, Box 5667, Pasadena, CA 91107, 1976. Film, 16mm, color, 15 minutes. $330.00 (rental $33.00).

*Eating On The Run.* Alfred Higgins Production, 9100 Sunset Boulevard, Los Angeles, CA 90069. Film, 16mm, color 15½ minutes. $305.00 (rental $31.00).

*Food Dollars and Sense.* Money Management Institute. Household Finance Corp., Prudential Plaza, Chicago, IL 60611, 1974. Filmstrip, audiocassette, 20 minutes. $4.50.

*Planning to Eat—A Guide to Saving Time, Money and Energy.* Tupperware Educational Services, Orlando, FL, 32802, 1977. Filmstrip, audiocassette, 13 minutes. $9.95.

*Winning the Grocery Game.* The Learning Seed, 21250 N. Andover Road, Kildeer, IL 60047, 1977. 2 filmstrips, activity guide, teacher reference. $64.00.

## UNIT 12—STORING FOODS TO PRESERVE NUTRIENTS

### Books

*The Berkeley Co-op Food Book.* Black, H. Bull Publishing Co., Palo Alto, CA, 1980. $7.95.

*Food and Your Well-Being.* Labuza, T. P. West Publishing Company, St. Paul, MN, 1977. Text, $17.95; instructor's manual and study guide, $9.50.

*Food for Today.* Kowtaluk, H. and Kopan, A. O. Charles A. Bennett Co., Inc. Peoria, IL, 1982. Text, $19.96; student guide, $3.96.

*Food. . . Your Choice: Home Economics Curriculum Level 4.* National Dairy Council, 6300 N. River Road, Rosemont, IL 60018, 1980. $45.00.

*Putting Food By.* Hertzberg, R., Vaughan, B. and Greene, J. The Stephen Greene Press, Brattleboro, VT, 1984 (paper $6.95).

### Booklet

"Conserving Nutrients in Fresh Fruits and Vegetables." Seelig, R. A. United Fresh Fruit and Vegetable Association, North Washington at Madison, Alexandria, VA 22314. No date. $.50.

### Audiovisuals

*Be Fair to Your Food.* Alfred Higgins Production, 9100 Sunset Boulevard, Los Angeles, CA 90069, 1982. Film, 16mm, color, 17 minutes. $310.00 (rental $31.00).

*Food Models.* National Dairy Council, 6300 N. River Road, Rosemont, IL 60018, 1974. $6.50 (small set); $9.00 (large set).

## UNIT 13—BUDGETING RESOURCES IN MEAL PLANNING

### Books

*Diet for a Small Planet.* Lappe, F. M. Ballantine Books, 201 E. 50th St., New York, NY 10022, 1982. $8.95.

*Energy, Food and You– An Interdisciplinary Curriculum Guide for Secondary Schools.* Washington State Environmental Education Office, 2000 NE Perkins Way, Seattle, WA, 98155-4033, 1977. $7.00.

*Food and Your Future*. White, R. B. Prentice-Hall, Inc., Englewood Cliffs, NJ 07632, 1979. $21.28.

*Meal Management Today*. Holmberg, R. Wadsworth Publishing Company, 10 Davis Drive, Belmont, CA 94002, 1983. $23.95.

*The Supermarket Handbook: Access to Whole Foods*. Goldbeck, N. and Goldbeck, D. The New American Library, New York, NY, 1974. $5.95.

### Booklets

"Conserving the Nutritive Value of Food." Government Printing Office, Superintendent of Documents, Washington, DC 20402, 1983. $2.25.

"Keys to Energy Efficiency (587-N)." Consumer Information Center, Pueblo, CO, 1984. Single copy free.

"Making Your Food Dollars Count." Superintendent of Documents, Government Printing Office, Washington, DC 20402, 1984. Set of 8 booklets. $2.00.

### Audiovisuals

*Buy Better*. Government Printing Office, Superintendent of Documents, Washington, DC 20402, 1984. Poster. $3.50.

*Chef Pennypincher's Shopping Guide*. Center for Science in the Public Interest, 1755 S Street, NW, Washington, DC 20009, 1980. Poster, $3.00.

*The Consumer and the Supermarket*. Barr Films, Box 5667, Pasadena, CA 91107, 1976. Film, 16mm, color, 15½ minutes. $330.00 (rental $33.00).

*Eat Better*. Government Printing Office, Superintendent of Documents, Washington, DC 20402, 1984. Poster. $3.50.

EFNEP Audio Cassette Programs: *#8—More from Your Money*. Media Services Audio-Visual Resource Center, 8 Research Park, Cornell University, Ithaca, NY 14850, 1982. Audio program on cassette, tape, script, supplementary handouts. $12.00.

*Food Dollars and Sense*. Money Management Institute. Household Finance Corp., Prudential Plaza, Chicago, IL 60601, 1974. Filmstrip, audiocassette, 20 minutes. $4.50.

*Planning to Eat—A Guide to Saving Time, Money and Energy*. Tupperware Educational Services, Orlando, FL, 32802, 1977. Filmstrip, audiocassette, 13 minutes. $9.95.

## UNIT 14—MENU PLANNING USING THE "DAILY FOOD GUIDE"

### Books

*American Wholefoods Cuisine*. Goldbeck, N. and Goldbeck, D. The New American Library, New York, NY, 1983. $8.95.

*Jane Brody's Nutrition Book*. Brody, J. Bantam Books, New York, NY, 1981. $7.95.

*Meal Management Today*. Holmburg, R. Wadsworth Publishing Co., 10 Davis Drive, Belmont, CA 94002, 1983. $23.95.

### Booklets

"Eating for Better Health." Superintendent of Documents, Government Printing Office, Washington, DC 20402, 1981. $3.50.

"Food—Home and Garden Bulletin #228. Superintendent of Documents, Government Printing Office, Washington, DC 20402, 1980. $6.00.

"Guide to Wise Food Choices." National Dairy Council, 6300 N. River Road, Rosemont, IL 60018, 1978. $ .35.

"Hassle-Free Guide to a Better Diet." Superintendent of Documents, Government Printing Office, Washington, DC 20402, 1980. $2.25 each; $15.00/100.

"Ideas for Better Eating: Menus and Recipes to Make Use of the Dietary Guidelines." Superintendent of Documents, Government Printing Office, Washington, DC 20402, 1981. $1.75.

### Audiovisual

*America Cannot Live by Junk Food Alone.* Tupperware Educational Services, P.O. Box 2353, Orlando, FL, 1979. Poster. $1.00.

## UNIT 15—MENU PLANNING FOR THE FAMILY

### Books

*The Family Health Cookbook.* White, A. and The Society for Nutrition Education. David McKay Co., New York, NY, 1980. $9.95.

*Food and Your Future.* White, R. B. Prentice-Hall, Inc., Englewood Cliffs, NJ 07632, 1979. $21.48.

*Keep It Simple.* Burros, M. Simon & Schuster, Inc., New York, NY, 1982. $7.95.

*Meal Management Today.* Holmberg, R. Wadsworth Publishing Company, 10 Davis Drive, Belmont, CA 94002, 1983. $23.95.

### Booklets

"Favorite American Recipes." Superintendent of Documents, Government Printing Office, Washington, DC 20402, 1974. $4.50.

"Food"—Home and Garden Bulletin #228. Superintendent of Documents, Government Printing Office, Washington, DC 20402, 1980. $6.00.

### Audiovisuals

*Advanced Grocery Shopping.* The Learning Seed, 21250 N. Andover Road, Kildeer, IL 60047, 1977. Two filmstrips, teacher reference activity guide. $65.00.

*Winning the Grocery Game.* The Learning Seed, 21250 N. Andover Road, Kildeer, IL 60047, 1977. Two filmstrips, activity guide, teacher reference. $64.00.

## UNIT 16—EVALUATING NUTRITION INFORMATION

### Books

*The Health Robbers.* Barrett, S. Charles Scribner's Sons, New York, NY, 1981. $13.95.

*Jane Brody's Nutrition Book.* Brody, J. Bantam Books, New York, NY, 1981. $7.95.

*The New Nuts Among the Berries.* Deutsch, R. Bull Publishing Co., New York, NY, 1977. $6.95.

*Nutrition Concepts and Controversies.* Hamilton, E. M. and Whitney, E. West Publishing Company, St. Paul, MN, 1985. $20.95.

### Booklets

"Books and Reference for School Teachers." The Nutrition Education Center. The Pennsylvania State University, Benedict House, University Park, PA 16802, 1981. $3.00.

"Preschool—Grade 12 Curriculum Recommended List." The Nutrition Education Center. The Pennsylvania State University, Benedict House, University Park, PA 16802, 1981. $5.00.

"Grades 7–12 Recommended Resource List: Audiovisuals." The Nutrition Education Center. The Pennsylvania State University, Benedict House, University Park, PA 16802, 1982. $3.00.

"Grades 7–12 Recommended Resource List: Print Materials." The Nutrition Education Center. The Pennsylvania State University, Benedict House, University Park, PA 16802, 1980. $3.00.

### Journals

*Environmental Nutrition.* Environmental Nutrition, 52 Riverside Drive, Suite 15-A, New York, NY 10024. $15.00/year.

*Nutrition and the M.D.* P. M. Inc., 14349 Victory Blvd., #204, Van Nuys, CA 91401. $36.00/year.

## UNIT 17—DIET AND DISEASE: OBESITY

### Books

*Food and Your Well-Being.* Labuza, T. P. West Publishing Company, P.O. Box 64526, 50 W. Kellogg Blvd., St. Paul, MN 55164-0526, 1977. Text $17.95; instructor's manual and study guide $7.50.

*Introductory Nutrition.* Guthrie, H. A. The C. V. Mosby Company, St. Louis, MO, 1983. $23.95.

*Nutrition, Weight Control and Exercise.* Katch, F. I. and McArdle, W. D. Lea & Febiger, Philadelphia, PA, 1983. $18.50.

*Thin from Within.* Osman, J. and Van, F. J Review and Herald Pub., 55 W. Oak Ridge Dr. Hagerstown, MA 21740, 1981. $6.95.

### Booklets

"Diet." Superintendent of Documents, Government Printing Office, Washington, DC 20402, 1981. $2.25.

"Food 2." American Dietetic Association, P.O. Box 91403, Chicago, IL 60693, 1982. $5.00.

"Food and Your Weight." Superintendent of Documents, Government Printing Office, Washington, DC 20402, 1977. $4.50.

"Obesity." Christakis, G. and Plumb, R. The Nutrition Foundation, 888 Seventeenth Street NW, Washington, DC 20006, 1966. Single copy free/additional copies, $ .25 each.

### Audiovisuals

*Exer-Guide: Health Benefits of Exercise.* Center for Science in the Public Interest, 1755 S Street, NW, Washington, DC 20009, 1981. Poster. $3.00.

*Food$ense—Reducing Diets.* Audiovisual Services, Special Services Building, The Pennsylvania State University, University Park, PA 16802, 1976. Videocassette, color, 8 minutes. $75.00 (rental $10.50).

*Good Loser: The Weight Control Game.* NASCO, 901 Jonesville Ave., Fort Atkinson, WI 53538. $17.50.

*Losing Weight with a Little Help from Your Friends.* Visual Media, 246 George Hart Hall, University of California, Davis, CA 95616, 1977. Slides with audiocassette. $41.25 (I)/$33.28 (II) (rental $7 per use).

## UNIT 18—DIET AND DISEASE: WORLD HEALTH PROBLEMS

### Books

*Diet for a Small Planet.* Lappe, F. M. Ballantine Books, 201 E. 50th St., New York, NY 10022, 1982. $8.95.

*The Feeding Web: Issues in Nutritional Ecology.* Gussow, J. D. Bull Publishing Company, Box 208, Palo Alto, CA, 1978. $14.95 (paper $11.95).

*Food, Energy, and Society.* Pimentel, D. and Pimentel, M. John Wiley & Sons, 605 Third Ave., New York, NY 10158, 1979. $16.95.

*Food: Where Nutrition, Politics and Culture Meet—An Activities Guide for Teachers.* Katz, D. and Goodwin, M. T. Center for Science in the Public Interest, 1755 S Street, NW, Washington, DC 20009, 1976.

*Introductory Nutrition.* Guthrie, H. A. The C. V. Mosby Company, St. Louis, MO, 1983. $23.95.

*Keep Earth Clean, Blue and Green: Environmental Activities for Young People.* Hennings, G. and Hennings, D. G. Citation Press, P.O. Box 7502, 2931 E. McCarty Street, Jefferson City, MO 65102.

## Booklets

"Hunger Awareness Dinner." Herald Press, 717 Walnut Ave., Scottsdale, PA 15683. $1.45.

"World Food Aid Needs and Availabilities, 1984." Superintendent of Documents, Government Printing Office, Washington, DC 20402, 1984. $5.50.

## Audiovisuals

*Beyond the Next Harvest.* Mass Media Ministries, 2116 N. Charles Street, Baltimore, MD 21218, 1978. Film, 16mm, 28 minutes, color. $300.00 (rental $25.00).

*Cross-World Food Puzzle.* Oxfam-America, 151 Broadway, Boston, MA 02116, 1985. Poster. $1.50.

*Ending Hunger; It's Possible; It's Happening.* American Friends Service Committee, 1979. Kit includes text, simulation game, case studies, issue study paper. $5.50.

*Toast.* Bullfrog Films, Inc. Oley, PA 19547, 1977. Film, 16mm, 12 minutes, color. $275.00 (rental, $30.00.)

# UNIT 19—DIETARY GUIDELINES FOR AMERICANS

## Books

*Nutrition Concepts and Controversies.* Hamilton, E. M. and Whitney, E. N. West Publishing Company, P.O. Box 64526, 50 W. Kellogg Blvd., St. Paul, MN 55164-0526, 1985. $20.95.

*Toward Healthful Diets.* National Academy Press, 2101 Constitution Avenue, NW, Washington, DC 20418, 1981. $8.50.

## Booklets

"Building a Better Diet." Superintendent of Documents, Government Printing Office, Washington, DC 20402, 1979. $28.00/100.

"Ideas for Better Eating: Menus and Recipes to Make Use of the Dietary Guidelines." Superintendent of Documents, Government Printing Office, Washington, DC 20402, 1981. $2.25.

"Nutrition and Your Health: Dietary Guidelines for Americans." Superintendent of Documents, Government Printing Office, Washington, DC 20402, 1981. $2.25 each; $27.00/100.

## Audiovisuals

*Eat Whole Grains.* Center for Science in the Public Interest, 1755 S Street, NW, Washington, DC 20009, 1982. Poster. $3.00.

*Even a Strong Body Can Be Diseased.* From: "Food for Health" Poster Set. Center for Science in the Public Interest, 1755 S Street, NW, Washington, DC 20009, 1979. $8.00 for set of 4 posters.

*Kernel of Wheat.* The Kansas Wheat Commission, 2630 Claflin, Manhattan, KS 66502. 1 poster, 50 handouts, free.

*Newtrition 7.* The Polished Apple, 3742 Scahorn Drive, Malibu, CA 90265, 1981. Filmstrip, audiocassette, 11 minutes. $49.75.

*Understanding the Dietary Guidelines Workshop Kit.* The Nutrition Education Center. The Pennsylvania State University, Benedict House, University Park, PA 16802. 56 color slides, audiocassette, handouts. $50.00 (15.00 rental).

# UNIT 20—DESIGNING A NATIONAL NUTRITION POLICY

## Books

*Am I Obligated to Be Well-Nourished? An Instructional Module.* Byrd-Bredbenner, C. and Mayer, S. Home Economics Education Program, Division of Occupational and Vocational Studies. The Pennsylvania State University, University Park, PA 16802, 1981. $6.75.

*Food and Your Well-Being*. Labuza, T. P. West Publishing Company, St. Paul, MN, 1977. Text $17.95; Instructor's Manual and Study Guide $9.50.

*The Great American Nutrition Hassle*. Hofmann, L. Mayfield Publishing Company, 285 Hamilton Ave., Palo Alto, CA 94301, 1978. $12.95.

*Introductory Nutrition*. Guthrie, H. A. The C. V. Mosby Company, St. Louis, MO, 1983. $23.95.

*The New Nuts Among the Berries*. Deutsch, R. Bull Publishing Company, New York, NY, 1977. $6.95.

*Nutrition in the Community: The Art of Delivering Services*. Frankle, Reva, T., and Owen, A. The C. V. Mosby Company, St. Louis, MO 63146, 1978. $22.95.

## Booklet

"Ideas for Better Eating: Menus and Recipes to Make Use of the Dietary Guidelines." Superintendent of Documents, Government Printing Office, Washington, DC 20402, 1981. $3.25.

## Journal

*Food and Nutrition: A Quarterly Periodical Exploring Food Assistance Programs and Issues*. Superintendent of Documents, Government Printing Office, Washington, DC 20402. $11.00 yearly.

# Answer Keys

## UNIT 1: METABOLISM: CALORIES IN, CALORIES OUT

SHEET 1-1:

(Answers will vary, depending on the weight of the cheese puffs and amount of water used.)

SHEETS 1-2 through 1-5:

1.

| Activity | Time Spent in Activity | Calories per Pound |
|---|---|---|
| Sleeping | 9 hours | 3.6 |
| Personal care (total) | 1/2 hour | 0.9 |
| Dressing | 15 minutes | 0.3 |
| Packing up and unpacking sleeping bags (like housework) | 15 minutes | 0.4 |
| Swimming | 1 hour, 45 minutes | 4.9 |
| Eating breakfast | 1/2 hour | 0.3 |
| Eating lunch | 1/2 hour | 0.3 |
| Eating snacks | 15 minutes | 0.15 |
| Eating dinner | 1 hour | 0.6 |
| Preparation and cleanup for meals (like housework) | 1 hour | 1.6 |
| Writing in daily diary | 15 minutes | 0.5 |
| Walking (3 mph) | 4 hours | 8.0 |
| Mountain climbing | 1 hour | 4.0 |
| Setting up camp (like housework) | 1 hour | 1.6 |
| Conversing | 2 hours | 1.6 |
| Standing (no activity) for a rest | 45 minutes | 0.45 |
| TOTAL | 24 hours | 29.20 |

2. Total calorie Output = 29.20 calories per pound × 100 pounds = 2,920 calories

3.

| | Food | Amount | Calories |
|---|---|---|---|
| Breakfast: | cereal, ready-to-eat | 1 ounce | 110 |
| | grape juice | 4 ounces | 85 |
| | orange | 1 | 65 |
| | bread, whole wheat (toasted) | 1 slice | 55 |
| | butter | 1/2 tablespoon | 50 |
| | egg, scrambled with butter | 1 | 95 |
| Lunch: | sandwich: bread, whole wheat | 2 slices | 110 |
| | peanut butter | 2 tablespoons | 180 |
| | chocolate chip cookies | 2 | 120 |
| | apricots, dried | 1/2 cup | 170 |
| | milk, nonfat dry | 1/3 cup powder & water | 80 |
| Snack: | apple | 1 | 80 |
| Dinner: | tuna casserole: | | |
| | tuna, canned | 1/2 cup | 160 |
| | noodles, enriched | 1 cup | 200 |
| | peas, canned | 1/2 cup | 60 |
| | carrots, raw | 1 whole | 35 |
| | milk, nonfat dry | 1/3 cup powder & water | 80 |
| | doughnut, cake | 1 | 165 |
| Snack: | popcorn (prepopped in hot air) with salt | 3 cups | 135 |

4. 2,035 calories
5. Calorie Input = 2,035
   Calorie Output = 2,920
6. Calorie input is less than calorie output. The difference is 885 calories.
7. Lose weight.
8. Increase calorie input by eating more. (Could also decrease calorie output, but this would not be practical.) Students may also give ideas about what foods could be added. For example, the afternoon snack could be increased by adding peanuts, raisins, and a glass of nonfat dry milk.
9. Carrying canned food may be too heavy. Fresh food such as eggs and butter may spoil. There is not enough milk as indicated by the "Daily Food Guide." One or two more cups of milk are needed.

QUIZ SHEET 1-1:

1. a
2. b
3. b
4. Accept any answer that includes an accurate definition of "calorie," that refers to foods as the sources of calories, and that refers to BMR, digestion and absorption, and physical activity as the uses of calories.

## UNIT 2: METABOLISM: BALANCING ENERGY INPUT AND ENERGY OUTPUT

SHEET 2-4:

**Case #1**

a. 1,375 calories
b. 40%
c. 550 calories
d. 9%
e. 50 calories
f. 600 calories
g. 198 calories
h. 2,173 calories

SHEET 2-5:

**Case #2**

a. 1,693 calories
b. 13%
c. 1,473 calories
d. 7%
e. 3.4°F
f. 351 calories
g. 1,824 calories
h. sedentary
i. 365 calories
j. 219 calories
k. 2,408 calories

SHEET 2-6:

**Case #3**

a. 50 years
b. 30 years
c. 3 decades
d. 1,764 calories
e. sedentary
f. 353 calories
g. 212 calories
h. 2,329 calories

QUIZ SHEET 2-1:

1. b
2. b
3. d
4. a
5. a
6. c

## UNIT 3: HOW FOOD PATTERNS DEVELOP

SHEET 3-2:

The following guide lists nutrients found in each food and includes the food group to which it belongs. Food groups are designated as follows: I = fruit/vegetable group; II = bread/cereal group; III = milk/cheese group; IV = meat/poultry/fish/beans group; V = fats/sweets/alcohol group.

SET 1

**Mexican Taco:**
taco shell—carbohydrate, protein, B vitamins, iron (II)
tomatoes—carbohydrate, vitamins A and C (I)
lettuce—carbohydrate, vitamins A and C (I)
cheese—calcium, riboflavin, protein, vitamins A, $B_6$, $B_{12}$, D (III)

**Southern Spoon Bread:**
cornmeal bread—carbohydrate, protein, B vitamins, iron (II)

**New England Clam Chowder:**
clams—protein, B vitamins, iron, phosphorus, unsaturated fats (IV)
potatoes—carbohydrate, vitamins A and C (I)
soup broth—protein, calcium, iron, phosphorus, B vitamins, Vitamin A (IV) or (I)

**Pennsylvania Dutch Scrapple:**
pork—protein, B vitamins, iron, phosphorus, saturated fats (IV)
cornmeal—carbohydrate, protein, B vitamins, iron (II)

SET 2

**Chili con Carne:**
hamburger—protein, B vitamins, iron, phosphorus, saturated fats (IV)
kidney beans—protein, B vitamins, iron, phosphorus (IV)
onions—carbohydrate, vitamins A and C (I)
tomato sauce—carbohydrate, vitamins A and C (I)

**Quiche Lorraine:**
pie shell—carbohydrate, protein, B vitamins, iron (II)
custard/egg mixture—protein, iron, phosphorus, calcium, riboflavin, Vitamin A, B vitamins, saturated fats (IV) or (III)
onions—carbohydrate, vitamins A and C (I)
cheese—calcium, riboflavin, protein, vitamins A, $B_6$, $B_{12}$, D (III)
bacon—protein, B vitamins, iron, phosphorus, saturated fats (IV)

**Cheese Ravioli:**
pasta squares—carbohydrate, protein, B vitamins, iron (II)
cheese—calcium, riboflavin, protein, vitamins A, $B_6$, $B_{12}$, D (III)
tomato sauce—carbohydrate, vitamins A and C (I)

**Irish Stew:**
lamb—protein, B vitamins, iron, phosphorus, saturated fats (IV)
potatoes—carbohydrate, Vitamin C (I)
onions—carbohydrate, Vitamin C (I)
carrots—carbohydrates, Vitamin A (I)

SET 3

**Beef Stroganoff:**
beef—protein, B vitamins, iron, phosphorus, saturated fats (IV)
mushrooms—carbohydrate (I)
onions—carbohydrate, Vitamin C (I)
sour cream—calcium, riboflavin, protein, vitamins A, $B_6$, $B_{12}$, D (III)
noodles—carbohydrate, protein, B vitamins, iron (II)

**Shrimp Egg Rolls:**
egg roll shell—carbohydrate, protein, B vitamins, iron (II)
shrimp—protein, B vitamins, iron, phosphorus, unsaturated fats (IV)
vegetables—carbohydrates, vitamins A and C, folacin, iron, magnesium, calcium (I)

**Curried Chicken:**
chicken—protein, B vitamins, iron, phosphorus, saturated fats (IV)
cream sauce—calcium, riboflavin, protein, vitamins A, $B_6$, $B_{12}$, D (III)
rice—carbohydrate, protein, B vitamins, iron (II)

**Beans with Rice:**
kidney beans—protein, B vitamins, iron, phosphorus (IV)
rice—carbohydrate, protein, B vitamins, iron (II)

SET 4

**Macaroni and Cheese:**
macaroni—carbohydrate, protein, B vitamins, iron (II)
cheese and milk sauce—calcium, riboflavin, protein, vitamins A, $B_6$, $B_{12}$, D (III)

**Bean Tostadas:**
beans—protein, B vitamins, iron, phosphorus (IV)
cornmeal tortilla—carbohydrate, protein, B vitamins, iron (II)
tomatoes—carbohydrate, vitamins A and C (I)
cheese—calcium, riboflavin, protein, vitamins A, $B_6$, $B_{12}$, D (III)

**Candied Yams:**
yams—carbohydrate, vitamins A and C (I)
brown sugar/butter sauce—carbohydrate, saturated fat (V)

**Carrot and Raisin Salad:**
carrots—carbohydrate, Vitamin A (I)
raisins—carbohydrate, iron (I)
salad dressing—saturated fat, Vitamin E (V)

SHEET 3-3:

| Factors: | Psychological | Social/family |
|---|---|---|
| | Cultural | Life style |
| | Geographic | Individual preference |
| | Religious | Nutritional |

(Examples will vary; students should supply examples that support the information provided in the "Teacher's Unit Introduction" for Unit 3.)

## UNIT 4: ANALYZING YOUR FOOD INTAKE

QUIZ SHEET 4-1:

1. Internal factors; external factors
2. Examples should be chosen from internal factors (such as blood glucose levels, fat cell size or number, brain messages) and external factors (such as the taste of food, food availability, time of day, social gatherings, sight and smell of food, food as an emotional outlet).
3. Any three of the following are acceptable answers: underweight, overweight, susceptibility to infection, decreased life expectancy, kidney problems, heart disease, gall bladder disease, increased blood pressure, diabetes, and arthritis.

## UNIT 5: THE VEGETARIAN WAY OF LIFE

SHEET 5-3:

1. False
2. Seventh-Day Adventists
3. Diet / Foods:

| | | | |
|---|---|---|---|
| Diet: | vegan | Foods: | only foods of plant origins |
| Diet: | lacto vegetarian | Foods: | foods of plant origins plus milk and milk products |
| Diet: | ovolacto vegetarian | Foods: | foods of plant origins plus milk, milk products, and eggs |

4. False
5. True
6. Meat-Poultry-Fish-Beans group

7. Beans-Nuts-Eggs group with the Bread-Cereal group
8. Calcium, Vitamin D, Vitamin $B_{12}$, iron

SHEET 5-5:

The following are sample answers. There are hundreds of possible answers.

| | |
|---|---|
| seeds + legumes | = hummous (chickpeas plus sesame seed butter)<br>lentil/sesame loaf<br>bread with seeds and soy flour |
| legumes + grains | = whole-grain bread made with soy flour<br>rice and lentil casserole<br>vegetarian chili (rice and kidney beans) |
| grains + milk/milk products | = sandwich and glass of milk<br>cheese sandwich<br>cheesey bulgur casserole |

QUIZ SHEET 5-1:

1. b
2. d
3. b
4. Answers will vary, but the menu should include all servings described on Sheet 5-4, "Vegetarian's Daily Food Guide."
5. Answers will vary depending on choices in question 4.

## UNIT 6: NUTRITION FOR THE EXPECTANT MOTHER

SHEET 6-5:

Answers can be justified on a positive basis (largest number of servings from four food groups is the best diet), or they can be justified on a negative basis (largest number of fats-sweets-alcohol is the poorest diet).

| BREAKFAST A | B | C |
|---|---|---|
| 1 bread-cereal<br>1/2 milk-cheese<br>1 fats-sweets-alcohol<br>2 | 1 fruit-vegetable<br>2 milk-cheese<br>1 bread-cereal<br>1 | 2 fats-sweets-alcohol<br>3 |
| **LUNCH A** | **B** | **C** |
| 2 fruit-vegetable<br>1 meat-poultry-fish-beans<br>1 bread-cereal<br>1 milk-cheese<br>1 | 2 fruit-vegetable<br>1 milk-cheese<br>1 fats-sweets-alcohol<br>2 | 1 meat-poultry-fish-beans<br>2 fats-sweets-alcohol<br>3 fats-sweets-alcohol<br>3 |
| **DINNER A** | **B** | **C** |
| 1/2 meat-poultry-fish-beans*<br>1 bread-cereal<br>1/2 milk-cheese<br>3 fats-sweets-alcohol<br>4 fats-sweets-alcohol<br>3 | 1 meat-poultry-fish-beans<br>2 fruit-vegetable<br>1 bread-cereal<br>1 milk-cheese<br>1 fats-sweets-alcohol<br>1 | 1 meat-poultry-fish-beans<br>1 fruit-vegetable<br>1 bread-cereal<br>2 fats-sweets-alcohol<br>2 |
| **SNACK A** | **B** | **C** |
| 2 fruit-vegetable<br>1/2 bread-cereal<br>1 milk cheese<br>1 | 2 fats-sweets-alcohol<br>3 | 1 fats-sweets-alcohol<br>1/2 fruit-vegetable<br>2 |

*Hot dogs have less protein and more fat than fresh meats.

SHEETS 6-6 through 6-7:

Diet B contains generally better food choices than Diet A. In Diet B the totals for each nutrient exceed the totals in Diet A. Although total calories are greater in Diet B, the total does not exceed the recommended number of calories during pregnancy. In addition to a comparison of nutrient content, it is notable that Diet A contains significant amounts of fats, sweets, alcohol, and caffeine, whereas Diet B does not.

**MENU A:**

| | Calories | Iron (mg.) | Calcium (mg.) | Protein (gm.) | Vitamin A (IUs) | Vitamin C (gm.) |
|---|---|---|---|---|---|---|
| BREAKFAST | | | | | | |
| 1 cup black coffee | 5 | 0.2 | T | 0 | 0 | 0 |
| 1 slice white toast | 70 | 0.6 | 21 | 2 | T | T |
| 1 Tbsp. peanut butter | 90 | 0.3 | 9 | 4 | 0 | 0 |
| MIDMORNING | | | | | | |
| 3 chocolate chip cookies | 180 | 0.6 | 12 | * | T | 0 |
| LUNCH | | | | | | |
| 2 slices cheese pizza | 280 | 2.0 | 178 | 10 | 502 | 6 |
| 1 glass (3½ oz.) red wine | 90 | 0.4 | 9 | * | 0 | 0 |
| MIDAFTERNOON | | | | | | |
| 28 potato chips | 320 | 1.0 | 22 | 4 | 0 | 8 |
| 1 12-oz. beer | 150 | T | 18 | 1 | 0 | 0 |
| DINNER | | | | | | |
| 1 alcoholic cocktail | 165 | – | – | – | – | – |
| 1/2 chicken breast | 195 | 1.0 | 10 | 29 | 100 | 0 |
| 1/2 cup corn, canned | 70 | 0.4 | 4 | 3 | 290 | 3 |
| EVENING | | | | | | |
| 1 12-oz beer | 150 | T | 18 | 1 | 0 | 0 |
| 1 cup popcorn, plain | 45 | 0.2 | 1 | * | 2 | 0 |
| TOTAL | 1,810 | 6.7 | 302 | 54 | 894 | 17 |

**MENU B:**

| | Calories | Iron (mg.) | Calcium (mg.) | Protein (gm.) | Vitamin A (IUs) | Vitamin C (gm.) |
|---|---|---|---|---|---|---|
| BREAKFAST | | | | | | |
| ½ cup oatmeal | 67 | 1.2 | 10 | 3 | 0 | 0 |
| 1 orange | 65 | 0.5 | 54 | 1 | 260 | 65 |
| 1 cup skim milk | 85 | 0.1 | 300 | 8 | 500 | 2 |
| 1 slice whole wheat toast | 55 | 0.5 | 23 | 3 | T | T |
| MIDMORNING | | | | | | |
| ½ cup grapes | 55 | 0.3 | 10 | * | 80 | 3 |
| 1/2 cup tapioca | 150 | 1.2 | 77 | 2 | 19 | 1 |
| LUNCH | | | | | | |
| 2 Tbsp. peanut butter | 180 | 0.6 | 18 | 8 | 0 | 0 |
| 2 slices whole wheat bread | 110 | 1.0 | 46 | 6 | T | T |
| 1 cup skim milk | 85 | 0.1 | 300 | 8 | 500 | 2 |
| 1 plum | 20 | 0.1 | 3 | * | 85 | 1 |

| | Calories | Iron (mg.) | Calcium (mg.) | Protein (gm.) | Vitamin A (IUs) | Vitamin C (gm.) |
|---|---|---|---|---|---|---|
| MIDAFTERNOON | | | | | | |
| 1-oz. slice, American cheese | 95 | 0.2 | 163 | 6 | 260 | 0 |
| 1 apple | 80 | 0.1 | 10 | * | 125 | 6 |
| DINNER | | | | | | |
| 1 pork chop | 330 | 3.3 | 11 | 26 | 0 | 0 |
| 1/2 cup broccoli | 20 | 0.6 | 68 | 2 | 1,937 | 70 |
| 1/2 cup french fries | 150 | 0.7 | 8 | 2 | T | 12 |
| 1 cup skim milk | 85 | 0.1 | 300 | 8 | 500 | 2 |
| 1 slice pumpkin pie | 290 | 1.2 | 106 | 6 | 2,467 | 3 |
| EVENING | | | | | | |
| 1 medium carrot | 35 | 0.6 | 30 | 1 | 8,910 | 6 |
| 1 package (1/4 cup) raisins | 125 | 0.9 | 23 | 1 | 7 | T |
| TOTAL | 2.082 | 13.3 | 1,560 | 91 | 15,650 | 173 |

SHEET 6-9

1. F Irritability, reduced attention span, restlessness, and hyperactivity are behavioral problems commonly identified in FAS.
2. F Growth deficiencies are evident at birth in infants with FAS.
3. T Mental deficiency symptoms of FAS may appear as a lower IQ score and may indicate learning difficulties or mental retardation.
4. F Alcohol in the mother's bloodstream passes on to the fetal blood without being diluted. The fetus's blood has the same alcohol content as the mother's blood because the fetus's own liver is too underdeveloped to break down the alcohol.
5. T Because alcohol travels in the blood, the alcohol contacts all body cells. However, the brain and nerve cells are the most affected by alcohol, and their reduced ability to function influences muscular control, judgment, and the senses.
6. F The risk of full FAS is greatest when alcohol consumption occurs during the first three months of pregnancy. The brain and central nervous system are developed early in fetal growth. This is evident when observing the appearance of a fetus in the early months of growth. The head and spinal cord are very prominent in early development.
7. F Definite limits of safe alcohol intake have not been determined. Presently, complete abstention from alcohol appears to be the safest route.
8. T See comments from #7.
9. F Some of the birth defects that have been identified as being characteristic of FAS may be caused by many other factors unrelated to alcohol consumption during pregnancy.
10. T See comments from #7. There may be critical periods of fetal development when a single exposure to alcohol has a detrimental effect. Many experts feel that a one-time binge at a critical developmental period may cause as much harm as daily moderate alcohol consumption.
11. F Approximately one in every twenty women of child-bearing age is alcoholic. These numbers have not been decreasing so there is a real concern about FAS affecting infants.
12. F Pure alcohol contains 7 calories per gram. Compare that to other energy-containing substances: protein—4 calories/gram; carbohydrate—4 calories/gram; and fat—9 calories/gram.

QUIZ SHEET 6-1:

1. a
2. d
3. c
4. Spinach, milk, carrots, whole-grain breads, and cheese are some examples of nutrient-dense foods. These foods have both significant levels of certain nutrients and also a fairly low number of calories. By consuming this type of food, a pregnant woman can obtain the nutrients she needs without consuming unnecessary calories.
5. c
6. Some doctors say that a definite risk occurs at about six average drinks per day. Others have shown that only two drinks per day consumed by the pregnant woman can cause her baby to be more irritable and restless. Babies of mothers who drink large amounts of alcohol may show signs of alcohol addiction at birth. Since we do not know the exact amount of alcohol that will harm a fetus, it is important to curtail the use of alcohol during pregnancy to no more than two drinks on any given day. FAS can be avoided by abstaining from alcohol while pregnant.
7. b

## UNIT 7: NUTRITION FOR INFANTS AND CHILDREN

SHEET 7-6:

1. breast milk, formula
2. bottle, breast
3. *Any of these:* designed for baby's special nutritional needs; protection from infections; always available and safe; can be less expensive; fewer allergies.
4. *Any of these:* other people cannot feed the baby; some women may feel embarrassed to breast-feed; some women are unwilling or physically unable to breast-feed.
5. *Any of these:* allows other people to feed the baby; allows mother to do other things.
6. *Any of these:* formula can be expensive; bottles and equipment must be sterilized and formula must be pre-

pared; the need for a safe, clean water supply; cow's milk in formula sometimes causes allergies; does not contain protection from allergies.

7. bottle-feeding
8. breast-feeding
9. cereal, fruits and vegetables, meats, finger foods, table foods
10. water, sugar, starch, fat, or other "fillers"; calories, nutrients
11. overcooking, long-term storage
12. love, rest, and good nutrition

SHEET 7-7:

1. (Selections of foods from the pocketboard.) Kim's diet should include all of the recommended number of servings from each of the food groups on Sheet 7-8. However, cheese, yogurt, and other milk products should be substituted for fluid milk.
2. (Selections of foods from the pocketboard.) Angela's lunch menus should ideally include one serving from each of the four food groups. However, a serving from the Meat-Poultry-Fish-Beans group does not have to be included if a serving from the Milk-Cheese group is included.

QUIZ SHEET 7-1:

1.

| **Age Range** | **Foods** |
|---|---|
| 6–8 months | strained meats |
| 4–6 months | cereals |
| 10–12 months | table foods |
| 4 –6 months | fruits, vegetables, and juices |
| 8–10 months | finger foods |

2. Answers will vary. Make sure the menu reflects the recommended number of servings.
3. b
4. a

## UNIT 8: NUTRITION FOR ADOLESCENTS, ADULTS, AND THE AGED

QUIZ SHEET 8-1:

1. d
2. b
3. Answers will vary. Accept any complete, well-written answers that support the viewpoints.
4. b
5. a

## UNIT 9: INTERPRETING INGREDIENT LABELS: NUTRITIVE FOOD ADDITIVES

SHEETS 9-6 through 9-7:

1. Preservative, nutritive, cosmetic, quality-giving
2. Cosmetic
3. Probably. If bread has to be shipped a long distance and stored for a length of time, it is probably necessary to add a preservative food additive like calcium propionate.
4. No. Bread will remain free of mold for about six days after baking if it is kept at room temperature.
5. Yes.
6. Bread that is enriched has more thiamin (4:2), riboflavin (3:2), niacin (3:2), and iron (4:2) than unenriched bread.
7. No. The reason you enrich a food is to put back nutrients lost during processing. Since you are not using the whole wheat kernel, you are not losing anything.
8. The levels of thiamin and niacin are the same for enriched and whole wheat bread. (Riboflavin and iron are lower than the values for enriched bread, but this is because more riboflavin and iron are added back in the enrichment process than was originally present.)
9. Chocolate, vanilla, caramel, or butterscotch flavors. Adding fruit such as bananas or strawberries will change the flavor of the milkshake.
10. *Answer depends on flavoring used:* Flavors are used mainly to make foods more appealing, not to change or improve the nutritional value of the food. Some flavors may increase the calories of the milkshake (chocolate sauce, caramel, or butterscotch). Sugar can also be considered a flavoring. Obviously, adding sugar will increase a food's calories. If foods such as fruit are added, the nutritional value will be increased.
11. People have different tastes. What is appealing to one person may not be appealing to another.
12. With food coloring or fruit juices such as raspberry.
13. *Answer depends on coloring used:* No, if food coloring is used. Yes, if fruit juice is added. Colors are used mainly to make foods more appealing, not to change or improve the nutritional value of the food. Like flavorings, some colors may increase the calories of the food. If colors from real food are added, this will tend to increase the nutritional value of the food.
14. If you like the new color of the shake.
15. Perhaps; different colors appeal to different people.
16. No
17. Those that increase the appeal of food (cosmetic additives).

SHEET 9-9:
**Name** Hardly Fortified Helen

# CHART E
# DIETARY CALCULATION CHART

| Name of Food and Amount Eaten | Calories | Pro (g) | Vit A (IU)* | Vit C (mg) | Thiamin (mg) | Riboflavin (mg) | Niacin (mg) | Calcium (mg) | Iron (mg) | Vit D (IUs)** |
|---|---|---|---|---|---|---|---|---|---|---|
| MILK-CHEESE GROUP | | | | | | | | | | |
| Milk, skim, 1 cup | 85 | 8 | 500 | 2 | 0.1 | 0.3 | 0.2 | 301 | 0.1 | 100 |
| Milk, skim, 1 cup | 85 | 8 | 500 | 2 | 0.1 | 0.3 | 0.2 | 301 | 0.1 | 100 |
| Milk, skim, 1 cup | 85 | 8 | 500 | 2 | 0.1 | 0.3 | 0.2 | 301 | 0.1 | 100 |
| SUBTOTAL | 255 | 24 | 1,500 | 6 | 0.3 | 0.9 | 0.6 | 903 | 0.3 | 300 |
| MEAT-POULTRY-FISH-BEANS GROUP | | | | | | | | | | |
| Peanut butter, 2 tbsp. | 175 | 8 | 0 | 0 | T | T | 4.8 | 18 | 0.6 | 0 |
| Peanuts, 1/4 cup | 210 | 9 | T | 0 | 0.1 | 0.1 | 6.2 | 27 | 0.8 | 0 |
| Chicken breast, 1/2 | 245 | 32 | 100 | 0 | 0.1 | 0.2 | 12.4 | 20 | 1.3 | – |
| SUBTOTAL | 630 | 49 | 100 | 0 | 0.2 | 0.3 | 23.4 | 65 | 2.7 | 0 |
| FRUIT-VEGETABLE GROUP | | | | | | | | | | |
| Banana, 1 | 100 | 1 | 226 | 12 | 0.1 | 0.1 | 0.8 | 4 | 0.1 | 0 |
| Raisins, 1/4 cup | 105 | 1 | 7 | T | T | T | 0.2 | 22 | 1.3 | 0 |
| Tossed salad, 1 cup | 30 | 2 | 2,279 | 26 | 0.1 | 0.1 | 0.7 | 48 | 1.1 | 0 |
| Potato, baked, 1 | 145 | 4 | T | 31 | 0.2 | 0.1 | 2.6 | 14 | 1.1 | 0 |
| SUBTOTAL | 380 | 8 | 2,512 | 69 | 0.4 | 0.3 | 4.3 | 88 | 3.6 | 0 |
| BREAD-CEREAL GROUP | | | | | | | | | | |
| Oatmeal, cooked, 1 cup | 135 | 5 | 0 | 0 | 0.2 | T | 0.1 | 22 | 1.4 | 0 |
| Bread, whole wheat, 2 slices | 110 | 5 | T | T | 0.1 | 0.1 | 1.2 | 44 | 1.0 | T |
| Bread, whole wheat, 2 slices | 110 | 5 | T | T | 0.1 | 0.1 | 1.2 | 44 | 1.0 | T |
| SUBTOTAL | 355 | 15 | 0 | 0 | 0.4 | 0.2 | 2.5 | 110 | 3.4 | 0 |

*To convert RDA for vitamin A to IUs, multiply μgRE by 5.
**To convert RDA for vitamin D to IUs, multiply μg by 40.

SHEET 9-9, *continued:*
**Name** Hardly Fortified Helen

## CHART E
## DIETARY CALCULATION CHART

| Name of Food and Amount Eaten | Calories | Pro (g) | Vit A (IUs)* | Vit C (mg) | Thiamin (mg) | Riboflavin (mg) | Niacin (mg) | Calcium (mg) | Iron (mg) | Vit D (IUs)** |
|---|---|---|---|---|---|---|---|---|---|---|
| FATS-SWEETS ALCOHOL GROUP | | | | | | | | | | |
| Margarine, 2 tsp. | 70 | * | 314 | 0 | T | T | 0.0 | 1 | 0.0 | – |
| Jelly, 1 tbsp. | 55 | 0 | 2 | 1 | T | T | T | 4 | 0.3 | 0 |
| Chocolate chip cookies, 2 | 120 | 1 | 6 | 0 | T | T | 0.2 | 8 | 0.4 | 6 |
| Gingerbread cake, 1 piece | 275 | 3 | 28 | 2 | 0.1 | 0.1 | 1.0 | 134 | 4.1 | 2 |
| Salad dressing, 1 tbsp. | 70 | * | T | 0 | T | T | T | 1 | 0.1 | – |
| Margarine, 2 tsp. | 70 | * | 314 | 0 | T | T | 0.0 | 1 | 0.0 | – |
| SUBTOTAL | 660 | 4 | 664 | 3 | 0.1 | 0.1 | 1.2 | 149 | 4.9 | 8 |
| GRAND TOTAL | 2,280 | 100 | 4,776 | 78 | 1.4 | 1.8 | 32 | 1,315 | 14.9 | 308 |
| Recommended Dietary Allowance | 2,100 | 46 | 4,000 | 60 | 1.1 | 1.3 | 14 | 1,200 | 18 | 400 |
| %RDA | 109% | 217% | 119% | 130% | 127% | 138% | 229% | 110% | 83% | 77% |

**Name** Fortified Frances

| Name of Food and Amount Eaten | Calories | Pro (g) | Vit A (IUs)* | Vit C (mg) | Thiamin (mg) | Riboflavin (mg) | Niacin (mg) | Calcium (mg) | Iron (mg) | Vit D (IU)** |
|---|---|---|---|---|---|---|---|---|---|---|
| MILK-CHEESE GROUP | | | | | | | | | | |
| Milk, skim, 1 cup | 85 | 8 | 500 | 2 | 0.1 | 0.3 | 0.2 | 301 | 0.1 | 100 |
| SUBTOTAL | 85 | 8 | 500 | 2 | 0.1 | 0.3 | 0.2 | 301 | 0.1 | 100 |
| MEAT-POULTRY-FISH-BEANS GROUP | | | | | | | | | | |
| Luncheon meat, 2 slices | 100 | 4 | T | 4 | 0.1 | T | 0.8 | 3 | 0.3 | 17 |
| Chicken breast, 1/2 | 245 | 32 | 100 | 0 | 0.1 | 0.2 | 12.4 | 20 | 1.3 | – |
| SUBTOTAL | 345 | 36 | 100 | 4 | 0.2 | 0.2 | 13.2 | 23 | 1.6 | 17 |

*To convert RDA for vitamin A to IUs, multiply µgRE by 5.
**To convert RDA for vitamin D to IUs, multiply µg by 40.

SHEET 9-9, *continued:*
**Name** Fortified Frances

## CHART E
## DIETARY CALCULATION CHART

| Name of Food and Amount Eaten | Calories | Pro (g) | Vit A (IUs)* | Vit C (mg) | Thiamin (mg) | Riboflavin (mg) | Niacin (mg) | Calcium (mg) | Iron (mg) | Vit D (IUs)** |
|---|---|---|---|---|---|---|---|---|---|---|
| FRUIT-VEGETABLE GROUP | | | | | | | | | | |
| Potato, baked, 1 | 145 | 4 | T | 31 | 0.2 | 0.1 | 2.6 | 14 | 1.1 | 0 |
| Tossed salad, 1 cup | 30 | 2 | 2,279 | 26 | 0.1 | 0.1 | 0.7 | 48 | 1.1 | 0 |
| SUBTOTAL | 175 | 6 | 2,279 | 57 | 0.3 | 0.2 | 3.3 | 62 | 2.2 | 0 |
| BREAD-CEREAL GROUP | | | | | | | | | | |
| Fortified cereal, 1 oz. | 110 | 2 | 5,000 | 60 | 1.5 | 1.7 | 20 | 40 | 18 | 400 |
| Bread, enriched white, 2 slices | 140 | 4 | T | T | 0.1 | 0.1 | 1.2 | 42 | 1.2 | T |
| SUBTOTAL | 250 | 6 | 5,000 | 60 | 1.6 | 1.8 | 21.2 | 82 | 19.2 | 400 |
| FATS-SWEETS-ALCOHOL GROUP | | | | | | | | | | |
| Pop-Tart, frosted, 1 | 220 | 3 | – | 7 | 0.3 | 0.3 | 2.5 | 25 | 2.5 | – |
| Fortified fruit drink, 8 oz. | 120 | 0 | 1,974 | 118 | 0.0 | 0.0 | 0.0 | 64 | T | 0 |
| Mayonnaise, 2 tbsp. | 200 | * | 78 | – | 0.0 | 0.0 | T | 6 | T | – |
| Fortified fruit drink, 8 oz. | 120 | 0 | 1,974 | 118 | 0.0 | 0.0 | 0.0 | 64 | T | 0 |
| Chocolate chip cookies, 2 | 120 | 1 | 6 | 0 | T | T | 0.2 | 8 | 0.4 | 6 |
| Fortified breakfast bar, 1 | 190 | 6 | 625 | 8 | 0.2 | 0.2 | 2.5 | 125 | 2.2 | 5 |
| Margarine, 2 tsp. | 70 | * | 314 | 0 | T | T | 0.0 | 1 | 0.0 | – |
| Salad dressing, 1 tbsp. | 70 | * | T | 0 | T | T | T | 1 | 0.1 | – |
| SUBTOTAL | 1,110 | 10 | 4,971 | 251 | 0.5 | 0.5 | 5.2 | 294 | 5.2 | 11 |
| GRAND TOTAL | 1,965 | 66 | 12,850 | 374 | 2.7 | 3.0 | 43.1 | 762 | 28.3 | 528 |
| Recommended Dietary Allowance (RDA) | 2,100 | 46 | 4,000 | 60 | 1.1 | 1.3 | 14.0 | 1,200 | 18.0 | 400 |
| %RDA | 94% | 143% | 321% | 623% | 245% | 231% | 308% | 64% | 157% | 132% |

*To convert RDA for vitamin A to IUs, multiply μgRE by 5.
**To convert RDA for vitamin D to IUs, multiply μg by 40.

QUIZ SHEET 9-1:

| | |
|---|---|
| 1. d | 7. a |
| 2. b | 8. c |
| 3. c | 9. b |
| 4. a | 10. b |
| 5. b | 11. d |
| 6. a | |

## UNIT 10: INTERPRETING INGREDIENT LABELS: COSMETIC FOOD ADDITIVES

SHEET 10-2:

Reaction #1: fruity
Reaction #2: banana

SHEET 10-3:

Reaction #1: bright red
Reaction #2: purplish brown

SHEETS 10-4 through 10-5:

Technically, there are no right or wrong answers to these worksheets. Students have the right to their own opinions about which foods they would like to eat. If their choices are substantiated with logical reasons, the students should be commended. However, the goal of this unit is to encourage students to select foods without cosmetic additives. Therefore, the following answers would be desirable.

1. a. Because choice (b) contains artificial colors and flavors. The additives listed in choice (a) are nutritive additives.
2. a. Because choice (b) contains artificial color.
3. b. Because choice (a) contains artificial coloring and flavoring. The natural flavorings in choice (b) are preferable because they contain components of real foods rather than their synthetic counterparts. Natural flavorings may add to the nutritive value of the food.
4. a. Because choice (b) contains bleaching agents which are cosmetic food additives used to add to consumer appeal. In addition, choice (a) contains, as its first ingredient, whole wheat flour, making it a more nutritious choice.
5. a. Because choice (b) contains artificial color, a cosmetic additive; whereas choice (a) uses carob powder, caramel, and paprika extract for coloring.

QUIZ SHEET 10-1:

| | |
|---|---|
| 1. b | 4. b |
| 2. d | 5. a |
| 3. d | 6. c |

## UNIT 11: GETTING THE MOST FOR YOUR FOOD DOLLAR

SHEET 11-2: **Protein**

| Food Source | Cost / Purchase Unit (1) | Amount Protein / Food Composition Unit (2) | Amount Protein / Purchase Unit (3) | Portion of Purchased Unit Consumed to Receive 1/2 U.S. RDA of Protein (4) | Cost of ½ U.S. RDA Protein (5) | Rank (6) |
|---|---|---|---|---|---|---|
| Bacon, fried crisp (low-quality) | $1.79/20 slices | 5 gm./2 slices | 50 gms./20 slices | .65 | $1.16 | 8 |
| Beef, regular ground, broiled (high-quality) | $1.69/lb. | 21 gm./3 oz. | 112 gms./lb. | .20 | $ .34 | 4 |
| Swiss cheese (high-quality) | $2.89/lb. | 8 gm./1 oz. | 128 gms./lb. | .18 | $ .52 | 6 |
| Milk, whole (high-quality) | $2.07/gal. | 9 gm./8 oz. | 144 gms./gal. | .16 | $ .33 | 3 |
| Tuna, light, oil-packed (high-quality) | $1.15/6½ oz. | 24 gm./3 oz. | 52 gms./6½ oz. | .43 | $ .49 | 5 |
| Liver, beef, fried (high-quality) | $ .99/lb. | 15 gm./2 oz. | 120 gms./lb. | .19 | $ .19 | 1 |
| Oatmeal, quick oats (low-quality) | $ .65/18 oz. | 5 gm./2.5 oz. | 36 gms./18 oz. | .90 | $ .59 | 7 |
| Eggs, Grade A, large (high-quality) | $ .99/doz. | 6 gm./1 egg | 72 gms./doz. | .31 | $ .31 | 2 |

SHEET 11-3: **Iron**

| Food Source | Cost / Purchase Unit [1] | Amount Iron / Food Composition Unit [2] | Amount Iron / Purchase Unit [3] | Portion of Purchased Unit Consumed to Receive 1/2 U.S. RDA of Iron [4] | Cost of 1/2 U.S. RDA Iron [5] | Rank [6] |
|---|---|---|---|---|---|---|
| Liver, beef, fried | $ .99/lb. | 5 mg./2 oz. | 40 mg./lb. | .23 | $ .23 | 2 |
| Beef, regular ground, broiled | $1.69/lb. | 2.7 mg./3 oz. | 14.4 mg./lb. | .63 | $1.06 | 8 |
| Peas, canned | $ .44/lb. | 4.2 mg./6 oz. | 11.2 mg./lb. | .80 | $ .35 | 3 |
| White bread, enriched | $ .79/22 slices | .7 mg./slice | 15.4 mg./22 slices | .58 | $ .46 | 5 |
| Corn flakes | $ .83/12 oz. | 1.8 mg./oz. | 21.6 mg./12 oz. | .42 | $ .35 | 4 |
| Graham crackers, 2½″ squares | $1.19/lb. | .4 mg./2 crackers (1/2 oz.) | 12.8 mg./lb. | .70 | $ .83 | 6 |
| Prune juice | $1.15/40 oz. | 10.5 mg./8 oz. | 52.5 mg./40 oz. | .17 | $ .20 | 1 |
| Raisins | $1.69/15 oz. | 1 mg./oz. | 15 mg./15 oz. | .60 | $1.10 | 7 |

Sheet 11-4:

## Calcium

| Food Source | 1 Cost / Purchase Unit | 2 Amount Calcium / Food Composition Unit | 3 Amount Calcium / Purchase Unit | 4 Portion of Purchased Unit Consumed to Receive 1/2 U.S. RDA of Calcium | 5 Cost of 1/2 U.S. RDA Calcium | 6 Rank |
|---|---|---|---|---|---|---|
| Milk, whole | $2.07/gal. | 288 mg./8 oz. | 4,608 mg./gal. | .11 | $ .23 | 3 |
| Milk, 2% butterfat | $2.05/gal. | 352 mg./8 oz. | 5,632 mg./gal. | .09 | $ .18 | 2 |
| Milk, evaporated | $ .49/13 oz. | 635 mg./8 oz. | 1,032 mg./13 oz. | .48 | $ .24 | 4 |
| Milk, nonfat, dry | $5.63/20 qts. | 300 mg./8 oz. | 24,000 mg./20 qts. | .02 | $ .11 | 1 |
| Cottage cheese, small curd | $ .79/12 oz. | 230 mg./8 oz. | 345 mg./12 oz. | 1.45 | $1.15 | 8 |
| Swiss cheese | $2.89/lb. | 262 mg./oz. | 4,192 mg./lb. | .12 | $ .34 | 5 |
| Processed cheese spread | $1.89/lb. | 160 mg./oz. | 2,560 mg./lb. | .20 | $ .37 | 6 |
| Ice cream, chocolate | $2.69/1/2 gal. | 194 mg./cup | 1,552 mg./1/2 gal. | .32 | $ .86 | 7 |

Sheet 11-5:

**Vitamin C**

| Food Source | Cost / Purchase Unit [1] | Amount Vitamin C / Food Composition Unit [2] | Amount Vitamin C / Purchase Unit [3] | Portion of Purchased Unit Consumed to Receive 1/2 U.S. RDA of Vitamin C [4] | Cost of 1/2 U.S. RDA Vitamin C [5] | Rank [6] |
|---|---|---|---|---|---|---|
| Orange | $ .99/8 | 66 mg./1 orange | 528 mg./8 | .06 | $ .06 | 3 |
| Orange juice, frozen, diluted, store brand | $1.29/64 oz. | 120 mg./8 oz. | 960 mg./64 oz. | .03 | $ .04 | 1 |
| Orange juice, frozen, diluted, name brand | $1.67/64 oz. | 120 mg./8 oz. | 960 mg./64 oz. | .03 | $ .05 | 2 |
| Broccoli, frozen | $ .53/10 oz. | 143 mg./10 oz. | 143 mg./10 oz. | .21 | $ .11 | 4 |
| Sauerkraut, canned, solids, and liquids | $ .39/16 oz. | 33 mg./7 oz. | 75 mg./16 oz. | .40 | $ .16 | 5 |
| Applesauce | $ .83/25 oz. | 3 mg./9 oz. | 8 mg./25 oz. | 3.75 | $3.11 | 7 |
| Prune juice | $1.15/40 oz. | 5 mg./8 oz. | 25 mg./40 oz. | 1.20 | $1.38 | 6 |

Sheet 11-6: **Vitamin A**

| Food Source | Cost / Purchase Unit [1] | Amount Vitamin A / Food Composition Unit [2] | Amount Vitamin A / Purchase Unit [3] | Portion of Purchased Unit Consumed to Receive 1/2 U.S. RDA of Vitamin A [4] | Cost of 1/2 U.S. RDA Vitamin A [5] | Rank [6] |
|---|---|---|---|---|---|---|
| Milk, whole | $2.07/gal. | 200 IUs/8 oz. | 3,200 IUs/gal. | .78 | $1.61 | 8 |
| Margarine, Vitamin A fortified | $ .57/lb. | 500 IUs/tbsp. | 16,000 IUs/lb. | .16 | $ .09 | 5 |
| Green beans, frozen | $ .55/9 oz. | 680 IUs/6 oz. | 1,020 IUs/9 oz. | 2.45 | $1.35 | 7 |
| Spinach, frozen, leaf | $ .89/20 oz. | 14,580 IUs/7 oz. | 41,657 IUs/20 oz. | .06 | $ .05 | 3 |
| Carrots, canned, sliced | $ .40/lb. | 15,220 IUs/6 oz. | 40,587 IUs/lb. | .06 | $ .02 | 2 |
| Liver, beef, fried | $ .99/lb. | 30,280 IUs/2 oz. | 242,240 IUs/lb. | .01 | $ .01 | 1 |
| Eggs, Grade A, large | $ .99/doz. | 590 IUs/1 egg | 7,080 IUs/doz. | .35 | .35 | 6 |
| Pumpkin, canned | $ .49/gal. | 14,590 IUs/9 oz. | 25,938 IUs/lb. | .10 | $ .05 | 4 |

QUIZ SHEET 11-1:

1. **Check marks for:** eating before you shop, using a shopping list, shopping alone, reading labels
2. **EC for:**

| | |
|---|---|
| blackberry jelly | canned buttercream frosting |
| granulated sugar | chocolate cake mix |
| nondairy creamer | maraschino cherries |
| maple syrup | ketchup |
| Red Hots | Lifesavers |

3. Convenience stores are located in neighborhoods and are usually open more hours than other food stores, which increases their prices. Also, convenience stores supply smaller packages, which are generally more expensive than the larger ones. Discount supermarkets are centrally located. This kind of store has fewer consumer conveniences like baggers and bags. It supplies economy-size packages and fewer brands. The discount store's prices are usually lower than regular supermarket prices.
4. Cost of nutrients in a serving.
5. How much of the food has to be eaten to receive the specified amount of that nutrient, and how palatable one type of food is compared to another type.

## UNIT 12: STORING FOODS TO PRESERVE NUTRIENTS

SHEET 12-1

| Case | Food | Nutrient | How Lost? |
|---|---|---|---|
| 1 | broccoli | Vitamin C | dissolved in water |
| 2 | apricots | Vitamin A | destroyed because of bruising and storage at room temperature |
| 3 | orange juice | Vitamin C | destroyed by air |
| 4 | spinach | Vitamin C calcium iron | dissolved in water |
| 5 | margarine | Vitamin A | destroyed by storage at room temperature |
| 6 | fruit punch | Vitamin C | destroyed by light, air, and temperature |

SHEET 12-5:

Students' answers will vary. The results of this experiment are dependent upon the atmospheric conditions and temperature of the storage area, as well as the original condition of the fresh food. Descriptors are given on Sheet 12-5, but accept any other reasonable answers. Check the food products to verify students' answers. An example of an acceptable group of answers is provided below:

| | Food Appearance/Color | Food Odor | Food Texture |
|---|---|---|---|
| Fresh banana | pale yellow, spotless | fruity, sweet, pleasing | soft, smooth, firm |

QUIZ SHEETS 12-1 through 12-2:

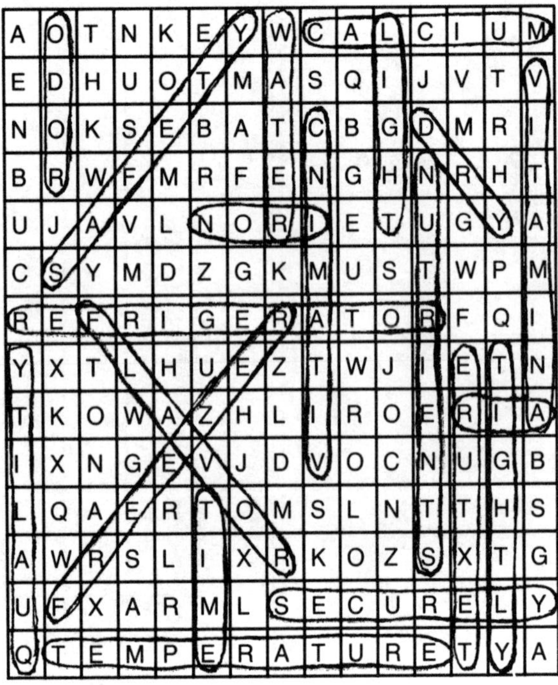


1. quality
2. safety
3. nutrients
4. dry
5. refrigerator
6. freezer
7. iron
8. calcium
9. Vitamin A
10. Vitamin C
11. temperature
12. time
13. air
14. water
15. light
16. tightly
17. securely
18. odor
19. color
20. texture
21. flavor

## UNIT 13: BUDGETING RESOURCES IN MEAL PLANNING

QUIZ SHEET 13-1:

1. Accept any answers that are well thought out.
   Sample answers:

| | |
|---|---|
| a. C, A | f. T, A, S |
| b. C, E | g. C, A, S |
| c. S | h. S, T |
| d. A | i. A |
| e. T, E | j. E |

2. d
3. b
4. d
5. a

## UNIT 14: MENU PLANNING USING THE "DAILY FOOD GUIDE"

SHEET 14-1:

Sample answers include the following:

**Seasonings:**

| | |
|---|---|
| basil | oregano |
| cinnamon | parsley |
| dill | pepper |
| garlic | salt |
| ketchup | soy sauce |
| mustard | vinegar |
| nutmeg | |

**Foods:**

Breads & Cereals
- flour
- oatmeal
- rice
- spaghetti

Fruits & Vegetables

| | |
|---|---|
| apples | orange juice |
| celery | peaches, canned |
| corn, canned | potatoes |
| eggplant | raisins |
| lemons | tomatoes, canned |
| lettuce | walnuts |
| onions | |

Milk & Milk Products
- powdered milk
- Swiss cheese

Meat & Meat Alternates
- beef, stewing cubes
- chicken, whole
- eggs
- lentils
- tuna, canned

Miscellaneous
- baking powder
- margarine

**Equipment:**

bowl, large
can opener
casserole dish, glass
cookie sheet
hand mixer
measuring cups and spoons
oven
pie pan
range
rolling pin
saucepans with lids (6″ and 8″)
skillet (10″)
spatula
spoon, large wooden

SHEET 14-4:

Answers will vary. Accept all answers without judgment. The purpose of this worksheet is to encourage students to explore their likes and dislikes in regard to personal food choices.

QUIZ SHEET 14-1:

1. c
2. c
3. a
4. b
5. c
6. a

## UNIT 15: MENU PLANNING FOR THE FAMILY

QUIZ SHEET 15-1:

1. d
2. Answers will vary. Accept any well-written paragraph that describes the "Family Profile."

## UNIT 16: EVALUATING NUTRITION INFORMATION

SHEETS 16-1 through 16-2:

| Claim Number | OK | Unreliable | Questions Answered "YES" from Sheet 16-3, "The Reliability Detector" |
|---|---|---|---|
| 1 | X | | |
| 2 | | X | 1, 8, 9 |
| 3 | | X | 2, 3, 6, 8 |
| 4 | X | | |
| 5 | | X | 8, 9 |
| 6 | | X | 1, 3 |
| 7 | | X | 1, 3 |
| 8 | X | | |
| 9 | | X | 1, 2 |
| 10 | | X | 3, 4, 5 |
| 11 | | X | 1, 2, 3, 6, 8 |
| 12 | | X | 3, 4, 5, 8, 11 |
| 13 | X | | |
| 14 | | X | 4, 5, 7 |
| 15 | | X | 1, 8 |
| 16 | | X | 1, 2, 3, 6 |

QUIZ SHEET 16-1:

1. Answers will vary but should include questions from Sheet 16-3. Samples include 1, 4, 8, 9.
2. b.

3., 4., 5. Answers will vary but should include reputable sources mentioned in this unit or in the "References/Resources" section for this unit. Sample answers include the following:

3. local dietitian
   family physician
   local health department
4. hospital dietitian
   American Heart Association
   American Dietetic Association (local chapter)
5. recommended nutrition textbook
   American Dietetic Association
   local dietitian

## UNIT 17: DIET AND DISEASE: OBESITY

SHEET 17-2:

Answers will vary. Sample answers are provided below:

**Health Problems:** Current Problem—shortness of breath. Future problems—diabetes, arthritis, hypertension, gout, menstrual abnormalities, reproductive problems, gallbladder disease, kidney disease, heart attack, stroke, some types of cancer, and complications during childbirth and surgery.

**Social problems:** Current problems—inability to participate in sports, withdrawal from friends, self-conscious about appearance. Future problems—difficulty in making new friends, inability or lack of desire to participate in many social events.

**Economic Problems:** Current problems—expense of new wardrobe, expense of diet books and foods, worry about employment due to appearance. Future problems—difficulty in obtaining employment in certain fields, expense of medical care.

**Barbara's principal problem:** Barbara used food as an emotional crutch when faced with the pressures of college. She also made excuses to avoid physical activity. This combination of excess calories and decreased exercise caused weight gain. Once overweight, she had trouble breaking a vicious cycle.

**General Weight-reduction plan:** Any plan must include decreasing caloric input and increasing caloric output while maintaining a well-balanced diet.

SHEET 17-4:

1. *False*. The primary cause of obesity is the consumption of more calories than are expended. For every 3,500 "extra" calories a person eats, a pound of fat is stored. Some people may have a tendency to gain weight more easily than others, but they are not doomed to being fat just because one or both of their parents are obese. They just have to eat fewer calories and/or exercise a little more.
2. *False*. Foods turn to fat when there are more calories taken in than the body needs regardless of who the individual is. For example, ingesting an extra ounce of hard cheese, a tablespoon of peanut butter, or one ounce of dry cereal (each worth about 100 calories) each day will result in a one-pound weight gain in 35 days. If overconsumption of food continues, any person will eventually become obese.
3. *False*. It is often the case that when people skip a meal, they overstuff themselves at the next meal and end up taking in as many or more calories than they would if they had eaten two smaller meals.
4. *False*. The purpose of reducing pills is generally to curb one's appetite so as to eat less. If, however, one takes reducing pills and continues to eat as much or more than usual, no weight will be lost. Reducing pills *do not* burn calories while one sits or sleeps, as many people are misled to believe. The best way to reduce is to eat less and exercise more.
5. *False*. In most cases, low-calorie breads are significantly higher priced. If one would carefully plan a reducing diet, being aware of calories contained in all foods, one would find that the "fat" culprits are not based around carbohydrates such as bread, but are in some of our other favorites, such as meats, cheese, salad dressing, nuts, and sweet desserts.
6. *False*. Toasting bread does not reduce the amount of calories contained in the bread.
7. *False*. It is dangerous and detrimental to restrict water intake during a weight-reduction diet. First, any weight loss caused by water restriction is immediately regained when one stops restricting water. Second, water restriction leads to dehydration. People who are dehydrated are tired and less likely to exercise, and exercise is an important part of any weight-reduction program. Water is a vital nutrient for *any* type of diet and is a good replacement for many high-calorie sweet beverages.
8. *False*. Candy enriched with vitamins supplies not only vitamins, but also extra calories in the way of refined sugar. One can receive just as many vitamins, as well as pleasure, by eating a balanced diet that follows the "Daily Food Guide." Candy enriched with vitamins is also devoid of fiber, an important substance to ingest, especially during weight loss and maintenance.
9. *False*. Small amounts of fat should be included in a weight-reduction diet. This will help an individual feel full (i.e., satisfied with intake at meals).
10. *False*. Sugar and starch are both carbohydrates and both provide the same number of calories. In fact, starch is broken down to sugar once it is inside our bodies. Starchy foods have an advantage over high-sugar foods in that the former often contribute fiber and greater amounts of other essential nutrients.
11. *False*. All of our foods, including high-protein foods (e.g., lean meat, poultry, fish) contain calories. Regardless of the source of our calories, anything taken in excess will be converted to fat.
12. *False*. Most gelatin desserts on the market today contain a large amount of sugar. While gelatin desserts may contain fewer calories than some other types of desserts (i.e., chocolate cake and ice cream), they cannot be considered nonfattening because they are indeed a source of calories. As mentioned before, any calories taken in *excess* will turn to fat.
13. *False*. On the average, walking 1 mile burns up only 100 calories. This amounts to 700 calories a week. To lose 1 pound of body fat, 2,800 more calories need to be expended in order to lose 1 pound of body fat in 1 week, provided that the amount of calories consumed is the same. (3,500 − 700 = 2,800) This is equivalent to walking 35 miles (or 5 miles each day) for a week.
14. *False*. Hamburger, hot dogs, and cheese contain a considerable amount of fat while bread and potatoes are very low in fat. Since fat provides 2-1/2 times as many calories per gram as does carbohydrate, the meat and cheese would provide more calories.
15. *False*. Both activities require one to use the same muscles. Running the mile uses the muscles more vigorously than walking. However, if one walks the mile, one uses the muscles for a longer length of time. It is the *distance* covered that is important, not whether one walks or runs it. Either way, about 100 calories is expended. (*See* Chart G)
16. *False*. In most cases, the label on the margarine package states that it contains the same amount of calories as butter (except for some diet margarines). Margarine, however,

contains no cholesterol and more unsaturated fats than butter, and it is a more desirable spread than butter for this reason.

17. *False.* Even when reducing, it is important to meet one's recommended dietary allowances for protein, vitamins, and minerals. Any diet that focuses on one particular group of foods, such as high-protein foods or low-carbohydrate foods, will not provide all of the essential nutrients. It also will not bring about such a tremendous weight loss that once it has been followed, an "anything goes" pattern of eating can be resumed. The best type of reducing diet is one that includes foods from all of the food groups in the "Daily Food Guide" but that reduces specific amounts of foods in each group. In this way, one can maintain the diet through a lifetime, without causing a risk to health.
18. *False.* Many people have been misled to believe that grapefruit possesses certain enzymes that convert fattening foods to fuel which is quickly burned by the body. While grapefruit is an excellent food to use in any diet, grapefruit by itself will not reduce a person's weight.
19. *False.* Because physical activity burns calories directly, it is a vital part of any weight-reduction/control program. Getting a moderate amount of exercise daily has actually been shown to help individuals to control their appetite.
20. *False.* It is not healthy to lose more than two pounds per week. It is also very difficult to lose weight at this rate, since one must expend 3,500 calories more than what is ingested to lose one pound.

SHEETS 17-5 and 17-6:

| | |
|---|---|
| A1, B9... | Body fat |
| A10, B1, C6 | Any 3 of these: adult-onset diabetes, arthritis, hypertension, gout, menstrual abnormalities, reproductive problems, gallbladder disease, heart attack, stroke, some types of cancer in females, kidney disease, complications during childbirth and surgery. |
| A2, B10, C1 | Any one of these: the cost of new clothing, trying various diets, health insurance, medical expenses, may be harder to obtain certain jobs. |
| B2, D1... | Any one of these: feeling like you are being rejected by peers, keeping to yourself, not participating in group activities. |
| A3, C7, D4 | 20 percent |
| B3, C2, D7 | Height-weight charts |
| A4, D10... | 156 |
| B4, C8, D2 | 180 |
| A5, C3, D5 | 3,500 |
| B5, D8... | Skinfold |
| A6, C9... | 1, 2 |
| B6, C4, D3 | Calories |
| A7, D6... | Fat |
| B7, D9... | They both contribute the same number of calories; all carbohydrates provide 4 calories per gram. |
| A8, C5... | New eating habits |
| B8, C10.. | They both burn approximately the same number of calories (*See* Chart G), although running burns slightly more calories than walking. Walking one mile burns 67 calories for a 100-pound person, while running one mile burns 83 calories. Remember to keep distance, and not speed, in mind. |
| A9 ....... | Exercise |

QUIZ SHEET 17-1:

1. c
2. b
3. d
4. b
5. a
6. a
7. a

## UNIT 18: DIET AND DISEASE: WORLD HEALTH PROBLEMS

QUIZ SHEET 18-1:

1. anemia
2. xerophthalmia
3. kwashiorkor
4. marasmus
5. goiter
6. anemia—iron
7. xerophthalmia—Vitamin A
8. kwashiorkor—protein
9. marasmus—calories
10. goiter—iodine

11., 12., 13. Stunted growth, increased susceptibility to infection, weight loss.

14. Answers will vary. Accept any well-written paragraph that describes a reasonable and logical solution.

## UNIT 19: DIETARY GUIDELINES FOR AMERICANS

QUIZ SHEET 19-1:

1. Accept any five of the Dietary Guidelines:
   #1 Eat a Variety of Foods
   #2 Maintain Ideal Weight
   #3 Avoid Too Much Fat, Saturated Fat, and Cholesterol
   #4 Eat Foods with Adequate Starch and Fiber
   #5 Avoid Too Much Sugar
   #6 Avoid Too Much Sodium
   #7 If You Drink Alcohol, Do So in Moderation
2. c
3. d
4. b
5. *Any or all of the following:* Obesity, heart disease, cancer, cerebrovascular disease or stroke, diabetes, high blood pressure, arteriosclerosis, cirrhosis of the liver.

## UNIT 20: DESIGNING A NATIONAL NUTRITION POLICY

QUIZ SHEET 20-1:

1. b
2. a
3. *Any two of these:* conflicting interests, politics, financial considerations.
4. He should identify the problem about presweetened cereals and make other people aware of the problem.
5. a
6. a